Community as Partner
THEORY AND PRACTICE IN NURSING

ELIZABETH T. ANDERSON, DrPH, RN, FAAN
Professor Emerita
The University of Texas Medical Branch
School of Nursing
Galveston, Texas

Honorary Member
Pan American Nursing and Midwifery Collaborating Centers
Global Network of World Health Organization Collaborating Centers
    for Nursing and Midwifery

JUDITH McFARLANE, DrPH, RN, FAAN
Parry Chair in Health Promotion and Disease Prevention
Texas Woman's University
College of Nursing
Houston, Texas

EDITION

6

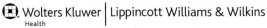
Wolters Kluwer | Lippincott Williams & Wilkins
Health
Philadelphia · Baltimore · New York · London
Buenos Aires · Hong Kong · Sydney · Tokyo

Acquisitions Editor: Hilarie Surrena
Product Manager: Helen Kogut
Editorial Assistant: Shawn Loht
Design Coordinator: Joan Wendt
Illustration Coordinator: Brett MacNaughton
Manufacturing Coordinator: Karin Duffield
Prepress Vendor: MPS Limited, A Macmillan Company

6th Edition

9 8 7 6 5 4 3 2

Printed in China

Library of Congress Cataloging-in-Publication Data

Anderson, Elizabeth T.
  Community as partner: theory and practice in nursing / Elizabeth T.
  Anderson, Judith McFarlane. — 6th ed.
     p. ; cm.
  Includes bibliographical references and index.
  Summary: "This user-friendly text is presented as a handbook for students and practicing nurses who work with communities to promote health. Community as Partner focuses on the essentials of practice with the community. Students will find this text helpful for the many examples of working with the community as partner. For over 20 years and five editions, this textbook has served undergraduate, RN to BS, and RN to MS students and graduate students alike as a framework for professional nursing practice in the community. Our intention is to keep the text basic and accessible to all who practice in the community. Using this text with distance education and virtual learning with Internet resources will enrich practice in any community. This sixth edition continues the philosophy of the authors by strengthening the theoretical base with new chapters on globalization and rural health. All other chapters have been revised and updated from the fifth edition. We continue with a series of chapters that takes the reader through the entire nursing process by using a real-life community as our example. The urban example is enhanced and expanded throughout the remainder of the book by selected aggregates which serve as exemplars of working with the community as partner as well."—Provided by publisher.
  ISBN 978-1-60547-855-5 (alk. paper)
  1. Community health nursing. I. McFarlane, Judith M. II. Title.
  [DNLM: 1. Community Health Nursing. 2. Health Promotion. 3. Nurse's
  Role. 4. Nursing Theory. WY 106 A546ca 2011]
  RT98.A533 2011
  610.73'43—dc22

                                                                          2010019255

Dedication

For inspiriting Community as Partner, *we wish to acknowledge communities everywhere...*

public health service areas;

rural villages;

shelters for battered women, the homeless, immigrants, migrants, and refugees;

workplaces;

faith groups;

schools...

and the nurses who work in partnership with them.

Community as Partner: Theory and Practice in Nursing *is dedicated to you.*

CONTRIBUTORS

Judith C. Drew, PhD, RN
Professor Emerita
The University of Texas Medical Branch
School of Nursing
Galveston, Texas

Nina M. Fredland, PhD, RN
Assistant Professor
University of Texas at Austin
School of Nursing
Austin, Texas

Julia Henderson Gist, PhD, RN
Visiting Assistant Professor
Arkansas Tech University
Russellville, Arkansas

Deanna E. Grimes, DrPH, RN, FAAN
Professor
The University of Texas Health Science
    Center-Houston
School of Nursing
Houston, Texas

David Hartley, MHA, PhD
Director
Maine Rural Health Research Center
Portland, Maine

Shirley F. Hutchinson, DrPH, RN
Associate Professor
Texas Woman's University
Houston, Texas

Bruce Leonard, PhD, RN, FNP, NP-C, BC
Associate Professor
The University of Texas Medical Branch
School of Nursing
Galveston, Texas

Ann T. Malecha, PhD, RN
Professor
Texas Woman's University
Houston, Texas

Robert W. McFarlane, PhD
Consulting Ecologist
Houston, Texas

Elnora P. Mendias, PhD, RN
Associate Professor
The University of Texas Medical Branch
School of Nursing
Galveston, Texas

Susan Scoville Walker, PhD, RN
Professor Emerita of Nursing
Texas A&M International University
Laredo, Texas

Teresa J. Walsh, PhD, RNC
Associate Clinical Professor
Texas Woman's University
Houston, Texas

Lynda Law Wilson, PhD, RN, FAAN
Professor, Assistant Dean for International
    Affairs
Deputy Director, WHO/PAHO Collaborating
    Center on International Nursing
University of Alabama at Birmingham
Birmingham, Alabama

Nancy Zamboras, RN, CCM, COHN-S
Occupational Health Associate
Chevron Phillips Chemical Company
The Woodlands, Texas

REVIEWERS

Laurel W. Boyd, MA, Med, RN
Assistant Professor
University of West Florida
Pensacola, Florida

L. Sue Gabriel EdD, MFS, MSN, RN
Assistant Professor
BryanLGH College of Health Sciences
Lincoln, Nebraska

Debbie Hooser, DNSc, RN
Associate Professor, Nursing
Baptist College of Health Sciences
Memphis, Tennessee

**Nancy N. Menzel, PhD, MS, APRN, BC,
    COHN-S, CNE, FAAOHN**
Associate Professor
University of Nevada, Las Vegas
Las Vegas, Nevada

Ruth G. Mullins, PhD, RN, CPNP
Professor of Nursing
California State University, Long Beach
Long Beach, California

**Patsy Ruppert Rider, MSN, BSN,
    APRN-BC**
Instructor in Clinical Nursing
The University of Texas at Austin School
    of Nursing
Austin, Texas

Shirley P. Smith, PhD, RN, CRNP
Assistant Professor
Duquesne University School of Nursing
Pittsburgh, Pennsylvania

PREFACE

This user friendly text is presented as a handbook for students and practicing nurses who work with communities to promote health. *Community as Partner* focuses on the essentials of practice with the community. Students will find this text helpful for the many examples of working with the community as partner. For over 20 years and five editions, this textbook has served undergraduate, RN to BS, and RN to MS students and graduate students alike as a framework for professional nursing practice in the community. Our intention is to keep the text basic and accessible to all who practice in the community. Using this text with distance education and virtual learning with Internet resources will enrich practice in any community.

This sixth edition continues the philosophy of the authors by strengthening the theoretical base with new chapters on globalization and rural health. All other chapters have been revised and updated from the fifth edition. We continue with a series of chapters that takes the reader through the entire nursing process by using a real-life community as our example. The urban example is enhanced and expanded throughout the remainder of the book by selected aggregates which serve as exemplars of working with the community as partner as well.

Part 1: Essential Elements for Healthy Partnerships

Part 1 of the book describes content areas basic to the practice of community health nursing. The areas encompassed include globalization, essentials of practice, theoretical foundations, epidemiology, environmental health, ethics, empowerment, cultural competence, health policy, informatics, and infectious diseases and disasters. Emphasis is on theory-based practice, with those theories critical to community as partner described and explicated.

Part 2: The Process

Part 2 covers the process of working with the community. The assessment chapter includes an introduction to the community-as-partner model which then serves as a framework for the remaining chapters in this section. One sample community is used to illustrate each step of the nursing process for community health nursing practice. The chapters guide the reader through processes of community assessment; data analysis; formulation of a community nursing diagnosis; and the planning, implementation, and evaluation of a community health program. Emphasis throughout is on understanding the community as a dynamic system that is more than the sum of its parts and in continual interaction with the environment.

Part 3: Practicing With Diverse Communities

Part 3 provides a number of examples in which nurses play a major role as partners in health promotion. Communities and aggregates in this section include marginalized groups, the workplace, rural populations, schools, faith communities, and the elderly.

Postscript

An editorial describing some of the roots of public health nursing is reproduced at the end of the book as both a reminder of our past and a beacon for the future.

Special Features

- **Learning Objectives** at the beginning of each chapter focus readers' attention on important chapter content.
- **Take Note** boxes highlight key concepts for readers as they go through the steps of the nursing process for a community.
- **Critical Thinking Questions** at the end of each chapter enable students to review and apply chapter content.
- **Further Readings** offer additional references on the chapter subject matter.

New to This Edition

New chapter (Chapter 1) on globalization. This chapter is in response to one of the most important factors affecting community health, that of globalization. The World Health Organization's Millennium Development Goals are included as are concepts of global health. How nurses can contribute to reducing global health challenges and promote Health for All is also part of this chapter.

New chapter (Chapter 21) on rural community nursing. We recognize that this is an important chapter to those in the field since many community health nurses practice in rural settings. Specific examples and theories related to rural health are included in this all-new chapter.

Internet Resources have moved from the book to the web site that accompanies the book to provide direct links to additional information and enhance distance learning. Visit the Point for even more resources!

Resources for Students

A variety of ancillary materials are available to support students and can be found online at http://thepoint.lww.com/Anderson6e.

Resources for Instructors

A comprehensive instructor's resource CD-ROM includes the following:

- A Test Generator, containing over 400 multiple choice questions
- PowerPoint presentations
- An Image bank, containing images from the text in formats suitable for printing, projecting, and incorporating into websites
- And more!

Resources for Instructors are also available online at http://thepoint.lww.com/Anderson6e

Elizabeth T. Anderson, DrPH, RN, FAAN
Judith McFarlane, DrPH, RN, FAAN

ACKNOWLEDGMENTS

Our colleagues who contributed to this edition have enriched both the book and our lives. Along with our families they have sustained this process and helped us to feel proud of our profession.

Community as Partner: Theory and Practice in Nursing could not have been written without the thoughts, critiques, and examples provided by our students and colleagues in public health.

The fine folks at Wolters Kluwer/Lippincott Williams & Wilkins, particularly Helen Kogut, have facilitated the process of doing this sixth edition so that it was an enjoyable experience.

We thank each of you.

Elizabeth T. Anderson
Judith McFarlane

CONTENTS

PART

1

Essential Elements for Healthy Partnerships

The World as Community: Globalization and Health

LYNDA LAW WILSON

LEARNING OBJECTIVES

This chapter introduces a global perspective to community health nursing, introducing the concepts of globalization, major global health challenges, and the role of the nurse in contributing to the goals of promoting global health equity and reducing health disparities.

After studying this chapter, you should be able to:

1. Discuss the concepts of global health and globalization.
2. Analyze the relationship between globalization and health.
3. Discuss major global health challenges.
4. Describe the contributions of the Millennium Development Goal (MDG) campaign to promoting global health.
5. Explore ways by which nurses can contribute to reducing global health challenges and promoting the goal of Health for All.

Introduction

*T*he world is indeed a global community, and this is an exciting time to be a nurse. There are unlimited opportunities to truly make a difference in promoting social justice, global health equity, and reducing health disparities for all of the world's peoples. Nurses provide 60% to 80% of the world's health care, although in some rural areas in Africa, nearly 85% of the health care is provided by nurses (World Health Organization Department of Human Resources for Health, 2008). Thus, it is critical that nurses have an awareness of key global health challenges, and the roles that they might play in addressing these challenges. One of the greatest challenges to global health that leads to health disparities is poverty and the associated problems related to lack of access to adequate food, water, shelter, and health care. The World Bank estimates that in 2005 about 1.4 billion people (or 25% of the population in the developing world) lived below the international poverty line of $1.25 a day. Although the percentage of the world's population living in poverty has declined from 52% in 1981 to 26% in 2005, there are significant disparities in the poverty rates among countries. The 50% poverty rate in sub-Saharan Africa, for example, has not changed since 1981 (World Bank, 2008). In addition to poverty, there are many other factors that contribute to health disparities including racial/ethnic status, presence of physical or mental disabilities, stigma associated with certain health problems such as mental illness or HIV/AIDS, and inequitable distribution of global resources, including funding for research to address global health problems. In 1990, it was estimated that only 5% of the world's research funds were used to address the health problems of low- and middle-income countries where 93% of the world's preventable deaths occur (Global Forum for Health Research, 2008). The term "10/90 gap" has been used to characterize this imbalance. Although the gap has narrowed in recent years, there remain significant disparities in spending for health and for health research between the rich and poor countries of the world.

T A K E   N O T E

"Health disparities are differences in the incidence, prevalence, mortality, and burden of diseases and other adverse health conditions that exist among specific population groups in the United States" (National Institutes of Health, 2006)

GLOBAL HEALTH AND GLOBALIZATION

In 1997, the Institute of Medicine in the United States published a landmark report that highlighted America's vital interest in global health. In this report, global health was defined as "health issues that transcend national boundaries, and may best be addressed by cooperative actions" (Institute of Medicine, 1997). Globalization is a term used to refer to the increasing economic, political, social, technological, and intellectual interconnectedness of the world. Changes in the economy in one part of the world quickly influence the markets in other countries. Similarly, emerging infectious diseases can quickly spread across the globe. Globalization is not a new phenomenon; however, the current phase of globalization is different from earlier phases because of the speed with which new technologies promote the sharing of information, resources, and people (Bauman & Blythe, 2008). The process of globalization has also been influenced by global trade policies and deregulation that facilitate the movement of products and people across national borders. These trade policies can have significant impacts on public health when products that are imported from countries with lax safety and monitoring standards are exported internationally. One example was the discovery of a problem in the food supply chain in China when many exported products were found to be contaminated with banned drugs or toxic chemicals (Ramzy & Yang, 2008).

With the growing strength of organizations such as the World Trade Organization (WTO) and trade pacts such as the North American Free Trade Agreement (NAFTA) with their emphasis on free trade, free financial markets, and economic profits, governments—especially those of resource-poor nations—find themselves losing the ability to define and control their own futures. Political scientists and sociologists warn of the declining strength of the "nation state" and the questionable future of international organizations such as the United Nations (UN) and its related units such as the World Health Organization (WHO). If many countries are weakening in relation to powerful international forces, what does this mean for the development of our local communities? How are they affected by the emphasis on profit—usually for a few privileged individuals and companies?

Globalization has both positive and negative effects on health. The positive effects include diffusion of ideas, technologies, and other innovations that leads to improvements in many areas such as availability of safe water, medications, and treatments for both acute and chronic health problems. Expansion of trade has resulted in increased living standards for many, especially for women (Abbot & Coenen, 2008). Another positive effect noted in the 2008 World Health Report is the emerging "global stewardship" that has been influenced by more international and global exchanges leading to growing recognition of common threats as well as opportunities, and a sense of growing solidarity and commitment to collaboration to promote global social justice and equity (World Health Organization, 2008e). Negative effects include increased crowding in urban areas, increased health problems (such as obesity and chronic disease) associated with adoption of unhealthy Western lifestyles, and faster transmission of infectious diseases associated with increased global travel and "so-called 'microbial hitchhikers'" (Abbot & Coenen, 2008). Examples include the 2003 outbreak of the Severe Acute Respiratory Syndrome (SARS) (Murphy, 2006), and the 2007 incident in which a U.S. citizen with extensively drug-resistant tuberculosis (XDR TB) failed to comply with medical orders and traveled on a commercial airplane to Paris, Athens, and then Rome for his honeymoon. The travel exposed more than 600 fellow passengers, requiring follow-up and tracking for testing and treatment as needed (Hitti, 2007).

Another negative effect of globalization is the "brain drain" that results from migration from lower-resource countries to higher-resource countries (World Health Organization Department of Human Resources for Health, 2008), and growing disparities between the "haves" and the "have-nots." Birdsall noted that globalization has resulted in benefits for those who are already ahead, namely, the high-resource countries, and within low- and middle-resource countries, those who are at the higher end of the socioeconomic spectrum (Birdsall, 2006). Abbott and Coenen noted that although increased access to information that is associated with globalization and advances in information and communication technology (ICT) has resulted in many benefits to health as well as education and social development, some societies find this open exchange of information threatening to their ideologies and social structures (Abbot & Coenen, 2008). These authors also noted that many groups who could most benefit from increased access to ICT are unable to enjoy these benefits because of challenges with limited access to ICT due to untrained personnel, and lack of infrastructure and resources.

MAJOR GLOBAL HEALTH PROBLEMS

Although there continue to be significant disparities in the global burden of disease, there has been considerable progress in leading health indicators (such as rates of infectious diseases, maternal and child mortality, or immunization coverage) over the past 30 years. The 2008 World Health Report noted that although 9.5 million children died in 2006, a total of 16.2 million children would have died that year if the child mortality rates remained the same as they were in 1978. Despite these improvements, there remain significant inequities in the global burden of disease, and many of these inequities are directly related to the effects of poverty and the inequitable distribution of the world's resources (World Health Organization, 2008c). The WHO is an excellent resource for information about the major causes of global morbidity and mortality.

TABLE 1.1

Top Causes of Death in the World

Cause	Deaths in Millions	Percentage of Deaths
Coronary heart disease	7.20	12.2
Stroke and other cerebrovascular diseases	5.71	9.7
Lower respiratory infections	4.18	7.1
Chronic obstructive pulmonary disease	3.02	5.1
Diarrhaeal diseases	2.16	3.7
HIV/AIDS	2.04	3.5
Tuberculosis	1.46	2.5
Trachea, bronchus, lung cancers	1.32	2.3
Road traffic accidents	1.27	2.2
Prematurity and low birth weight	1.18	2.0

Source: World Health Organization (2008d).

In 2008, the WHO published a report comparing the global burden of disease in both high-income as well as low- and middle-income countries in the six WHO regions (Africa, the Americas, Eastern Mediterranean, Southeast Asia, and Western Pacific). In this report, WHO defined high-income countries as those with gross national income per capita in 2004 as more than $10,066. Low- and middle-income countries were those with gross national income per capita less than this amount. The global burden of disease is defined as "the disability-adjusted life year (DALY), which is a time-based measure combining years of life lost due to premature mortality and years of life lost due to time lived in states of less than full health" (World Health Organization, 2008b). Table 1.1 lists the top 10 causes of death across all regions of the world, and Table 1.2 illustrates 10 key facts reported in the 2008 WHO report on the Global Burden of Disease (World Health Organization, 2008b).

These global data provide important guidance for nurses and other health workers in identifying priorities for programs to address the most pressing health needs, but it is also important for nurses to be familiar with the specific problems in the communities where they practice. Nurses also need to be aware of new and emerging health problems associated with infectious diseases, climate change, and other factors such as potential threats to public health security resulting from industrial accidents, natural disasters, bioterrorism, or other health emergencies.

Infectious Diseases

The HIV/AIDS pandemic has had a devastating effect in many countries since it was first identified in the 1980s. In 2007, there were 33.2 million people living with HIV, and there were 2.1 million deaths. Sub-Saharan Africa is the region with the highest rate of HIV/AIDS, and AIDS is the leading cause of death in this region. Sixty-eight percent of adults and 90% of children infected with HIV live in this region (Joint United Nations Program on HIV/AIDS and World Health Organization, 2007). Other emerging infections are caused by newly evolved strains of pathogens (such as multiple drug–resistant tuberculosis, *Staphylococcus aureus*, or chloroquine-resistant malaria), or newly recognized infections such as the Sudden Acute Respiratory Syndrome (SARS) (Jones et al., 2008; Murphy, 2006). In a recent analysis of the emergence of 335 global infectious diseases that were reported from 1940 to 2004, Jones et al. reported that 22.8% of these diseases were vectorborne, and that the incidence

TABLE 1.2

Ten Facts about the Global Burden of Disease

Around 10 million children under the age of 5 die each year	The WHO estimates that nearly all of these deaths are preventable with low-cost interventions such as primary care to treat diarrhea and respiratory infections, and with integrated health systems
Cardiovascular diseases are the leading causes of death in the world	The WHO estimates that 80% of premature deaths from cardiovascular heart disease and strokes could be prevented through appropriate diets, physical exercise, and avoiding the use of tobacco
HIV/AIDS is the leading cause of adult death in Africa	Inadequate health systems and limited access to care are major barriers in reducing deaths due to HIV/AIDS
Population aging is contributing to the rise in cancer and heart disease	There is a need to prepare health systems and caregivers to cope with the elderly and their associated chronic illnesses and other health problems
Lung cancer is the most common cause of death from cancer in the world	The WHO estimates that smoking is responsible for 80% of lung cancer, and thus efforts to reduce smoking would have a significant effect on lung cancer deaths
Complications of pregnancy account for almost 15% of deaths in women of reproductive age worldwide	The WHO estimates that each year more than 500,000 women die from preventable complications during pregnancy or childbirth
Mental disorders such as depression are among the 20 leading causes of disability worldwide	Lack of mental health services is a major problem worldwide. The WHO estimates that less than 25% of persons with depression have access to adequate treatment and health care.
Hearing loss, vision problems, and mental disorders are the most common causes of disability	There are many international organizations that are excellent resources for promoting appropriate services and protecting the rights of persons with disabilities, including the World Federation of the Deaf (www.wfdeaf.org), Disabled Persons International (http://v1.dpi.org/lang-en/), Rehabilitation International (http://www.riglobal.org/), the International Disability Alliance (http://www.internationaldisabilityalliance.org)/, and the World Blind Union (http://www.worldblindunion.org/en)/
Road traffic injuries are projected to rise from the ninth leading cause of death globally in 2004, to the fifth in 2030	This problem could be reduced by the use of seat belts and helmets (for motorcycle riders and bikers), and reduction of driving under the influence of drugs or alcohol
Undernutrition is the underlying cause of death for at least 30% of all children under the age of 5	The WHO estimates that nearly 20 million children worldwide are severely malnourished, increasing their risk of acquiring infections and reducing their ability to resist such infections

Source: World Health Organization (2008a).

of these diseases corresponded to climate anomalies that occurred during the 1990s, lending support to the hypothesis that global warming and climate change may lead to the emergence of these types of diseases (Jones et al., 2008).

Climate Change

Although the specific health effects of climate change and global warming continue to be debated, it is likely that there will be shifts in patterns of disease in the coming decades that are attributable at least in part to the effects of climate change. There are several ways in which climate change might influence health outcomes including the following: (a) changes in intensity of extreme heat waves, floods, and droughts; (b) changes in air pollutants and allergens; (c) alterations in ecosystems, water, and food supplies that in turn influence the incidence of infectious diseases as well as nutritional status; and (d) population displacement due to rising sea-levels (Patz, Campbell-Lendrum, Gibbs, & Woodruff, 2008). Luber and Hess, from the United

States Centers for Disease Control, identified the following potential health effects of climate change: (a) the elderly and other vulnerable groups will be at greatest risk for exposure to catastrophic weather events such as hurricanes and extreme heat; (b) increased flooding will result in possible food and water shortages and may lead to mass migration, "environmental refugees, and regional tension and conflict"; (c) persons affected by disasters and economic problems due to ecosystem and climate changes will be vulnerable to mental health stresses; and (d) and many vectorborne diseases may become more frequent and widespread (Luber & Hess, 2007).

Threats to Global Public Health Security

In today's world, it is essential that countries work together to minimize risks from disease outbreaks or health hazards related to factors such as natural disasters, infectious disease outbreaks, bioterrorism incidents, or other emergencies. Recognizing the importance of such global cooperation, the 2007 World Health Report was devoted entirely to the issue of global public health security in the 21st century (World Health Organization, 2007). It is important that every nurse be familiar with plans in his/her local community for dealing with potential threats to public health security, since nurses will be first key responders to any such threats.

MILLENNIUM DEVELOPMENT GOALS

In a historic meeting in New York in September 2000, representatives of 189 UN member states met and endorsed a plan called the Millennium Declaration, which has been described as "a new vision for humanity." The Millennium Declaration is a set of eight goals and specific targets under each goal designed to reduce poverty, reduce global inequities, and promote health and social welfare of the world's citizens (United Nations, 2008). This plan, named the Millennium Development Goals (MDG) report, outlined eight broad goals and specific targets for each goal, that were to be achieved by the year 2015. The eight goals, along with specific targets, are listed in Table 1.3, and these goals have served as guiding principles for both public and private organizations that focus on addressing global health and social welfare issues.

Each year the UN issues an MDG report to summarize the progress in addressing the eight goals. The 2007 report summarized the progress made on each of the eight goals at the midpoint of the 15-year target period. In the introduction to this report, Ban Ki-Moon, the Secretary General of the UN, noted that, "So far, our collective record is mixed. The results presented in this report suggest that there have been some gains, and that success is still possible in most parts of the world. But . . . there is a clear need for political leaders to take urgent and concerted action, or many millions of people will not realize the basic promises of the MDGs in their lives (United Nations, 2008)." This section highlights some of the key indicators of progress that were noted in the 2007 MDG report, and also describes the use of microfinance as a key strategy that has been used in many low-resource countries to reduce poverty and thereby enhance health and well-being.

Goal 1: Eradicate Extreme Poverty and Hunger

The 2007 MDG report indicated that although global poverty rates have decreased since 1990, there are still significant disparities, and the rates are highest in sub-Saharan Africa where 41.1% of people live on less than $1 per day (United Nations,

TABLE 1.3

Millenium Development Goals

Goal	Targets
Eradicate extreme hunger and poverty	Target 1: Halve, between 1990 and 2015, the proportion of people whose income is less than $1 a day Target 2: Halve, between 1990 and 2015, the proportion of people who suffer from hunger
Achieve universal primary education	Target 1: Ensure that, by 2015, children everywhere, boys and girls alike, will be able to complete a full course of primary schooling
Promote gender equality and empower women	Target 1: Eliminate gender disparity in primary and secondary education preferably by 2005 and in all levels of education no later than 2015
Reduce child mortality	Target 1: Reduce by two thirds, between 1990 and 2015, the under-five mortality rate
Improve maternal health	Target 1: Reduce by three quarters, between 1990 and 2015, the maternal mortality ratio
Combat HIV/AIDS, malaria, and other diseases	Target 1: Have halted by 2015 and begun to reverse the spread of HIV/AIDS Target 2: Half halted by 2015 and begun to reverse the incidence of malaria and other major diseases
Ensure environmental sustainability	Target 1: Integrate the principles of sustainable development into country policies and programs and reverse the loss of environmental resources Target 2: Halve, by 2015, the proportion of the population without sustainable access to safe drinking water and basic sanitation Target 3: To improve the lives of at least 100 million slum dwellers by 2020
Develop a global partnership for development	Target 1: Address the special needs of the least developed countries, landlocked countries and small island developing states Target 2: Develop further an open, rule-based, predictable, nondiscriminatory trading and financial system Target 3: In cooperation with developing countries, develop and implement strategies for decent and productive work for youth Target 4: In cooperation with the private sector, make available the benefits of new technologies, especially information and communications

Source: United Nations (2008).

2008). The poverty rates actually increased between 1990 and 2005 in many areas in Western Asia, in the Commonwealth of Independent States (CIS), and in the transition states of Eastern Europe. The 2007 MDG report concluded that if present trends continue, the first MDG goal will be met by 2015. One strategy that has shown much promise in reducing poverty, and thereby contributing to improvements in health status, has been the use of microfinance programs to provide the poor with access to financial services including savings plans and opportunities for low-interest loans to stimulate income-generating businesses. Pronyk, Hargreaves, and Morduch (2007) reported that the repayment rates across these programs are often greater than 95%, and that programs generally recover most of their administrative costs through user fees and interest rates. There were more than 3,000 such programs providing services to 113 million clients (84% women) by the end of 2005. In 2006, Muhammad Yumus and the Grameen Foundation won the Nobel Peace Prize in recognition of their use of microfinance as a means to reduce poverty, improve health, and stimulate social change. Poor village women in Bangladesh who received microloans were able to purchase cell phones and become Village Phone

Operators (VPOs), selling calls to their neighbors and increasing access to the outside world. This access in turn stimulated local businesses and had other community benefits as the VPOs earned enough money to invest in the education, health, and nutrition of their children and families (Grameen Foundation). The VPO model has been implemented in much of Africa and is viewed as a tool to promote sustainable development, as "wealth has impacted health" (Abbot & Coenen, 2008).

Goal 2: Achieve Universal Primary Education

Although enrollment in primary education increased in developing countries from 80% to 88% between 1990 and 2005, there is still much to be done in order to achieve the second MDG goal by 2015. In sub-Saharan Africa, for example, 30% of children who are of primary school age are not in school (United Nations, 2008). Given the strong correlation between education and health, there is a need to strengthen programs to ensure that all children have access to quality educational programs.

Goal 3: Promote Gender Equality and Empower Women

The 2007 MDG report included some encouraging statistics to indicate that women's involvement in politics and in leadership positions is increasing. In 2007, the percentage of women representatives in parliaments increased to 17% (compared to 13% in 1990), although much of women's work remains unpaid (United Nations, 2008). Because women are often the major family caregivers and assume primary responsibility for health care decisions, there is a clear relationship between health and the goal of promoting gender equity and women's empowerment.

Goal 4: Reduce Child Mortality

Although there have been significant improvements in child mortality rates, particularly in deaths due to measles, there continue to be wide disparities and in 2005, it was estimated that there were 10.1 million deaths among children under the age of 5. Child mortality is closely related to poverty, AIDS, malaria, and to wars and conflicts (United Nations, 2008).

Goal 5: Improve Maternal Health

The 2007 MDG report noted that there have been significant improvements in maternal mortality rates in middle-income countries since 1990, but the rates continue to be unacceptably high in many countries in sub-Saharan Africa and in Asia (United Nations, 2008). Key strategies to improve maternal health include increased access to prenatal care, to skilled birth attendants, and the prevention of teen and unplanned pregnancies.

Goal 6: Combat HIV/AIDS, Malaria, and Other Diseases

The 2007 MDG report indicated that although the prevalence of HIV has leveled off in the developing world, deaths from AIDS continue to increase in sub-Saharan Africa where it is estimated that only 28% of patients with HIV who need treatment have access to treatment. The President's Emergency Program for AIDS Relief (PEPFAR), an initiative of the United States Government that was launched in 2004, has provided significant funding for medications, care, and treatment of patients with HIV, targeting 15 countries with the highest rates of HIV (see http://www.pepfar.gov/). Gender imbalances continue to contribute to increasing numbers of women, including married women, becoming infected. Clearly there is a need to strengthen programs for prevention, treatment, and support to address the HIV pandemic.

Malaria remains a significant cause of morbidity and mortality throughout the world, although there have been substantial improvements in malaria control programs since 1990. One of the most effective prevention strategies is the use of insecticide-treated bed nets, since the mosquitoes that cause malaria typically bite only between dusk and dawn. Unfortunately, the use of bed nets is still limited in many areas. In sub-Saharan Africa, it is estimated that only 5% of children under the age of 5 sleep under these bed nets. There is also an urgent need to increase access to appropriate medicines to treat malaria, and to address the problem of resistance to many of the traditional antimalarial medications (United Nations, 2008).

Other infectious diseases also present considerable threats in many countries. Such diseases include tuberculosis, cholera, measles, typhoid, polio, guinea worm, diarrheal diseases, and upper respiratory infections. There has been notable progress in reducing the incidence of many of these infections. For example, between 2000 and 2006, there was a 91% reduction of deaths due to measles in Africa (http://www.globalhealth.org/infectious_diseases/).

Goal 7: Ensure Environmental Sustainability

The 2007 MDG report noted some encouraging data related to the seventh goal, as the international community has increased the amount of protected land and expanded the development and use of cleaner energy technologies such as biofuels and hydroelectric power. Despite these gains, however, the report noted that half of the developing world still lacks basic sanitation, and that expanded migration to urban areas has resulted in increasing numbers of slum dwellers. The report concluded that extraordinary global collaboration and cooperation will be needed in order to achieve the seventh goal by 2015 (United Nations, 2008).

Goal 8: Develop a Global Partnership for Development

It is clear that achieving the MDGs will require global partnership and collaboration, and increased commitment to international aid by high-resource countries. The 2007 MDG report noted that there has been some progress in lowering the debt service burden of low-resource countries; however, only five countries have reached or exceeded the UN target of allocating 0.7% of their gross national income to development aid (Denmark, Luxembourg, the Netherlands, Norway, and Sweden) (United Nations, 2008). One of the targets associated with the eighth MDG was to make available the benefits of increased technology and communication. The 2007 MDG report noted that access to technology has increased, particularly for mobile cell phones, and that although Internet use is growing, it remains low throughout most of the developing world. Abbott and Coenen (2008) provided an excellent review of the relationships between globalization, health, and the use of ICT, identifying numerous opportunities for nursing to contribute "in this flattening and increasingly interconnected world" (page 238). Such opportunities include using ICT to (a) provide educational and collaborative learning programs; (b) deliver nursing and health care using telenursing or telehealth services; (c) develop interoperable Electronic Health Record Systems (EHRS) to facilitate sharing data and to improve clinical decision making; (d) facilitate knowledge management and utilization to promote evidence-based practice; and (e) develop collaborative partnerships and communities of practice (CoPs) involving nurses throughout the world. One such CoP is the Global Alliance for Nursing & Midwifery (GANM), which was initiated by the WHO Department of Human Resources for Health, the WHO Office for Nursing & Midwifery, and the Johns Hopkins University School of Nursing Collaborating Center for Nursing Knowledge & Information Management. Membership in the GANM is free and open to nurses and midwives throughout the world. There are currently more than 1,500 members from 123 countries, who share knowledge and best practices, participate in continuing education, and have access to library resources (Abbot & Coenen, 2008). Another example of a CoP is the Network for Nurses in Child Health (Red Internacional de Enfermeria en Salud Infantil, Red ENSI), one of more than 15 specialty nursing networks that has been promoted by the Pan American Health Organization (PAHO) (Harrison et al., 2008). This network has coordinators from every country in Latin America and from Spain and the United States. Participants hold virtual meetings using Internet technology, facilitated by the PAHO/WHO Collaborating Center on International Nursing at the University of Alabama at Birmingham, and also share information via email correspondence and a website (http://www.enfermeriainfantil.org/R-ENSI/). A third example of using ICT for global networking is the Nightingale Initiative for Global Health (NIGH). The NIGH was established in 2003 and has two goals: (a) to globally unite 10 million nurses through the Internet and through developing regional groups around the world to promote a healthier world by 2020; and (b) to demonstrate the significance of nursing's contribution to global health. A key strategy to achieving this goal is the creation of the web-based Nightingale Global Alliance Campaign for a Healthy World (www.nightingaledeclaration.net). A final example of how ICT can facilitate information management and sharing, even when access to Internet and other technologies are limited, is the eGranary Digital Library, a collection of digital resources (such as web pages, articles, clinical practice guidelines, and other media), that can be accessed in areas where Internet connectivity is limited. The eGranary project is coordinated by the University of Iowa with support from many global partners including the WHO, universities, and private corporations. The nursing collection has been developed with input and recommendations from nurses all over the world (http://www.widernet.org/digitallibrary).

OTHER OPPORTUNITIES FOR NURSES TO CONTRIBUTE TO GLOBAL HEALTH AND THE GOAL OF "HEALTH FOR ALL"

In addition to using ICT to facilitate global partnerships and collaboration as described in the previous section, there are many other ways in which nurses can make significant contributions to global health at the local, national, and international levels. This final section will highlight four additional opportunities for nurses to "make a difference" in global health: (a) supporting primary health care initiatives; (b) helping to address challenges associated with the global nursing shortage and international nurse migration; (c) promoting global health equity through leadership and involvement in health policy development; and (d) participating in international exchanges and collaborations.

Primary Health Care

The year 2008 marked the 60th anniversary of the WHO and the 30th anniversary of a famous declaration supporting the essential role of primary health care in achieving the goal of global health equity, the Alma Ata Declaration (WHO report, 2008e). The

TABLE 1.4

Eight Essential Elements of Primary Health Care

In the globalized 21st century, community health nurses committed to primary health care need to focus on

1. Education for the identification and prevention/control of prevailing health problems
2. Proper food supplies and nutrition
3. Adequate supply of safe water and basic sanitation
4. Maternal and child care, including family planning
5. Immunization against the major infectious diseases, prevention and control of locally endemic diseases
6. Appropriate treatment of common diseases using appropriate technology
7. Promotion of mental health
8. Provision of essential drugs

Alma Ata Declaration was the result of a meeting of delegates from 134 nations of the world, plus representatives from nongovernmental organizations (NGOs) officially accredited by WHO, in what was then known as Alma Ata, USSR (now Almaty, Kazakhstan). In that historic meeting, the nations of the world committed themselves and their resources to the achievement of health for all by the year 2000 through primary health care. The 2008 WHO report (Primary Health Care: Now More than Ever) reflected the ongoing commitment to the Alma Ata Declaration and identified four reforms necessary to achieving the "Health for All" goal: (a) universal access to social health protection; (b) service delivery reforms to reorganize health services around people's needs and expectations; (c) public policy reforms; and (d) leadership reforms to promote more inclusive and participatory leadership. The eight elements essential to the primary health care approach reflect the priorities identified in 1978 at Alma Ata (Table 1.4). Nurses are the backbone for provision of primary health care services. Although applied differently around the world, these elements remain valid for all countries, at all levels of socioeconomic development.

Addressing Challenges Associated With the Global Nursing Shortage and International Nurse Migration

Numerous professional and governmental organizations have identified the critical shortage of nurses in countries around the globe as a major challenge to providing adequate health care services. The American Academy of Nursing's Expert Panel on Global Health published a White Paper in 2007 (Rosenkoetter & Nardi, 2007), addressing many of these challenges and reviewing the factors that contribute to the shortage and to the unequal global distribution of nurses. The average number of nurses per 100,000 people ranges from 10 to 1,000, with the ratios in Europe nearly 10 times higher than the ratios in many countries in Africa and Southeast Asia. Factors that contribute to the shortage in low-resource countries include challenges related to HIV/AIDS, high-stress work environments, gender-based discrimination and violence, and international migration of nurses. Many high-resource countries, faced with their own nursing shortages, contribute to this problem by recruiting nurses from lower-resource countries, further compounding the problem (Dovlo, 2005; Simpson, 2004). In addition to participating in efforts to address the nursing shortage at the local level (promoting the profession of nursing, helping to recruit young people into the profession, and working to strengthen retention of nurses in the workplace), nurses can join international efforts to promote ethical practices in international nurse recruitment. During the World Health Assembly in 2004, the WHO adopted a resolution (WHA57.19) addressing "International Migration of Health Personnel: A Challenge for Health Systems in Developing Countries" (http://www.who.int/gb/ebwha/pdf_files/WHA57/A57_R19-en.pdf). This resolution included a series of recommendations including international collaboration to collect information to monitor migration patterns and identify effects of such migration, strengthening mechanisms to train sufficient numbers of health care workers, and developing a code of practice on international recruitment of health personnel. More recently, the WHO has developed a "Global Code of Practice for the International Recruitment of Health Personnel" (http://apps.who.int/gb/ebwha/pdf_files/EB124/B124_13-en.pdf).

Promoting Global Health Equity through Leadership and Policy Development

The first step in making a contribution to global health equity involves developing a global perspective and awareness of important global health issues, and then finding ways to make a personal contribution to addressing these issues. Smith identified several questions that could help guide nurses in finding ways by which they could make such contributions, and suggested that some of the strategies outlined in the Academy of Nursing White Paper on Global Nursing and Health could provide a useful road map (Smith, 2006). Such strategies include promoting ethical models of nurse recruitment, incorporating more global health content into nursing curricula, supporting appropriate-technology distance-learning initiatives, and supporting legislation that supports *global* health research. Walker and Elberson suggested that organizational leaders have a responsibility to facilitate changes that will promote collaboration among organizational members and suggested that the use of technology can facilitate these leadership initiatives (Walker & Elberson, 2005).

Participating in International Exchanges and Collaborations

We all have much to learn from one another, and participation in international exchanges and collaborative projects can facilitate this learning. There are many ways to facilitate these types of exchanges. Spry described the goal of the International Networking Committee of the Association of periOperative Registered Nurses (AORN) to welcome and engage international attendees at the AORN annual conference (Spry, 2008). Leite de Silva identified the need for "emancipating education" for nurses that would prepare them to know about local and global reality and develop culturally competent practice (Leite de Silva, 2008). McAuliffe and Cohen reviewed 79 articles that were published in English describing international educational or research exchanges, and concluded that although such exchanges provide valuable opportunities for learning and for knowledge development, there is a need for the further development of theoretical models to guide such exchanges (McAuliffe & Cohen, 2005). These authors also suggested that faculty and student exchanges are most useful when they address priorities identified by the host country, and when they ensure that the projects increase the capacity of nurses in the host countries. Baumann and Blythe (2008) noted that the trend towards globalization of higher education in nursing brings both benefits and challenges (Bauman & Blythe, 2008). One of the challenges is the need for mechanisms to compare different educational qualifications of nurses against global standards. These authors noted several initiatives that have begun to address this challenge including the Code of Good Practice in the Provision of Transnational Education adopted by the European Union in 2001 and Guidelines on Quality Provision in Cross-Border Education developed by the United Nations Educational, Scientific, and Cultural Organization (UNESCO).

Summary

Nurses today have multiple and exciting opportunities to truly make a difference in addressing health disparities and promoting the goal of "Health for All." The world is indeed a community, and each nurse is a global citizen. We can begin by embracing the Nightingale Declaration of Commitment for a Healthy World by 2020:

"We, the nurses and concerned citizens of the global community, hereby dedicate ourselves to achieve a healthy world by 2020.

We declare our willingness to unite in a program of action, to share information and solution and to improve health conditions for all humanity—locally, nationally and globally.

We further resolve to adopt personal practices and to implement public policies in our communities and nations—making this goal achievable and inevitable by the year 2020, beginning today in our own lives, and in the life of our nations and in the world at large."

Source: © 2004. Nightingale Declaration of Commitment for a Healthy World by 2020. Used with permission of the Nightingale Initiative for Global Health. Available at http:// www.nightingaledeclaration.net

Critical Thinking Questions

1. Describe the relevance of one of the Millenium Development Goals to the community in which you live. How would you promote that goal to your own community? What types of data would you need to present your "case"?

2. Climate change affects everyone worldwide. Describe one major "natural disaster" that may be connected to climate change that had an impact on your community recently. What were the effects? Who was affected? How were nurses involved in the aftermath of that disaster?

3. Consider the recommendations of this chapter about how you can be involved in making a difference in global health. What does being a "global citizen" mean to you? Where can you go to find international opportunities for nurses?

4. Explore the websites listed at the end of this chapter. How can you use the information about global issues in your own practice?

● REFERENCES

Abbot, P. A., & Coenen, A. (2008). Globalization and advances in information and communication technologies: The impact on nursing and health. *Nursing Outlook*, 56(5), 238–246.

Bauman, A., & Blythe, J. (2008). Globalization of higher education in nursing. *OJIN: Online Journal of Issues in Nursing*, 13(2).

Birdsall, N. (2006). *The world is not flat: Inequality and injustice in our global economy*. Helsinki, Finland: United Nations University World Institute for Development Economics Research. WIDER Annual Lecture 9.

Dovlo, D. (2005). Taking more than a fair share? The migration of health professionals from poor to rich countries. *PLoS Medicine*, 2(5), 376–379.

Global Forum for Health Research. (2008). The 10/90 gap: Now. Retrieved December 19, 2008, from http://www.globalforumhealth.org/About/10-90-gap

Grameen Foundation. Village phone: Connecting technology and innovation. Retrieved January 2, 2009, from http://www.grameenfoundation.org/what_we_do/technology_programs/village_phone/

Harrison, L., Montenegro, G., Malvares, S., Astudillo, M., Behn, V., & Bertolozzi, M. R., et al. (2008). The network for nursing in child health. *Pediatric Nursing*, 34(2), 113–116, 138–139.

Hitti, M. (2007). Officials seeking more than 600 passengers on patient's flight; patient feeling well in hospital. *WebMD Health News*.

Institute of Medicine. (1997). *America's vital interest in global health*. Washington, D.C.: National Academy Press.

Joint United Nations Program on HIV/AIDS and World Health Organization. (2007). *AIDS epidemic update*. Geneva, Switzerland: Joint United Nations Program on HIV/AIDS and world Health Organization (J. U. N. P. o. H. A. a. w. H. Organization).

Jones, K. E., Patel, N. G., Levy, M. A., Storeygard, A., Balk, D., & Gittleman, J. L., et al. (2008). Global trends in emerging infectious diseases. *Nature*, 451, 990–993.

Leite de Silva, A. (2008). Nursing in the era of globalisation: Challenges for the 21st century. *Revista Latino-americana de Enfermagem*, 16(4), 787–790.

Luber, G., & Hess, J. (2007). Climate change and human health in the United States. *Journal of Environmental Health*, 70(5), 43–46.

McAuliffe, M. S., & Cohen, M. Z. (2005). International nursing research and educational exchanges: A review of the literature. *Nursing Outlook*, 53(1), 21–25.

Murphy, C. (2006). The 2003 SARS outbreak: Global challenges and innovative infection control measures. *OJIN: The Online Journal of Issues in Nursing*, 11(1).

National Institutes of Health. (2006). *Strategic research plan and budget to reduce and ultimately eliminate health disparities. Vol. 1, Fiscal years 2002–206*. Bethesda, MD: National Institutes of Health.

Patz, J., Campbell-Lendrum, D., Gibbs, H., & Woodruff, R. (2008). Health impact assessment of global climate change: Expanding on comparative risk assessment approaches for policy making. *Annual Review of Public health*, 29, 27–39.

Pronyk, P. M., Hargreaves, J. R., & Morduch, J. (2007). Microfinance programs and better health: Prospects for sub-Saharan Africa. *Journal of American Medical Association*, 298(16), 1925–1927.

Ramzy, A., & Yang, L. (2008). Tainted-baby-milk scandal in China. Retrieved December 18, 2008, from www.time.com/time/world/article/0,8599,1841535,000.html.

Rosenkoetter, M. M., & Nardi, D. A. (2007). American academy of nursing expert panel on global nursing and health: White paper on global nursing and health: Academia Americana de Enfermeria, Panel de Expertos en Enfermeria Global y Salud: Documento de Opinion en Enfermeria Global y Salud. *Journal of Transcultural Nursing*, 18(4), 305–315.

Simpson, R. L. (2004). Global informing. Impact and implications of technology in a global marketplace. *Nursing Administration Quarterly*, 28(2), 144–149.

Smith, B. A. (2006). The role of nursing leaders in global health issues and global health policy. *Nursing Outlook*, 54(6), 309–310.

Spry, C. (2008). Global perspectives. International sharing: What's in it for us? *AORN Journal*, 88(3), 443.

United Nations. (2008). *Millenium Development Goals Report*. New York: United Nations.

Walker, P. H., & Elberson, K. L. (2005). Collaboration: Leadership in a global technological environment. *Online Journal of Issues in Nursing*, 10(1).

World Bank. (2008). Poverty at a glance. Retrieved December 19, 2008, from http://web.worldbank.org/WBSITE/EXTERNAL/TOPICS/EXTPOVERTY/EXTPA/0, contentMDK:20040961~isCURL:Y~menuPK:435040~pagePK:148956~piPK:216618~ theSitePK:430367,00.html.

World Health Organization. (2007). *The World Health Report 200—A safer future: Global public health security in the 21st century*.

World Health Organization. (2008a). 10 facts on the global burden of disease. Retrieved December 19, 2008, from http://www.who.int/features/factfiles/global_burden/en/.

World Health Organization. (2008b). Global burden of disease (definition). Retrieved December 19, 2008, from http://www.who.int/topics/global_burden_of_disease/en/.

World Health Organization. (2008c). Global burden of disease, 2004 update. Geneva, Switzerland: World Health Organization.

World Health Organization. (2008d). The top 10 causes of death. Retrieved December 19, 2008, from http://www.who.int/mediacentre/factsheets/fs310/en/print.html.

World Health Organization. (2008e). *World Health Report 2008: Primary health care now more than ever*. Geneva, Switzerland: World Health Organization.

World Health Organization Department of Human Resources for Health. (2008). *Report of the global consultation on an implementation framework for scaling up nursing and midwifery capacity*. Geneva, Switzerland: World Health Organization.

Internet Resources can be found on the**Point** at http://thepoint.lww.com/Anderson6e.

Community Health Nursing: Essentials of Practice

Elizabeth T. Anderson

LEARNING OBJECTIVES

This chapter continues the conceptual basis of community as partner. As such, it introduces the key concepts of community health nursing and public health nursing.

After studying this chapter, you should be able to:

1. Describe the historical development of community health nursing.
2. Define community health nursing in the 21st century.
3. Identify the domains of community health nursing competency.
4. Describe nursing roles in the community.

Introduction

*T*he second decade of the 21st century is bustling with phenomenal opportunities and challenges for health care delivery and community health nursing. There is no better time to be a community health nurse. The discussion that follows represents some reflections on what we believe will characterize the practice of community health nursing in the 21st century. We use the term *community health nursing* to denote the practice of nursing by professional nurses who have been educated in the processes of population-based nursing and whose principal client is the aggregate community.

In the past, population-based nursing was referred to as public health nursing. Public health nurses usually worked in health departments. This chapter uses the term *community health nurse*, which was adopted in recent years and intended to be more inclusive of population-based nursing practiced in a variety of community settings, including schools, worksites, shelters, health departments, and a multitude of others, some of which will be discussed in Part 3 of this book. You will encounter both terms, public health nursing and community health nursing, during your education and practice. Titles and practice settings are not as relevant as the nature of the practice itself. This chapter discusses the essence and diversity of that practice.

Until now the majority of your nursing education has focused on individual behavior. The theoretical basis for your nursing care has included knowledge about chemistry, physiology, pharmacology, and so on. Community health nursing, too, relies on that basic knowledge, but is also based on theories about populations. Hence, you will discover in subsequent chapters the concepts of epidemiology, demography, ethics, environment, culture, and policy. To understand why these theories are important to the community health nurse, let's begin with a bit of history.

REFLECTIONS ON THE PAST

Reflecting on the historical contributions of community health nurses is both instructive and inspirational. Examining our roots allows us to take the best from the past in order to shape the future. Community health nurses can gain motivation and direction from the work of Lillian Wald, Lavinia Dock, and Margaret Sanger who "make up nursing's 'distinguished history of concern . . . for social justice'" (Bekemeier & Butterfield, 2005, p. 153) and who, more than 100 years ago, " . . . grew indignant from witnessing the destructive health outcomes of institutionalized poverty and of gender and ethnic inequalities" (Bekemeier & Butterfield, 2005, p. 153). Observing rapid industrialization, large concentrations of people moving into cities, unsanitary environmental conditions, poor housing, poverty, misuse of child labor, infectious diseases, and short life expectancy, Lillian Wald and Mary Brewster were moved to action. Together, they founded the Henry Street Settlement House in New York City. There they lived and worked among the people, teaching hygiene practices, visiting the sick in homes, and crusading for better health care in all aspects of the community. Lillian Wald recognized the intertwining of health status, environmental sanitation, and social and political forces. Her work targeted the root causes of ill health, which meant that she had to take on institutions, politics, and social policy to effect change for the improvement of the community's health. Lillian Wald had an exceptional ability to inform and convince people of the need for social change (Backer, 1993). Wald first coined the term public health nurse and is regarded as the "mother of public health nursing" in the United States. Her contributions include establishing nursing schools, advocating for better housing, working to change child labor laws, teaching preventive practices, advocating occupational health nursing, and improving the education of public health nurses, to name a few (Coss, 1989; Feld, 2008).

With the discovery of antibiotics in the 1940s and vaccines for mass immunizations in conjunction with tremendous improvements in environmental sanitation, the United States experienced a considerable decline in morbidity and mortality due to communicable diseases. According to the Centers for Disease Control and Prevention (CDC), public health is credited with adding 25 years to the life expectancy of people in the United States. In addition, the CDC has identified ten great achievements of public health in the 20th century that have contributed to this increase in longevity (CDC, 1999). These achievements are listed in Box 2.1. Public health nurses were at the forefront of ensuring that these great achievements were carried out in the community.

Beginning in the 1960s, as communicable diseases declined, attention turned to the prevention of chronic diseases and related risk factors such as cigarette smoking and dietary fat. Community health nurses working in health departments focused attention on screening, case finding, home visiting to individual clients, and health

BOX 2.1

TEN GREAT PUBLIC HEALTH ACHIEVEMENTS IN THE 20TH CENTURY

1. Immunizations
2. Improvements in motor vehicle safety
3. Workplace safety
4. Control of infectious diseases
5. Decline in deaths from heart disease and stroke
6. Safer and healthier foods
7. Healthier mothers and babies
8. Family planning
9. Fluoridation of drinking water
10. Recognition of tobacco as a health hazard

Source: Centers for Disease Control and Prevention. (1999). Ten great public achievements— United States, 1900–1999. *Morbidity and Mortality Weekly Report*, 48(12), 241–243.

education activities related to disease prevention. This trend continued into the early 1980s when the focus of health shifted somewhat to health promotion, prompted by the Health for All era established by the World Health Organization (WHO, 1978). However, the 1990s were marked by considerable emphasis on clinical care and high-tech medicine as ways to increase life span in the United States. Health departments began to emphasize clinical care, such as prenatal care, family planning, treatment of communicable diseases, and immunizations, particularly for citizens without access to basic preventive services. The 1990s can also be characterized as the era in which the high cost of health care in the United States became a major concern of policymakers.

In recent years, official agencies have become more involved in direct clinical care, and community health nursing has focused on clinical and illness care or "clinic" roles and functions, assigning less importance to family- and community-focused roles and functions. This shift was primarily in response to the reimbursability of clinical services. Now public health is shifting back to its "roots" and is focusing more on disease prevention, health promotion, and assurance that care is provided, rather than providing one-on-one care. To respond to the challenges facing community health nursing in the future, we must understand the changes occurring in health-care delivery, including directions for population-based health.

COMMUNITY HEALTH NURSING IN THE UNITED STATES: THE CONTEXT

Past debates about health-care reform largely ignored the contributions of population-based community health, concentrating almost entirely on clinical care, with the exception of immunizations. Mechanisms to deliver and pay for illness care are driving current health-care system changes. The debate really ought to be about what can be done to make our population the healthiest rather than how we can best pay for illness. Some elected officials have been reluctant to fund health-promotion services at the levels needed, but it takes excellent health promotion to minimize the cost of illness care. Health promotion results in wellness.

TABLE 2.1

Essential Public Health Services and Selected Nursing Activities

Essential Public Health Services	Selected Nursing Activity
1. Monitor health status to identify community health problems.	Participate in community assessment; identify potential environmental hazards.
2. Diagnose and investigate health problems and hazards in the community.	Understand and identify determinants of health and disease.
3. Inform, educate, and empower people about health issues.	Develop and implement community-based health education.
4. Mobilize community partnerships to identify and solve health problems.	Explain the significance of health issues to the public and participate in developing plans of action.
5. Develop policies and plans that support individual and community health efforts.	Develop programs and services to meet the needs of high-risk populations as well as members of the broader community.
6. Enforce laws and regulations that protect health and ensure safety.	Regulate and support safe care and treatment for dependent populations such as children and the frail elderly.
7. Link people to needed personal health services and ensure the provision of health care when otherwise unavailable.	Establish programs and services to meet special needs.
8. Ensure a competent public health and personal health-care workforce.	Participate in continuing education and preparation to ensure competence.
9. Evaluate effectiveness, accessibility, and quality of personal and population-based health services.	Identify unserved and underserved populations in communities.
10. Research new insights and innovations solutions to health problems.	Participate in early identification of factors detrimental to the community's health.

Source: Association of State and Territorial Directors of Nursing. (2000). *Public health nursing: A partner for healthy populations.* Washington, DC: American Nurses Association.

Community health in the 21st century must offer integrated services and activities that focus on minimizing threats to health, promoting wellness, and then focusing on illness management.

To improve the health of communities community health nurses need to focus on the ten essential public health services (Table 2.1). The essential public health services provide a fundamental framework by describing the public health activities that should be undertaken in all communities. The essential services provide a working definition of public health and a guiding framework for the responsibilities of local public health systems. Table 2.1 includes both the essential services as well as a selected nursing activity for each. These essential services comprise an impressive list, and each service can be used to direct community health nursing practice in a diversity of settings.

In addition to the services, community health practice is focused on prevention rather than illness care. The levels of prevention—primary, secondary, and tertiary—are described in Chapter 3.

COMMUNITY HEALTH NURSING PRACTICE

The focus of this text is on populations and systems as you will see from our selected model as well as the exemplars described in Part 3. As the basis for your practice, as with any professional role, you are expected to be familiar with the scope and standards of practice. Developing the statements has been an iterative process with input from the Quad Council as well as numerous nurses in practice, education, and research. The American Nurses Association published the scope and standards using the term public health nursing (American Nurses Association, 2007).

The four organizations of the Quad Council (the American Nurses Association, Council of Community, Primary, and Long-Term Care; American Public Health Association—Public Health Nursing Section; Association of Community Health Nurse Educators; and Association of State and Territorial Directors of Nursing) met over time to describe community health nursing more clearly. Their definition of public health nursing is as follows:

> *Public health nursing is the practice of promoting and protecting the health of populations using knowledge from nursing, social, and public health sciences (American Public Health Association, Public Health Nursing Section 1996). The practice is population-focused with the goals of promoting health and preventing disease and disability for all people through the creation of conditions in which people can be healthy.*
>
> *Although practicing in a variety of public and private organizations, all public health nurses focus on one or more populations. A population may be defined as those living in a specific geographic area (e.g., neighborhood, community, city, or county) or those in a particular group (e.g., racial, ethnic, age, disease) who experience a disproportionate burden of poor health outcomes.*
>
> *(American Nurses Association, 2007, p. 5)*

The Quad Council described the competencies required of public health nurses in eight domains to advance the goal of promoting and protecting the health of the population. Underpinning these competencies are the eight principles of public health nursing (Box 2.2). The competencies are divided into Generalist/Staff Public Health Nurse and Manager/Consultant/Program Specialist/Executive to reflect two levels of preparation—baccalaureate and masters. Competencies under each level are divided into individuals and families or populations/systems. We can use these principles and competencies to guide our practice of community health nursing, regardless of the setting.

BOX 2.2

THE EIGHT PRINCIPLES OF PUBLIC HEALTH NURSING

1. The Client or "unit of care" is the population.
2. The primary obligation is to achieve the greatest good for the greatest number of people or the population as a whole.
3. The processes used by public health nurses include working with the client(s) as an equal partner.
4. Primary prevention is the priority in selecting appropriate activities.
5. Selecting strategies that create healthy environmental, social, and economic conditions in which populations may thrive is the focus.
6. There is an obligation to actively reach out to all who might benefit from a specific activity or service.
7. Optimal use of available resources to assure the best overall improvement in the health of the population is a key element of the practice.
8. Collaboration with a variety of other professions, organizations, and entities is the most effective way to promote and protect the health of the people.

Source: American Nurses Association. (2007). *Public health nursing: Scope and standards of practice.* Silver Spring, MD: The Association.

BOX 2.3

FACTORS SHAPING 21ST CENTURY HEALTH

Health care "reform"
Demographics
Globalization
Poverty and growing disparities
Violence, injuries, and social disintegration

FACTORS INFLUENCING COMMUNITY HEALTH NURSING IN THE 21ST CENTURY

All health professions are being influenced by the changes occurring in our health care system. Some relevant factors shaping 21st century community health are summarized in Box 2.3 and are elaborated below.

Health Care Delivery System

All aspects of health care need to become increasingly community based and population focused. The present focus of change in health care delivery centers on cost containment. Competition based on market forces is a major driver in the emerging health care system. Large, integrated health systems are rapidly developing with mergers of large hospitals, physician practice groups, nursing home care facilities, home health agencies, and other specialty groups. All of these factors create the challenge of balancing the needs of the individual within the broader social context. The increase in managed care organizations has meant fewer individual patients for health departments (and less revenue) in prenatal, well-child, and family planning clinics. This change means that the Medicaid population is cared for by managed care groups and there is less need for health department clinical services.

One innovative program aimed at our fragmented system serves as an example of how health professionals can partner to affect the health of our citizens. This program, Turning Point, was begun in 1997 with funding from the Robert Wood Johnson Foundation and additional funding from the W. K. Kellogg Foundation. Threats to our nation (bioterrorism and emerging infectious diseases, along with obesity, violence, and tobacco-related illnesses) require a strong public health system, and currently, 23 states practice the philosophy of Turning Point. It behooves community health nurses to be aware of such innovations and to support those that prove effective in improving health. Tools for improving practice and collaboration are readily available through the W.K Kellogg Foundation website [www.wkkf.org], and positive outcomes, such as the establishment of local health departments to cover all of Nebraska, for example, are being reported regularly (Berkowitz, Nicola, Lafronza, & Bekemeier, 2005).

Demographics

Many countries with very large populations have shown great progress in lowering their birth rates. However, the very size of their current populations means that, in absolute terms, their populations will continue to increase for many years. As large numbers of young people become sexually active, they, in turn, will place greater pressures on local health services, schools, and employers. In the United States, certain ethnic and cultural groups with young populations are presenting similar challenges to local education and social service systems.

Family structures and living arrangements are also changing rapidly in much of the world. Fewer people live in traditional family groups or have extended family support networks. The stress that often results from these changes, along with the growing disruption of traditional cultural patterns, is another factor adding to the erosion of social support systems and people's burden of disease.

Two significant demographic factors shaping the future of community health nursing and all health care are age and increasing ethnic diversity. Studies predict that by 2040, one out of five Americans will be 65 years or older. The graying of America will continue to shift the focus of medical care from acute to chronic illness and challenge the development of new and effective health promotion strategies for this population. Quality of life, not merely a long life, will become the priority. There is no debate about the growing ethnic diversity of this country. Changes in immigration laws and differential fertility rates and age patterns among minority groups have dramatically altered the ethnic makeup of the United States. Nationwide, Asians and Pacific Islanders will constitute the fastest growing ethnic group, but Hispanics will comprise the largest ethnic "minority" group. These changes have many social and health implications for community health nursing.

Globalization

The major factor affecting communities today and in the foreseeable future is the phenomenon known as globalization. Globalization represents a global market that brings together capital, technology, and information across borders to create what some call a global village. When global financial markets go up or down, when trade agreements are negotiated, when recessions threaten the countries that purchase the products made in our towns and communities, we and our communities can be in danger. When recession or political instability occurs in other countries, foreign companies often lower their prices to make their products more competitive. They are able to do this and still make a profit because the levels of local unemployment create conditions in which those competing for jobs are willing to work for less and less. When this happens over a period of time and is widespread, companies and factories, once considered sources of stable employment in our communities, frequently close their U.S. operations and move to countries where salaries are lower and labor laws are weak or nonexistent. Anyone doubting this trend needs only to look at the labels on the clothes, electrical appliances, toys, food, flowers, and other merchandise in our local stores.

With the growing strength of organizations such as the World Trade Organization (WTO) and trade pacts such as the North American Free Trade Agreement (NAFTA) with their emphasis on free trade, free financial markets, and economic profits, governments—especially those of resource-poor nations—find themselves losing the ability to define and control their own futures. Political scientists and sociologists warn of the declining strength of the "nation state" and the questionable future of international organizations such as the United Nations (UN) and its related units such as the World Health Organization (WHO). If many countries are weakening in relation to powerful international forces, what does this mean for the development of our local communities? How are they affected by the emphasis on profit—usually for a few privileged individuals and companies?

Globalization, however, can have many positive consequences in our lives. New technologies bring almost instant communication with other parts of the world. Today, mobile phones, many connected to satellites, bring nearly instant access to previously remote areas. Cyberspace, with its Internet electronic mailing lists and chat rooms, allows us to learn of other people's realities—their dreams, needs, and challenges. In education, for example, there is a proposal "to launch the iNet Global Village program. This program includes a series of activities and events aimed at preparing today's school children to become competent and productive citizens in a world that is increasingly global and virtual" (Zhao, 2006).

How can these same advances in technology and information be used by communities in their struggles for social justice and equity for all?

Poverty and Growing Disparities

Although it is true that many of us have improved our standard of living, nearly half the world's population still lives on less than $2 per day, and approximately 1.4 billion people are living in extreme poverty—more than one-quarter of the population of developing countries. (World Bank, 2008). People's health and well-being suffer the most when they are unable to secure appropriate employment and can no longer access adequate "social safety nets" and supportive services.

T A K E   N O T E

"Health disparities are differences in the incidence, prevalence, mortality, and burden of diseases and other adverse health conditions that exist among specific population groups in the United States" (National Institutes of Health, 2006, p. 1).

Wherever people live, poverty has been identified as a major cause of malnutrition and illness, thus undermining the efforts of health workers and health services. Whether at home or at work, the poor are often more exposed to pollution and other health risks than others. They frequently eat poorly, whether in quantity or in quality, and are more likely to smoke tobacco and be exposed to other harmful substances. Differences such as these are found throughout the world, including in the United States.

But poverty is not the only disparity. Additional disparities identified are geographic and racial or ethnic. Lack of health insurance is a major disparity. Today, the number of uninsured Americans is reported to be between 45.7 million (U.S. Census Bureau, 2007) and 86.7 million or one in three Americans under 65 (Families USA, 2009).

Devoting entire issues of nursing journals to the topic reflects the importance of health disparities in the United States. *Nursing Outlook*, the Official Journal of the American Academy of Nursing, published a special issue on health disparities (American Academy of Nursing, 2005). The same year *Advances in Nursing Science (ANS)* and *Nursing Research* collaborated on a call for manuscripts addressing the problem. Editor Chinn of ANS reminds us that there is a long history of nurses reaching out to the underserved and advocating policies to improve health (Chinn, 2005). Recall earlier in the chapter when we spoke of Lillian Wald and others. May our legacy also represent our future.

Violence, Injuries, and Social Disintegration

Violence takes many forms and ranges from highly visible armed conflict and teen street gangs, to the 4 million women and girls sold into sexual slavery each year, to the estimated 25% to 30% of all women who experience domestic violence, and to the 130 million women who are victims of genital mutilation. Entertainment media have long been able to produce extremely violent movie scenes and games in which the aim is to kill. In the United States, powerful groups have made easy access to guns a "right." Although it is very difficult to establish a cause-and-effect relationship between the number of guns available, the violence of the entertainment media, and the number of gun-related crimes committed by younger and younger people, communities have become increasingly concerned about violence. They are also concerned about the weakening of human relationships—in families, between generations, and in communities—that often result in social disintegration.

Internationally, the UN Convention on the Elimination of all Forms of Discrimination against Women (CEDAW) was created in 1979 as an important tool for all those who seek to end abuse of women and girls. The American Nurses Association is one of some 168 professional, religious, civic, and community organizations that support ratification of this International Bill of Rights for Women (Convention on the Elimination of all Forms of Discrimination retrieved December 30, 2009 at http://www.un.org/womenwatch/daw/cedaw/). Being aware of such documents and promoting their adoption is a way the community health nurse can serve as an advocate.

TAKE NOTE

"Health is a social, economic and political issue and, above all, a fundamental right. Inequality, poverty, exploitation, violence, and injustice are at the root of ill health and the death of poor and marginalized people" (People's Health Movement, 2003, p. 5).

CHALLENGES FOR THE FUTURE

Community health nurses in the future need to stretch themselves and go far beyond traditional nursing practice in conventional medical and health services. They will continue to be teachers, advocates, monitors, catalysts, and enablers. They will be scientifically and technically skilled. They will be knowledgeable about economics, politics, and global issues. But, most of all, they will be partners with communities at local, regional, national, and international levels. Amelia Maglacas, Chief Nurse Scientist of the WHO at the time, pointed out that enabling people to increase control over and to improve their health will continue to be an integral part of all nurses' roles. This new partnership, involving nurses, communities, and their environments, involves a common search, based on personal choice and social responsibility, for a healthier future (Maglacas, 1988). Her words continue to ring true for community health nurses.

Summary

This chapter has provided you with an overview of the role of the community health nurse and introduced you to factors influencing that role. Essential theories will be elaborated in subsequent chapters. Awareness of the global factors that affect health and of the essentials of community health nursing will arm you with the tools and knowledge to work toward improving health in communities everywhere.

Critical Thinking Questions

1. Review the 10 essential public health services. How could managed care organizations benefit from having a public health nurse on staff?

2. What health concerns in your community have resulted in death, disease, or injury? How could population-based community health nursing help prevent these problems?

3. Identify three factors that impinge on the health of the community in which you live. Prioritize these factors in terms of their impact and give the rationale for your choices.

● REFERENCES

American Academy of Nursing. (2005). Special Issue: Health disparities. *Nursing Outlook*, 53(3), 107–166.

American Nurses Association. (2007). *Public health nursing: Scope & standards of practice*. Silver Spring, MD: The Association.

American Public Health Association, Public Health Nursing Section. (1996). *Definition and role of public health nursing*. Washington, DC: Author.

Association of State and Territorial Directors of Nursing. (2000). *Public health nursing: A partner for healthy populations*. Washington, DC: American Nurses Association.

Backer, B. A. (1993). Lillian Wald: Connecting caring with action. *Nursing and Health Care*, 14(3), 122–129.

Bekemeier, B., & Butterfield, P. (2005). Unreconciled inconsistencies: A critical review of the concept of social justice in 3 national nursing documents. *Advances in Nursing Science*, 28(2), 152–162.

Berkowitz, B., Nicola, R., Lafronza, V., & Bekemeier, B. (2005). Turning point's legacy. *Journal of Public Health Management and Practice*, 11(2), 97–100.

Centers for Disease Control and Prevention. (1999). Ten great public health achievements—United States, 1900–1999. *Morbidity and Mortality Weekly Report*, 48(12), 241–243.

Chinn, P. L. (2005). From the Editor: Nursing activism and scholarship to address health disparities. *Advances in Nursing Science*, 28(3), 193.

Coss, C. (1989). *Lillian Wald: A progressive activist*. New York, NY: Feminist Press.

FamiliesUSA. (2009). Retrieved December 26, 2009 at http://www.familiesusa.org

Feld, M. N. (2008). *Lillian Wald: A biography*. Chapel Hill, NC: The University of North Carolina Press.

Maglacas, A. M. (1988). Health for all: Nursing's role. *Nursing Outlook*, 36(2), 66–71.

National Institutes of Health. (2006). *Strategic research plan and budget to reduce and ultimately eliminate health disparities. Vol. 1, Fiscal years 2002–2006*. Bethesda, MD: Author. Retrieved December 26, 2009 from http://seer.cancer.gov/publications/disparities/md_defining.pdf

People's Health Movement. (2003). *Preamble to the People's Charter for Health*. Berkeley, CA, and Decatur, GA: Hesperian Foundation and Doctors for Global Health (co-conveners of the US Circle of the People's Health Movement).

U.S. Bureau of the Census. Retrieved December 26, 2009 at http://www.census.gov/compendia/statab/

World Bank. (2008). Poverty data: A supplement to World Development Indicators 2008. Washington, D.C.: World Bank. Accessed December 26, 2009 at http://siteresources.worldbank.org/DATASTATISTICS/Resources/WDI08supplement12 16.pdf

World Health Organization. (1978, September). *Report of the international conference on primary health care*. Geneva, Switzerland: Author.

Zhao, Y. (2006). iNet global village [concept paper], March 19, 2006, Michigan State University. Retrieved December 26, 2009 at http://www.ssat-inet.net/PDF/iNet%20Global%20Village%20concept%20paper.pdf

Internet Resources can be found on the Point at http://thepoint.lww.com/Anderson6e.

Epidemiology, Demography, and Community Health

JUDITH MCFARLANE

LEARNING OBJECTIVES

After studying this chapter, you should be able to:

1. Interpret and use basic epidemiologic, demographic, and statistical measures of community health.
2. Apply principles of epidemiology and demography to the practice of community health.

Introduction

*E*pidemiology and demography are sciences for studying population health. To promote, restore, and maintain the health of populations, the community health professional integrates and applies concepts from these fields. Use of the epidemiologic process can significantly enhance community health practice, providing both a body of knowledge and a methodology for investigating health problems and evaluating health services. This chapter introduces epidemiologic and demographic concepts that are essential for the practice of community health nursing.

EPIDEMIOLOGY

The term *epidemiology* originates from the Greek terms *logos* (study), *demos* (people), and *epi* (upon)—literally, "the study of what is upon the people." Epidemiology is concerned with the distribution and determinants of health and diseases, morbidity, injuries, disability, and mortality in populations. Population in this context refers to people with a common characteristic such as gender, age, and place of residence. Although epidemiologic investigations examine conditions in population groups, it is important to remember that a population consists of individuals, each of whom is a person with a particular condition.

   Epidemiology is the study of the distribution and determinants of health-related states or events in specified populations and the application of this study to improve health. Epidemiology is a quantitative discipline based on principles of statistics and research methodologies. Epidemiologic studies have made a significant contribution to the identification of risk factors, such as smoking and lung cancer. In addition, epidemiologic studies identify modifiable risk factors for heart disease resulting in lifestyle changes for individuals along with changes in public health policy. Thus, epidemiologic research methods are a powerful tool for investigating health-related events.

Early epidemiologic studies were concerned chiefly with the control of epidemics (an outbreak of an illness beyond the levels expected in a population). John Snow's study of a cholera epidemic in London in 1853 is a classic in epidemiologic history. At that time, the mode of transmission of cholera was unknown. Snow suspected it was spread by contaminated water. Applying epidemiologic principles, Snow determined that death rates from cholera were highest in areas served by two specific water-pumping systems. He learned that the water from these systems came from portions of the Thames River into which London sewage was discharged. Thus, this early epidemiologist was able to identify a waterborne mode of transmission of cholera and determine measures to control its spread (Snow, 1936).

Many epidemiologic studies have a disease morbidity/mortality focus; however, the dimensions of health and well-being extend beyond these components. Epidemiology as practiced today has expanded its scope to include investigation of lifestyles, health-promotion strategies, injury, environmental conditions, and other factors that influence health. Public health practitioners use the knowledge gained from the epidemiologic process to guide decision making and aid in developing and evaluating interventions for health promotion and disease prevention. The epidemiologic process is analogous to the nursing process in that critical analysis is required to gain further insight into public and community health issues.

Descriptive Epidemiology

Descriptive epidemiology focuses on the distribution of frequencies and patterns of health events with groups in a population. Descriptive studies examine disease patterns and other health-related phenomena according to "person" (who is affected?), "place" (where were they affected?), and "time" (when were they affected?). Descriptive statistics provide data, information, and insight into the characteristics present in a group or population with a disease or the absence of disease in unaffected groups or populations. The question addressed is, "Are there characteristics present in the affected population that are not present in the unaffected population?" For example, why are breast cancer rates lower in women who have had children and breast-fed them than in women who have not had children? Descriptive statistics provide epidemiologic studies with data to develop rates, ratios, and proportions of morbidity and mortality statistics for use in public health and vital statistics. Data from descriptive studies suggest hypotheses for further testing and usually involve some form of quantification and statistical analysis. Descriptive studies generally precede analytic studies.

Analytic Epidemiology

In contrast to descriptive epidemiology, analytic epidemiology seeks to identify associations between a particular disease or health problem and its etiology. Analytic studies are directed toward finding answers to the "how" and "why" of health and disease to determine causality. Analytic studies are concerned with the determinants of disease and seek to identify the causes of the problem. They test hypotheses or seek to answer specific questions and can be retrospective or prospective in design.

DEMOGRAPHY

Demography (literally, "writing about the people," from the Greek *demos* [people] and *graphos* [writing]) is the statistical study of human populations with reference to size and density, distribution, and vital statistics. Demographic statistics provide information about significant characteristics of a population that influence community needs and the delivery of health care services. Demographic studies (i.e., demographic research) provide descriptions and comparisons of populations according to the characteristics of age, race, sex, socioeconomic status, geographic distribution, and birth, death, marriage, and divorce patterns. Demographic studies often have health implications that may or may not be addressed by the investigators. The census of the U.S. population is an example of a comprehensive descriptive demographic study conducted every 10 years.

LEVELS OF PREVENTION IN COMMUNITY HEALTH PRACTICE

The concept of prevention is a key component of modern community health practice. In popular terminology, prevention means inhibiting the development of disease before it occurs. For the community health practitioner, three levels of prevention—primary, secondary, and tertiary—guide practice.

Primary prevention applied to a generally healthy population precedes disease or dysfunction. Primary prevention is divided into two component areas: (1) general health promotion such as nutrition, hygiene, exercise, and environmental protection and (2) specific health promotion, which includes immunizations and the wearing of protective devices to prevent injuries. If a disease is environmentally induced, primary prevention can prevent a person's exposure to the environmental factor involved and thereby prevent development of the disease. Prevention is difficult to measure and demonstrate empirically; however, it is less costly both in terms of human suffering and in terms of economic expenditures than crisis intervention and treating disease and disabilities after they have occurred.

Secondary prevention is the early detection and treatment of adverse health conditions. The goal of secondary prevention is to detect and treat a problem at the earliest possible stage when disease or impairment already exists. Secondary prevention may result in the cure of illnesses that would be incurable at later stages, the prevention of complications and disability, and confinement of the spread of communicable diseases. Examples of secondary prevention include blood pressure screening for hypertension, audiometric testing for hearing impairment, skin test for tuberculosis, and phenylalanine test for phenylketonuria in infancy. On a community basis, early treatment of people with infectious disease, such as a sexually transmitted disease (STD), may protect others from acquiring infection and thus provides secondary prevention for infected people and primary prevention for their potential contacts.

Tertiary prevention is employed after diseases or events have already resulted in morbidity. The purpose of tertiary prevention is to limit disability and to rehabilitate or restore the affected people to their maximum possible capacities. Examples of tertiary prevention include physical therapy for stroke victims, social support programs for recovering alcoholics, exercise programs for heart attack victims, and mental health counseling for rape victims.

The goal of intervention at each of the three levels of prevention is to prevent the progression process. To plan appropriate methods of primary, secondary, and tertiary prevention, the community health nurse must initially assess the current health status of the community.

DESCRIPTIVE MEASURES OF HEALTH

Demographic Measures

Certain human characteristics, or demographics, may be associated with wellness or illness. Age, race, gender, ethnicity, income, and educational level are important demographics that may affect health outcomes. For example, men are more likely than women to develop certain heart diseases, and African-American women are more likely than Caucasian women to deliver low-birthweight infants (usually defined as infants weighing less than 2500 g at birth). To plan for the health of a community, the nurse must be familiar with the demographic characteristics of the community and with the health problems associated with those characteristics.

Morbidity and Mortality

Although epidemiology describes the distribution and determinants of both wellness and illness states, wellness is difficult to measure. Therefore, many measures of "health" are expressed in terms of morbidity (illness) and mortality (death). An excellent source of morbidity and mortality data, by state and for select cities, is the Centers for Disease Control and Prevention, *Morbidity and Mortality Weekly Report* (http://www.cdc.gov/mmwr).

Incidence

The incidence of any health or disease condition refers to the number of people in a population who develop the condition during a specified period of time. Incidence rates measure the rate at which people without a disease develop the disease during a specific period of time (i.e., the number of new cases of a disease in a population over a period of time). Mathematically, incidence rate over a period of time is expressed as:

$$\frac{\text{Number of new cases of disease}}{\text{Total population at risk}} \times 100,000$$

The incidence rate uses the frequency of new cases in the numerator. The denominator for incidence rates is the population at risk. For example, to calculate the incidence rate of postmenopausal breast cancer, women who are still premenopausal would not be a part of the population at risk. Incidence is particularly important for analytic epidemiologic research because it allows the estimation of risk necessary to assess causal association (relative risk). The calculation of incidence generally requires that a defined population initially free of the disease in question must be followed over a period of time in what is called a prospective (forward-looking) study.

Prevalence

The prevalence of a disease or condition refers to the total number of people in the population who have the condition at a particular time. Thus, prevalence may be calculated in a "one-shot" cross-sectional (slice of time) or retrospective (backward looking) study. Mathematically, prevalence is expressed as:

$$\frac{\text{Number of existing cases of disease}}{\text{Number in total population}} \times 100,000$$

Prevalence, therefore, examines the extent of morbidity in a community and is influenced by the rate of new cases, the number of existing cases, effective new treatment modalities, and deaths. It can be classified as period prevalence (existence during a period of time, such as 32% of children at Camp North had diarrhea between June 10 and June 25) or point prevalence (a specific point in time, such as 10% of children at Camp North had diarrhea on June 15).

Understanding Incidence and Prevalence

Measures of incidence and prevalence provide different information. To understand the relationship between incidence and prevalence, consider the number of passengers on a train. The number of passengers represents prevalence (existing disease, old and new cases); the number of boarding passengers represents incidence (new cases of disease); passengers who get off the train represent individuals who either recover or die. Both the number of new cases entering and the number of individuals with disease who leave either through death or through recovery from the illness influence prevalence. The number of passengers on board will increase if the number of boarding passengers (new cases) is high, if the number of passengers exiting is low (fewer deaths or increased survival rate due to new treatment), or both occur. Conversely, prevalence will decrease when the number of new cases is low or when individuals die or persons are cured of disease or both.

Consider another example. You read about an increase in the prevalence of a certain type of cancer; this increase may mean that there are a higher number of people with this type of cancer in the population. This higher number may be due to more new cases (in other words, increased incidence) or because people with this type of cancer are living longer. In either case, the community may need to allocate additional resources toward cancer identification and treatment.

Ratios, Proportions, and Rates

In epidemiologic studies, data and statistics make comparison possible among populations. Therefore, it is necessary to convert raw data into ratios, proportions, and rates to provide a more valid description of health problems. A *ratio* is simply one number divided by another in which there is no specified relationship between the numerator and denominator. For example, of 1,000 motorcycle fatalities, 950 victims are male and 50 are female. The sex ratio is the number of males compared to the number of females (950/50 or 19 males to 1 female).

In contrast, a *proportion* is one number divided by another in which the numerator is a subset of the denominator (i.e., it is included in the denominator) and is expressed as a percentage. Using the same data, you can calculate the proportion of males to females. Of 1,000 motorcycle fatalities, 950 are male and 50 are female. What percentage of fatalities is male? A proportion is expressed by the formula $X/(X + Y)$; thus, the percentage of males to females would be 950/1,000 multiplied by 100, which equals 95%. Neither ratio nor proportion has a population base or specific unit of time.

Because epidemiology is the study of population health, statistical measures must relate the occurrence of a health condition to the population at risk. To assess the probability that one group is at higher risk than another, rates are calculated. *Rates* measure the amount of disease, injury, disability, or death within a unit of the population and within a unit of time. Rates express a mathematical relationship in which the *numerator* relates to the number of persons experiencing the condition, and the *denominator* expresses the population at risk or the total number of persons who have the possibility of experiencing the condition. Rates improve the ability to make comparisons because they reduce the standard of comparison to a common denominator, the unit size of the population. For example, the crude death rates for heart disease in Florida and Texas were 288.0 and 190.0 per 100,000 persons, respectively. It appears that the death rate is higher in Florida compared to Texas. This difference may be due to population characteristics (e.g., age differences between the states) that can affect mortality experiences. Later in this chapter, specific rates are discussed that can be calculated for a subgroup of persons, such as death rate for heart disease in Florida and Texas for persons over the age of 65.

Do not confuse rates with other proportions that do not use the population at risk as the denominator. For example, the death rate from cancer is not the same as the proportion of deaths from cancer. In each, the numerator is the number of deaths from cancer. However, the denominator differs. In the death rate, the denominator represents all people at risk of dying from cancer. Therefore, the cancer death rate is an expression of the risk of dying from cancer. In the proportion of deaths, also called proportionate mortality rate (PMR), the denominator is the total number of deaths from all causes. Mathematically, the PMR is expressed as:

$$\frac{\text{Number of deaths due to a specific cause}}{\text{Total number of deaths from all cases}} \times 100$$

Therefore, the proportionate cancer mortality simply describes the proportion of deaths attributable to cancer. For example, if the PMR of heart disease is 37%, this indicates that 37% of all deaths, regardless of age, sex, or race, are related to diseases of the heart. However, this statistic provides no indication of the rate for heart disease.

Calculation of Epidemiologic Rates

Rates are calculated by the formula:

$$\text{Rate} = \frac{\text{Number of people experiencing condition}}{\text{Population at risk experiencing condition}} \times K$$

K is a constant (usually 1,000 or 100,000) that allows the ratio, which may be a very small number, to be expressed in a meaningful way. The concept of rates can be understood more easily by applying this formula to the calculation of the infant mortality rate (IMR), which estimates an infant's risk of dying during the first year of life.

Example of a Rate: The Infant Mortality Rate

The IMR is usually calculated on a calendar year basis. The number of infant deaths (deaths before the age of 1 year) during the year is divided by the number of live births (infants born alive) during that year. The numerator represents the number of infants experiencing the "condition" of dying in the first year of life, and the denominator represents the population of infants at risk for dying in the year.

If within a given year 34,400 infant deaths and 4,084,000 live births were reported for the United States, these data would provide the numerator and denominator to calculate the IMR. Applying the formula for a rate, one would divide the numerator 34,400 by 4,084,000 and obtain a value of 0.0084, which would indicate that 0.0084 of the infants died during the first year of life. To obtain a meaningful rate, it is necessary to multiply by a constant, in this case 1,000, and find that 8.4 infants per 1,000 live births died during the first year of life (i.e., the IMR was 8.4 infant deaths per 1,000 live births). This IMR would be calculated as follows:

$$\frac{34,400}{4,084,000} \times 1,000 = 8.4 \text{ infant deaths per live births}$$

Interpretation of Rates

Rates enable researchers to compare different populations in terms of health problems or conditions. To assess if one community is at greater or lesser risk for the problems or conditions, compare the rates for the community with rates from similar communities, from the state, or from the United States as a whole.

Caution is required in interpreting rates. Like most statistical measures, rates are less reliable when based on small numbers. This is important when assessing relatively infrequent events or conditions or communities with small populations.

The majority of rates are based on data from a calendar year, which may also present some difficulties. Populations may increase or decrease during a calendar year. To adjust for population changes over the year, the midyear population estimate is generally used because the population at risk cannot be determined accurately.

Commonly Used Rates

Box 3.1 summarizes a number of important rates. Note that the measures of natality and mortality are, in essence, measures of incidence of the conditions of "being born" and "dying." Study the various ways in which the denominator, or population at risk, is determined in different rates.

Crude, Specific, and Adjusted Rates

Rates can be broken down into three categories: crude, specific, and adjusted. Rates computed for a population as a whole are *crude rates*. When calculating deaths in the total population, irrespective of age, the rate obtained is the *crude mortality rate* or crude death rate. With the crude mortality rate, there is no allowance for the age distribution of the population or comparisons between populations with different age groups.

Subgroups of a population may have differences not revealed by the crude rates. Rates calculated for subgroups are *specific rates*. Specific rates relate to demographic factors such as age, race, and gender, or they may refer to the entire population but be specific for some single cause of death or illness. For example, to eliminate the effects of different age structures in the population of comparison, the age-specific death rate would be appropriate. Mortality rates for specific diseases such as heart disease relate to a specific cause of death, any subgroup or any age, race, gender, religion, or for an entire population. Information gained from specific rates can aid in identification of groups at increased risk within the population and facilitate comparisons between populations that have different demographic compositions.

In comparing populations with different distributions of a factor known to affect the health condition of interest, the use of *adjusted rates* may be appropriate. An

COMMONLY USED RATES

Measures of Natality

$$\text{Crude birth rate} = \frac{\text{Number of live births during time interval}}{\text{Estimated midinterval population}} \times 1{,}000$$

$$\text{Fertility rate} = \frac{\text{Number of live births during time interval}}{\text{Number of women aged 15–44 at midinterval}} \times 1{,}000$$

Measures of Morbidity and Mortality

$$\text{Incidence rate} = \frac{\text{Number of new cases of specified health conditions during time interval}}{\text{Estimated midinterval population at risk}} \times 1{,}000$$

$$\text{Prevalence rate} = \frac{\text{Number of current cases of specified health condition at a given point in time}}{\text{Estimated population at risk at same point}} \times 1{,}000$$

$$\text{Crude death rate} = \frac{\text{Number of deaths during time interval}}{\text{Estimated midinterval population}} \times 1{,}000$$

$$\text{Specific death rate} = \frac{\text{Number of deaths in subgroup during time interval}}{\text{Estimated midinterval population of subgroup}} \times 100{,}000$$

$$\text{Cause-specific death rate} = \frac{\text{Number of deaths from specified cause during time interval}}{\text{Estimated midinterval population}} \times 100{,}000$$

$$\text{Infant mortality rate} = \frac{\text{Number of deaths of infants aged} <1 \text{ year during time interval}}{\text{Total live births during time interval}} \times 1{,}000$$

$$\text{Neonatal mortality rate} = \frac{\text{Number of deaths of infant aged} <28 \text{ days during time interval}}{\text{Total live births during time interval}} \times 1{,}000$$

$$\text{Postneonatal mortality rate} = \frac{\text{Number of deaths of infants aged} \geq 28 \text{ days but} <1 \text{ year during time interval}}{\text{Total live births during time interval}} \times 1{,}000$$

$$\text{Maternal mortality rate} = \frac{\text{Number of deaths from puerperal cases during 1 year}}{\text{Number of live births during same year}} \times 100{,}000$$

adjusted rate is a summary measure in which statistical procedures remove the effect of differences in the composition of the various populations. In essence, adjustment produces an estimate of what the crude rate would be if the populations were identical in respect to the adjusted factor. Rates are adjusted for age, race, gender, or any factor or combination of factors suspected of affecting the rate. Adjusted rates are helpful in making community comparisons, but they are imaginary: Caution is necessary when interpreting.

ANALYTIC MEASURES OF HEALTH

As discussed previously, rates describe and compare the risks of dying, becoming ill, or developing other health conditions. In epidemiologic studies, it is also desirable to determine if health conditions are associated with, or related to, other factors. The research findings may provide the theoretical foundation by which preventive actions are identified (e.g., the linking of air pollution to health problems has led to environmental controls). To investigate potential relationships between health conditions and other factors, analytic measures of community health are required. In this section, three analytic measures are discussed: *relative risk*, *odds ratio*, and *attributable risk*.

Relative Risk

To determine if a relationship or association exists between a health condition and a suspected factor, it is necessary to compare the risk of developing the health condition for the population exposed to the factor with the risk for the population not exposed to the factor. The relative risk (RR) expresses the risk ratio of the incidence rate of those exposed (e.g., smokers) and those not exposed to the suspected factor (e.g., nonsmokers). The relative risk indicates the benefit that might accrue to the person if the risk factor is removed. In this situation, calculation of the relative risk illustrates how much the risk for the smoker increases compared with nonsmokers. The relative risk only applies to studies that determine incidence (prospective data). Relative risk is used to make causal inferences, such as *smoking causes lung cancer*. Relative risk can be calculated as follows:

$$RR = \frac{\text{Incidence among those exposed}}{\text{Incidence rate among those not exposed}}$$

The relative risk indicates whether the rate in the exposed population is higher than the rate in the nonexposed population and, if so, how many times higher. A high relative risk in the exposed population suggests that the factor is a risk factor in the development of the health condition. Relative risk does not indicate that someone with the factor will develop the disease. It is important to note that risk estimates are probability statements; therefore, (1) all those exposed to the factor do not develop the disease but merely have an increased probability of doing so and (2) some people who have not been exposed to the factor will develop the disease. A relative risk of 1.0 means the risk of disease among the exposed is no different from the risk of disease among the nonexposed. A relative risk of 2.0 implies that risk is twice as high, whereas a relative risk of 0.5 indicates that the exposure factor is associated with half the risk of disease. For example, if the relative risk of postmenopausal breast cancer among women who breast-fed is 0.8, then breastfeeding can be considered a protective factor for postmenopausal breast cancer.

Internal and External Risk Factors

The concept of relative risk applies when one group of people clearly is exposed and another is not exposed to an external factor such as cigarette smoke, exercise, or foods high in saturated fat. However, it may be confusing to see relative risks applied to internal factors such as age, race, or gender. Nevertheless, as can be seen in the following example, people also are "exposed" to intrinsic factors that may carry as much risk as extrinsic ones.

Relative Risk: Homicide

Sinauer, Bowling, Moracco, Runyan, and Butts (1999) studied female homicide (termed femicide) over a 5-year period in North Carolina and found the overall homicide rate was 6.2 per 100,000. However, among young (aged 15 to 33 years) black females (women exposed to the two intrinsic factors of age and race), the rate was 19.5 per 100,000, compared to 5.4 homicides per 100,000 for white women of the same age. With this information, one can calculate a relative risk. Among young black women (those "exposed" to the intrinsic condition of being young and black), the rate was 19.5 per 100,000, and among young white women (those "not exposed" to the condition of being young and black), the rate was 5.4 per 100,000. Thus, the relative risk of homicide for young black women compared to young white women is calculated as follows:

$$RR = \frac{19.5 \text{ per } 100,000}{5.4 \text{ per } 100,000} = 3.61$$

In other words, the risk of dying from homicide was three and one half times greater for black women than for white women. Clearly, race is a risk factor. Race cannot be altered, but the information provided by this analysis can be used to plan protective services for the population at greatest risk.

Odds Ratio

Calculation of the relative risk is straightforward when incidence rates are available. Unfortunately, not all studies are prospective as is required for the computation of incidence rates. In a retrospective study, the relative risk is approximated by the *odds ratio*.

As shown in Table 3.1, the odds ratio is a simple mathematical ratio of the odds in favor of having a specific health condition when the suspected factor is present and the odds in favor of having the condition when the factor is absent. The odds of having the condition when the suspected factor is present are represented by *a/b* in

TABLE 3.1

Crosstabulation for Calculation of Odds Ratio

	Health Condition		
	Present	**Absent**	**Total**
Exposed to factor	*a*	*b*	*a + b*
Not exposed to factor	*c*	*d*	*c + d*
Total	*a + c*	*b + d*	*a + b + c + d*

TABLE 3.2

Toxic Shock Syndrome Cases among 156 Tampon Users

	Toxic Shock Syndrome		
Brand of Tampon Used	Present	Absent	Total
Suspected brand	30	30	60
Other brands	12	84	96
Total	42	114	156

Data from CDC. (1980). Follow up on toxic shock syndrome. *Morbidity and Mortality Weekly Report, 29*(37), 441–445.

the table. The odds of having the condition when not exposed to the factor are c/d. The odds ratio is thus:

$$\frac{a/b}{c/d} = \frac{ad}{bc}$$

An example frequently cited in epidemiologic literature is that of toxic shock syndrome (TSS). When TSS, a severe illness involving high fever, vomiting, diarrhea, rash, and hypotension or shock, first occurred, it was neither practical nor ethical to consider cases only on a prospective basis. Therefore, existing cases were compared retrospectively with nonexisting cases or controls. Early studies noted an association between TSS and tampon use and suggested that users of a specific brand of superabsorbent tampon might be at especially high risk. To clarify the issue, researchers analyzed data from TSS cases and controls, all of whom used tampons. TSS data in Table 3.2 can be used to calculate the odds ratio for users of the specific brand of tampon.

$$\text{Odds ratio} = \frac{ad}{bc} = \frac{30(84)}{30(12)} = 7$$

An odds ratio of 1.0 implies that the odds of exposure are equal and suggest that a particular exposure is not a risk factor for the disease of study. Users of the specific brand of tampons were seven times more likely to develop TSS than were tampon users of other brands. Based on the results of studies, the brand was removed from the market.

Relative Risk and Odds Ratio: Caution in Interpretation

A high odds ratio or relative risk must be regarded with appropriate concern; however, the finding should not obscure the potential involvement of other factors. As illustrated in Table 3.2, 12 people in the sample had TSS although they did not use the specific brand of tampon. In other words, this product was not the sole cause of TSS. Subsequent research showed that certain superabsorbent materials in tampons or certain aspects of tampon use foster growth of *Staphylococcus aureus*, the probable causal organism in TSS (Centers for Disease Control and Prevention [CDC], 1980, 1981, 1983; Davis, Chesney, Ward, LaVenture, & the Investigation and Laboratory Team, 1980).

Attributable Risk and Attributable Risk Percentage

Another measure of risk is *attributable risk* (AR), which measures the difference between the incidence rates for those exposed and those not exposed to the risk factor.

The measure estimates the excess risk attributable to exposure to the risk factor. It shows the potential reduction in the overall incidence rate if the factor is eliminated. The AR is calculated by subtracting the incidence among those unexposed to a risk factor (nonsmokers) from those who were exposed (smokers):

AR = incidence rate in exposed group *minus* incidence rate in nonexposed group

AR usually is further quantified into attributable risk percentage:

$$\frac{AR}{\text{Incidence rate in exposed group}} = 100$$

This provides an estimate of the percentage of occurrences of the health condition that is potentially preventable if the risk factor is eliminated. For example, studies of the relation between physical inactivity and mortality from coronary heart disease (CHD) have shown that the attributable risk associated with physical inactivity was 35% (CDC, 1993). Thus, improved physical activity has the potential to reduce CHD mortality.

Point Estimate and Confidence Intervals

Relative risks and odds ratios provide a point estimate (a number) that identifies whether those in the exposed group will develop the disease or condition when compared to those not exposed. To apply the point estimate to decisions of community health, it is important to understand the relationship of the point estimate to the number one (1.0), and the range of numbers within the confidence interval (CI).

A point estimate is the mathematical calculation derived from the data, such as a relative risks or odds ratio. Relationship of the point estimate, such as a relative risk of 3.0, to the number one (1.0) allows you to determine whether an association exists between the exposure and the condition. As you learned earlier, a risk of 1.0 means the person has no added risk. A risk of less than 1.0 suggests some protection from the exposure and a relative risk above 1.0 suggests increased risk of the disease or condition from the exposure.

After establishing the point estimate and the position of the relative risk in relationship to 1.0, you must also assess the CI or range of point estimates around the relative risk. Most studies report a 95% CI. The relationship is statistically significant *only* if the entire CI is *above* or *below* 1.0 (Brucker, 2005). For example, a relative risk may be 5.0, but the 95% CI is reported as 0.45 to 10.8. The CI crosses, or encompasses, the number 1.0. Therefore, the association is not significant. However, the relative risk of 0.21 with a 95% CI of 0.10 to 0.45 would be statistically significant, as the CI does not cross or encompass 1.0. In a study by McFarlane, Campbell, Sharps, and Watson (2002), the odds ratio for murder or attempted murder of women abused during pregnancy was 3.08 with 95% CI of 1.86 to 5.10. The CI did not include 1.0; therefore, the women abused during pregnancy were three times as likely to be murdered or have an attempt made on their life compared to women not abused during pregnancy.

Cause and Association

Ultimately, community health professionals hope to determine causes of adverse health conditions so steps can be taken to improve health. In view of the complexity of the human body and human behavior, establishing causality is very difficult. Therefore, investigations of population health generally examine relationships or associations between variables. The *variables* are the characteristics or phenomena (such as age, occupation, or physical exercise) and the health conditions (such as heart disease) being studied.

Variables and Constants

An important requirement in any study is that the factors studied must have the potential to vary from person to person. If a factor cannot vary, it is not a variable but a *constant*. It is impossible to establish an association between a constant and a variable because the constant, by definition, cannot change when the variable changes. Thus, a study that looks only at men cannot establish an association between gender and, for example, heart disease; the study has made gender a constant. A study that looks only at people with heart disease cannot establish an association between heart disease and any other variable; heart disease has become a constant in the study.

Control or Comparison Groups

To ensure that associations between variables can be examined, control groups or comparison groups are essential. A study of heart disease might compare people with the disease with a control group of people without the disease. An investigation of a new treatment would study people who receive the treatment and a control group of people who do not receive the treatment.

Independent and Dependent Variables

The *dependent variable* is the outcome or result that the investigator is studying. The dependent variable can change (e.g., health status, knowledge, and behavior). The *independent variable* is the presumed "cause" of or contributor to variation in the dependent variable. For example, in the heart disease study cited earlier (CDC, 1993), physical inactivity, the independent variable, contributes to heart disease, the dependent variable. An independent variable may be a naturally occurring event or phenomenon such as level of usual physical activity, exposure to ultraviolet radiation, and type of employment, or it might be a planned intervention such as an exercise program, a medication, and a support group. An independent variable might also be an intrinsic quality such as age, race, gender, or genes. (Note that these intrinsic qualities, although they cannot vary within an individual, can vary from person to person; thus, they are studied as independent variables.)

Confounding Variables

When an association exists between variables, it is tempting—but incorrect—to assume that one variable causes the other. If, for example, a study found that communities with low salaries for public health workers had high crime rates, one could not conclude that low public health salaries lead to high crime rates. Common sense suggests that economic conditions might influence both salaries and crime (i.e., economic conditions intervene in the study and confound the results). Here is another example: Driving without seatbelts increases the risk of a fatal automobile accident. However, nonusers of seatbelts are likely to speed, and speeding is another cause of automobile fatalities. Therefore, some of the apparent benefits of seatbelts relate to differing driving speeds of users and nonusers of seatbelts. In this example, speeding is a confounding variable. Any factor that may influence a study's results is an extraneous, intervening, or confounding variable.

Criteria for Determining Causation

Association does not imply causation. If an association is found between variables, it means the variables tend to occur or change together (parallel increase or decrease); it does not prove that one variable causes the other. The first question to ask is whether a statistical relationship exists between the two factors. Before an association is assessed for possibility that it is causal, other explanations such as chance, bias, and confounding variables are considered. Statistical methods alone, however, cannot establish proof of a causal relationship in an association. Because of the possibility of confounded results, very strict criteria for determining causation exist. An association must be evaluated against all of the criteria; the more criteria that are met, the more likely it is that the association is causal. However, an association may meet all the criteria for causation and later be shown to be spurious (false or factitious association) because of factors that were not known at the time the study was done. For this reason, investigators must interpret results with great caution; they rarely consider a cause "proven." Six widely used criteria for evaluating causation are the following:

1. *The association is strong.* The strength of the relationship is usually measured statistically with relative risk or, alternatively, the odds ratio. The higher the relative risk or odds ratio, the greater the likelihood that the association is causal.
2. *The association is consistent.* The same association exists repeatedly in other studies, in other settings, and with other populations. The more the association appears under diverse circumstances, the more likely it is to be causal in nature.
3. *The association is temporally correct.* The hypothesized cause of the health condition must occur before the onset of the condition (i.e., exposure to the risk factor must precede the onset of disease). This criterion is definitely essential. It is the first and most important variable—if exposure did not precede the onset, the remaining facts are irrelevant because exposure could not have caused the disease.
4. *The association is specific.* The hypothesized cause should be associated with relatively few health conditions. Specificity measures the degree to which one particular exposure produces one specific disease—the uniqueness of the relationship. If the biologic response is variable, it is less likely to be causal.
5. *The association is not the result of a confounding variable.* Although not all potential intervening variables are identified, the alternate explanations for the association are examined carefully before considering an association causal.
6. *The association is plausible and consistent with current knowledge.* Any disease or injury causation association must be congruent and compatible with current biomedical and scientific knowledge and information. This depends on the state of scientific information at a given time. An association that contradicts current scientific views must be evaluated very carefully. However, associations may be inconsistent with current knowledge simply because current knowledge is not as advanced as a new discovery.

SOURCES OF COMMUNITY HEALTH DATA

To be an effective community health practitioner, it is essential to interpret and use data from various sources. This section reviews important sources of data.

Census

The census is probably the most comprehensive source of health-related data for the United States. Every 10 years, the Bureau of the Census enumerates the U.S. population and surveys it for basic demographics. Census data provide a wealth of information about a community's characteristics such as age, race, and sex, along with other factors such as employment, income, migration, and education. Traditionally, epidemiologists have used the census of the population as a reliable source for denominators in the calculation of rates.

Census information is analyzed and reported for the nation as a whole and in progressively smaller regions down to municipalities, census tracts, and blocks. Results are also reported in regions known as standard metropolitan statistical areas (SMSA). Census data are available online at http://www.census.gov. Only a limited number of questions are asked of the entire population. More detailed surveys are taken of selected samples of the population.

Although census data are comprehensive, bias does occur. For example, people may answer personal questions dishonestly. Perhaps more significantly, the census underrepresents low-income residents, minorities, and transients. These people are more difficult to locate, enumerate, and tend to be less likely to respond to census surveys.

Vital Statistics

Data that describe legally registered events such as births, deaths, marriages, and divorces are called vital statistics. Government agencies collect vital statistics on an ongoing basis. The CDC's National Center for Health Statistics collects and publishes vital statistics from individual states. Health professionals can use the data in examining trends over time and in establishing health improvement plans. The data are available on the Internet at http://www.cdc.gov/nchs. The U.S. Public Health Service also gathers data from the states and publishes annual volumes, along with periodic reports on specific topics.

Beginning researchers tend to consider vital statistics "hallowed" because they are, after all, legal data. However, legality does not guarantee validity. For example, a person's race sometimes differs on birth and death certificates, and the manner in which cause of death is recorded on death certificates is inconsistent. The numbers of unmarried but cohabiting couples also demonstrate that marriage and divorce records are also not completely valid measures of reality. Despite their limitations, vital statistics are often the best available data.

Notifiable Disease Reports

The CDC/U.S. Public Health Service reports data collected by state and local health departments on legally reportable diseases and periodically requests voluntary reporting of nonnotifiable health conditions of special interest. Notifiable diseases are frequently referred to as reportable diseases. Criteria to determine if a disease is notifiable are (1) the ability of the disease to cause death and (2) the communicability of the disease. Notification to public health officials of diseases posing a threat to large populations provides an initial starting point for local epidemiologic investigations. The concept of surveillance is essential to identification and control of notifiable diseases. Surveillance is the systematic collection of data pertaining to the occurrence of specific diseases, the analysis and interpretation of these data, and the dissemination of information about the data. The CDC weekly publication, *Morbidity and Mortality Weekly Report* (MMWR), is a valuable resource for community health practice.

The major deficiency of this category of data for epidemiologic research purposes is the possible incompleteness of population coverage. Even legally mandated disease reports may not be representative of all cases of the disease. Thus, valid descriptions of the disease as it exists in the community may not be accessible. In practice, health care providers may also fail to complete the required reporting form.

Vital Record Linkage

Vital record linkage connects data and information contained in two or more medical, morbidity, or mortality records, and other vital event records. Record linkage systems provide excellent sources of information on the courses of diseases, demographic data, health care services utilization, fertility, maternal health issues, child health concerns, chronic disease tracking, and the natural history of specific disease or morbidity-related events. Record linkage is facilitated by the advent of modern computers. This system offers a potentially rich source of information and may facilitate research on measures of public health.

Medical and Hospital Records

Medical and hospital records provide valuable information for community health research. First, these records, however, do not provide a completely representative or valid picture of community health. Not all clients with health problems receive medical attention, so medical records are obviously biased. Second, medical documentation is not always complete. Finally, hospitalized patients are also more likely to have coexistent illnesses. This phenomenon, called Berkson's bias, creates the likelihood of finding a false association between the two illnesses.

Autopsy Records

Autopsy records have a very severe inherent bias: The patient may have been so ill that death occurred. Autopsies are not performed for all deaths. Autopsy records include a disproportionate number of cases of violent death and people for whom the cause of death was unknown until after autopsy (e.g., the manifestation of the illness was unusual). People who do not sanction autopsy are underrepresented. These factors influence the validity and representativeness of the findings of any study using autopsy records.

National Electronic Disease Surveillance System

The National Electronic Disease Surveillance System (NEDSS) provides an integrated surveillance system that transmits public health laboratory and clinical data via the Internet. This process improves the nation's ability to identify and track emerging infectious diseases and potential bioterrorism attacks. Therefore, NEDSS is of particular importance to state health departments in investigating outbreaks and monitoring disease trends in that it is used for surveillance and analysis of notifiable diseases. For further information, visit http://www.cdc.gov/nedss.

SCREENING FOR HEALTH CONDITIONS

Screening can be defined as the presumptive identification of unrecognized disease or defects by the administration of tests, examinations, or other procedures that can be applied rapidly. Screening tests do not provide a conclusive diagnosis of a disease but rather identify asymptomatic people who may unknowingly have a health problem. Anyone who shows evidence of symptoms of a disease through a screening program should have further medical diagnostic testing. The purpose of screening is to rapidly and economically identify people who have a high probability of having (or developing) a particular illness so they can be referred for definitive diagnosis and treatment.

Considerations in Deciding to Screen

Screening goes further than identifying groups at risk for illness; it identifies individuals who may actually have an illness. Screening carries an ethical commitment to continue working with these people and to provide them access to diagnostic and treatment services. In general, screening should be conducted only if

- Early diagnosis and treatment can favorably alter the course of the illness
- Definitive diagnosis and treatment facilities are available, either through the screening agency or through referral
- The group being screened is at risk for the illness (in other words, the group is likely to have a high prevalence of the illness)
- The screening procedures are reliable and valid

Screening Test Reliability and Validity

Reliability (precision) refers to the consistency or repeatability of test results; *validity* refers to the ability of the test to measure what it is supposed to measure. A few considerations specific to screening tests are discussed below.

Test Reliability

A reliable screening test yields the same result even when administered by different screeners. Training for all screening personnel involved in the test is essential. Lack of reliability may suggest that the screeners are administering the test in an inconsistent manner.

Test Validity: Sensitivity and Specificity

To be valid, a screening test must distinguish correctly between those people who have the condition and those who do not. This ability to distinguish is measured by the test's sensitivity and specificity, as shown in Table 3.3.

Sensitivity is the ability of a test to correctly identify people who have the disease (i.e., to call a true positive "positive"). A test with high sensitivity will have few false negatives.

Specificity is the ability of a test to identify correctly people who do not have the disease, or to call a true negative "negative." If a test is not specific, people who do not actually have the disease will be referred for additional diagnostic testing. A test with high specificity has few false positives.

Ideally, a screening test's sensitivity and specificity should be 100%; in practice, however, screening tests vary in this regard. As shown in Table 3.3, sensitivity, or the true-positive rate, is the complement of the false-negative rate, and specificity, or the

TABLE 3.3

Sensitivity and Specificity of a Screening Test

	Reality	
Screening Test Results	**Diseased**	**Not Diseased**
Positive	True positive	False positive
Negative	False negative	True negative
Total	Total diseased	Total not diseased

$$\text{Sensitivity (true-positive rate)} = \frac{\text{True positives}}{\text{Total diseased}}$$

$$\text{Specificity (true-negative rate)} = \frac{\text{True negatives}}{\text{Total not diseased}}$$

$$\text{False-negative rate} = \frac{\text{False negatives}}{\text{Total diseased}} \text{ or } 1 - \text{Sensitivity}$$

$$\text{False-positive rate} = \frac{\text{False positives}}{\text{Total not diseased}} \text{ or } 1 - \text{Specificity}$$

true-negative rate, is the complement of the false-positive rate. Thus, as sensitivity increases, specificity decreases. Therefore, decisions regarding screening test validity may require uncomfortable compromises, as discussed in the following section.

Decision Making in Screening: Practical and Ethical Considerations

In a community health setting, a screening program is necessary for a deadly disease that is curable only if detected early. The two tests available are one with a high sensitivity and low specificity and one with high specificity and low sensitivity. One must make a decision as to which test should be selected. To save the most lives, high sensitivity is essential (i.e., a low rate of false negatives [people who have the disease but are not detected by the screening test]). However, if one selects the test with high sensitivity, its low specificity means that one will have a high rate of false positives (people who do not have the disease but whom the test falsely identifies as having it). With increased numbers of false positives, many people could be alarmed needlessly, resulting in unnecessary expenses by overreferral of people who are disease-free. Which test would you choose? Why?

How does the situation differ when one is screening for a deadly disease, but the diagnostic and treatment facilities in the community are already overloaded and further budget cuts are projected? To minimize unnecessary referrals of false positives, the test with high specificity would be preferable. However, due to the low sensitivity of this test, it will be necessary to weigh the benefits of a low false-positive rate against the ethics of a high false-negative rate. Is it justifiable to lull the undetected diseased people into a false—and potentially fatal—sense of security? Which test would you select in this situation? Why?

Decisions regarding screening involve seeking the most favorable balance of sensitivity and specificity. Sometimes, sensitivity and specificity can be improved by adjusting the screening process (e.g., adding another test or changing the level at which the test is considered positive). At other times, evaluating sensitivity and specificity may result in a decision not to conduct a screening program because the economic costs of overreferral or the ethical considerations of underreferral outweigh the usefulness of screening. An understanding of the principles discussed in this section will help you make informed decisions regarding community screening.

EPIDEMIOLOGIC APPROACHES TO COMMUNITY HEALTH RESEARCH

Epidemiologic models guide investigators in examining the determinants of population health. This section describes three models and explains how each might guide the approach to the same problem.

Application of each model is illustrated using the problem of an increase in the IMR in a hypothetical community. The IMR is a particularly important health index that health professionals should understand even if their main concern is not maternal or child health. Because infant mortality is influenced by a variety of biologic and environmental factors affecting the infant and mother, the IMR is both a direct measure of infant health and an indirect measure of community health as a whole.

The Epidemiologic Triangle

The epidemiologic triangle or agent–host–environment model is a traditional view of health and disease developed when epidemiology was concerned chiefly with communicable disease. The model, however, is applicable to other health conditions. In the model, the *agent* is an organism capable of causing disease. The *host* is the population at risk for developing the disease. The *environment* is a combination of physical, biological, and social factors that surround and influence both the agent and the host. The epidemiologic triangle is used to analyze the role and interrelatedness of each of the factors (i.e., the influence, reactivity, and effect each factor has on the other two). According to this model, the agent, host, and environment can coexist. Disease and injury occur only when there is an interaction or altered equilibrium between them.

Figure 3.1 shows the triangle in its normal state of equilibrium. Equilibrium does not signify optimum health but simply the usual pattern of illness and health in a population. Any change in one of the factors (agent, host, or environment) will result in disequilibrium—in other words, a change in the usual pattern.

How could this model guide the investigation of increased infant mortality? To understand this, one must consider the three facets of the model.

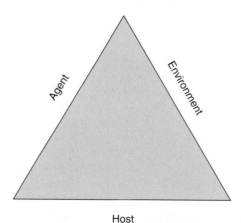

Host

Figure 3.1   The epidemiologic triangle is the traditional view, showing health and disease as a composite state of three variables.

Agent

If one thinks of the epidemiologic triangle model from an infectious disease perspective, it might appear that the investigation should focus on types of infections as agents that cause infant deaths. However, major causes of infant mortality in the United States include prematurity and low birthweight, birth injuries, congenital malformations, sudden infant death syndrome (SIDS), accidents, and homicides. Therefore, an investigator may try to determine whether there has been a change in any of the other agents.

Host

The characteristics of the host (the infant population) will be the second area of assessment. This assessment involves examining infant birth and death patterns in terms of age, ethnicity, sex, and birth weight. These characteristics have been shown to be important risk factors for infant mortality. By studying these factors, it may be possible to identify groups of infants who are at particularly increased risk of dying.

Environment

Lastly, the environment is assessed. The mother is a significant part of the infant's prenatal and postnatal environment. Therefore, the investigators will analyze birth and infant mortality patterns according to factors such as maternal age, ethnicity, parity (number of previous live births), prenatal care, and education or socioeconomic status. Analysis of these factors, which are also related to infant mortality, will help provide further identification of at-risk groups. Other conditions in the environment also need to be considered. For instance, has migration into the community from other areas increased? Has adult morbidity or mortality, particularly among pregnant women, increased? Have there been changes in health services, policies, personnel, funding, or other factors that could affect infant health?

Practical Application

The analysis of these three areas—the agent, host, and environment—should provide information regarding groups at risk for increased infant mortality and a means of reducing a risk factor. Thus, the epidemiologic triangle, although it was designed with a communicable disease orientation, can provide a useful guide for studying the multifaceted problem of infant mortality, along with other health problems.

The Person–Place–Time Model

In an epidemiologic study, variables can be considered in terms of person (who is affected), place (where affected), and time (when affected) relationships. The person–place–time model examines the characteristics of the people affected (the host in the triangle model), the place (environment) or location, and the time period involved (which could relate to the agent, host, or environment). In studying infant mortality according to this model, infant and maternal factors are considered traits of "person." Aspects of "place" are such factors as whether the community is rural or urban and affluent or poor. Aspects of "time" include seasonal or age-specific patterns or trends in mortality.

The Web of Causation

The web of causation (MacMahon & Pugh, 1970) views a health condition as the result not of individual factors but of complex interrelationships of numerous factors interacting to increase or decrease the risk of disease. The essence of this concept is the multifactorial nature in that a number of interrelated variables are almost always involved in the cause of a particular outcome. The web of causation attempts to identify all the possible influences on the health and illness processes. Creating the web identifies the most direct causes of conditions, factors contributing to those causes, factors influencing each of these factors, and so on.

Synergism and Factors in the Web

Central to the web of causation model is the concept of *synergism*, wherein the whole is more than the sum of its separate parts. For example, the effects of a *Shigella* infection of the infant, combined with the effects of poverty, youth, and low educational level of the mother, are more deleterious to infant health than the sum of the effects of the individual risk factors.

Use of the web of causation may result in a more expansive study of infant mortality than one guided by other models. Ideally, investigators using this model first identify all factors related to infant mortality. Next, they identify factors that are related to each of these factors. These two comprehensive steps provide the outline for the web of causation for infant mortality. Finally, the investigators examine the relationships among all the identified components of the web and attempt to determine the most feasible point of intervention to improve infant mortality in the community. Figure 3.2 depicts a web of causation for infant mortality.

Practical Application

This multifaceted approach taken in the web of causation model addresses the concept of causation in a manner consistent with current knowledge of human health. However, it may be overwhelming to carry out in everyday practice. In fact, it is more common to examine only a portion of the web, acknowledging that other relationships exist. Thorough examination of one portion of the web may provide sufficient information for initiation of useful actions to improve community health.

Models: Guides to Investigation and Practice

In this section, three models, each providing a slightly different approach to a community health problem, have been discussed. As you continue to study community health, you will find other models that can guide your practice. There is no one

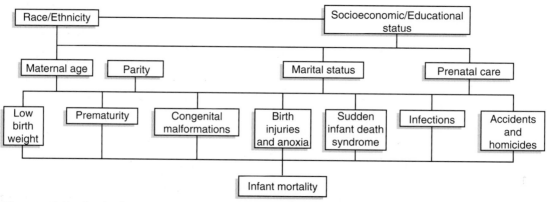

Figure 3.2 A web of causation for infant mortality, based on information available from birth and death certificates.

"correct" model; as you gain experience, you will be able to choose or adapt those that are most appropriate for your work.

Summary

In this chapter, you have learned about demography (the broad science of population) and epidemiology (the specific science of population health). We have discussed examples of how these two sciences can guide community health nursing practice. Now, you should be able to apply epidemiologic and demographic principles to your community health practice. For more detailed information on epidemiology and demography, consult the References and Further Readings sections at the end of the chapter, and the Internet Resources that can be found on thePoint website (http://thepoint.lww.com/Anderson6e).

Critical Thinking Questions

1. Centerville, located in Anderson County, has a population of 30,000. Centerville has an infant mortality rate (IMR) of 11 per 1,000. Anderson County has a population of 300,000 with an IMR of 6 per 1,000. During the last year, the maternal mortality rate (MMR) for Centerville was 9 per 100,000, whereas in Anderson County the rate was 7 per 100,000. How would the community health nurse interpret these data?
   a. Does the IMR in Centerville reflect a problem? If so, why?
   b. Does the MMR indicate a problem? If so, why?
   c. What does the IMR and MMR indicate about the health status of Centerville and Anderson County?

2. Select a health issue such as asthma, domestic violence, or cardiovascular disease, which affects a large number of people. Draw a web of causation that connects the different factors that may result in this health condition. Identify where the community health nurse can intervene.

3. An epidemiologic study investigates smoking as a contributing factor to lung cancer. The findings of the study are as follows: a relative risk ratio of 3.5 in the exposed group (smokers), an odds ratio of 4.0, and an attributable risk of 10 cases per 100 people in 10 years. Which of the three measures of association would have significant implications for designing a prevention plan? Explain the rationale for your selection.

4. Incidence and prevalence rates provide different information about the same health condition.
   a. Which rate provides the most useful information about the risk of illness? Explain your answer.
   b. If you were a health agency administrator, in what situations would incidence rates be helpful to you?
   c. Under what situations would prevalence rates be helpful to the community health team?

5. You are an administrator in a community health center. A screening program is necessary for a deadly disease, which is *curable* only if detected early. The tests available are one with a *high sensitivity* and *low specificity* and one with *high specificity* and *low sensitivity*. You must make a decision as to which test would be more appropriate.
   a. What are your concerns with the test with high specificity and low sensitivity?

    b. What are the consideration in the selection of the test with high sensitivity and low specificity?

6. Does fast food cause weight gain? A recent research study reported that eating at a fast-food restaurant two or more times a week was associated with a 10-pound weight gain over a 2-year period based on a relative risk of 2.5 (95% CI of 1.5 to 4.8).

    a. Is the research finding statistically significant?

    b. Does eating fast food cause obesity?

    c. Is the risk of weight gain increased or decreased for someone who eats two or more times a week at fast-food restaurants?

    d. What is the magnitude of increased risk compared to the average person: 2.5 times, 2.5%, or 25%?

● REFERENCES

Brucker, M. C. (2005). Providing evidence-based care: You can understand research and use it in practice. *AWHONN Lifelines*, 9(1), 47–55.

Centers for Disease Control and Prevention. (1980). Follow up on toxic shock syndrome. *Morbidity and Mortality Weekly Report*, 29(37), 441–445.

Centers for Disease Control and Prevention. (1981). Toxic shock syndrome—United States, 1970–1980. *Morbidity and Mortality Weekly Report*, 30, 25–33.

Centers for Disease Control and Prevention. (1983). Update: Toxic shock syndrome—United States. *Morbidity and Mortality Weekly Report*, 32, 398–400.

Centers for Disease Control and Prevention. (1993). Public health focus: Physical activity and the prevention of coronary heart disease. *Morbidity and Mortality Weekly Report*, 42, 398–400.

Davis, J. P., Chesney, P. J., Ward, P. J., LaVenture, M., & the Investigation and Laboratory Team. (1980). Toxic shock syndrome: Epidemiologic features, recurrence, risk factors, and prevention. *New England Journal of Medicine*, 303, 1429–1435.

McFarlane, J., Campbell, J., Sharps, P., & Watson, K. (2002). Abuse during pregnancy and femicide: Urgent implications for women's health. *Obstetrics and Gynecology International*, 99(7), 27–36.

MacMahon, B., & Pugh, T. F. (1970). *Epidemiology: Principles and methods*. Boston, MA: Little, Brown, & Co.

Sinauer, N., Bowling, J. M., Moracco, K. E., Runyan, C. W., & Butts, J. D. (1999). Comparisons among female homicides occurring in rural, intermediate, and urban counties in North Carolina. *Homicide Studies*, 3(2), 107–128.

Snow, J. (1936). *Snow on cholera, being a reprint of two papers by John Snow, M.D., together with a biographical memoir by B. W. Richardson, M.D., and an introduction by Wade Hampton Frost, M.D.* New York: The Commonwealth Fund.

■ FURTHER READINGS

Aschengrau, A., & Seage, G. R. (2008). *Essentials of epidemiology in public health* (2nd ed.). Boston, MA: Jones & Bartlett.

Chernick, K. M., & Friis, R. (2003). *Introductory biostatistics for the health sciences*. Hoboken, NJ: Wiley.

Cravens, G., & Mair, J. L. (1977). *The black death*. New York: Dutton.

Crichton, M. (1969). *The Andromeda strain*. New York: Alfred A. Knopf.

Dunne, T. L. (1978). *The scourge*. New York: Coward, McCann, & Geohegan.

Everitt, B. (2003). *Modern medical statistics: A practical guide*. London: Oxford University Press.

Fowler, J., Jarvis, P., & Chevannes, M. (2002). *Practical statistics for nursing and health care* . New York: Wiley.

Friis, R., & Sellers, T. (2009). *Epidemiology for public health practice* (4th ed.). Sudsbury, MA: Jones & Bartlett.

Merril, R., & Timmreck, T. (2006). *An introduction to epidemiology*. Boston, MA: Jones & Bartlett.

Savitz, D. (2003). *Interpreting epidemiologic evidence: Strategies for study design and analysis*. New York: Oxford University Press.

Selvin, S. (2004). *Statistical analysis of epidemiologic data* (3rd ed.). New York: Oxford University Press.

Internet Resources can be found on the**Point** at http://thepoint.lww.com/Anderson6e.

Environment and the Health of Communities

ROBERT W. MCFARLANE

Introduction

> *Environmental health is the promotion of safe, healthful living conditions and protection from environmental factors that may adversely affect human health or the ecologic balances essential to long-term human health and environmental quality, whether in the natural or man-made environment. These factors include but are not limited to air, food, soil, and water contaminants; radiation; toxic chemical exposure; disease vectors; worksite hazards; and habitat alterations. (Institute of Medicine, 1995)*

Florence Nightingale emphasized the importance of clean and safe environments for proper recovery to health (Nightingale, 1969). Her emphasis was on pure air, pure water, efficient drainage, cleanliness, and light.

Good health lies in recognizing that each of us is part of a wider web of life. No one person or community is an independent entity. Each is intimately linked to the environment, frequently in ways we have never imagined. Thus, the environment influences health, directly and indirectly, through subtle, indirect pathways. Conversely, human activities affect the health of the environmental system. One aspect of human ecology is the study of these linkages. Let's explore the ways in which interconnections, transport mechanisms, and constant change combine to affect health.

POLLUTION

Pollutants are the residues of things humans make, use, and throw away. Nondegradable pollutants either do not degrade or degrade very slowly in the natural environment. Biodegradable pollutants can be rapidly decomposed by natural processes unless input exceeds decomposition or dispersal capacity. Degradable pollutants that provide energy or nutrients may increase the productivity of an ecosystem by providing a subsidy when the rate of input is moderate. However, high rates of input can cause productivity to oscillate, whereas additional input may poison the system completely.

When any pollutant is introduced into the environment, we must be concerned about both the fate of the pollutant (where it goes and how it gets there) and its effect on humans or any of the ecosystems on which we depend. We must always keep in mind that any effects that pollutants have on other species are early-warning signals that something is amiss in the ecosystem and that humans may well be the next to be affected.

Major Pollutant Mechanisms

Living organisms have a hierarchical organization. Atoms link to form molecules, then macromolecules and cells are created. Cells link to form tissues, then organs and organ systems, and finally an independent organism. Numbers of self-replicating organisms create populations. Interacting populations of different kinds create an ecologic community, combining with the flow of nutrients and energy to form an ecosystem. Unicellular and multicellular organisms capable of photosynthesis combine carbon dioxide and water with sunlight to create complex carbon molecules, store energy, and release oxygen to the atmosphere. The photosynthesizing green plants and algae are eaten by myriad creatures, large and small, which are also eaten, in turn, by others. This pattern of consumption creates a food web, with links in numerous directions. Each exchange constitutes a trophic level within the food web. At each level, the consumer builds nutrients into its own body, burns most of the consumed energy for its own existence, and stores a small portion of the energy. In this manner, the self-organizing ecosystem creates an efficient mechanism for gathering and moving nutrients and energy from one organism to another. Pollutants are incorporated into this distribution system as readily as nutrients. Five pollutant mechanisms are of particular concern: transport, transformation, bioaccumulation, biomagnification, and synergism.

Transport

Transport of the pollutant, once it is introduced into the environment, is generally accomplished by way of wind patterns or aquatic systems. Pollutants can be dispersed aerially as particulates or in a gaseous state; they can travel long distances before falling to earth as dust or being carried in rain water. Ironically, the construction of increasingly tall smokestacks to relieve local pollution generally results in greater dispersal, thus enlarging the area affected without diminishing the amount of pollutant released. Once air pollutants have settled to earth, they frequently continue their movement by traveling along waterways. After a single heavy rainfall, storm water runoff can mobilize more suspended particulates than may be transported during the rest of the year. Dissolved pollutants may be transported long distances before settling onto the bottom sediments through some precipitatory mechanism.

Pollutants generally exert greater influence on aquatic ecosystems than on terrestrial environments. Air pollutants may enter a person's lungs or settle on vegetation and then be eaten with the plants. Water, though, is nature's best solvent, and many pollutants go into solution in aquatic ecosystems, with the result that aquatic animals and plants live in a weakly polluted "soup." Many chemicals enter the biota directly through the skin or across gill surfaces, because there is no escape from a dissolved pollutant. The effects of a given one-time polluting event, such as an accidental spill, are, therefore, exerted for a longer time in aquatic than terrestrial ecosystems. Not only is a greater portion of the pollution incorporated into and cycled within the biotic nutrient pool, but material that settles into the sediment can also be resuspended and redistributed with every major storm event. The dispersion of pollutants is also more restricted in aquatic than in terrestrial systems because movement is always downstream, until the pollutants reach the ocean. The efficacy of ocean transport has been demonstrated by the ubiquitous spread of several insecticides throughout the world; their area of distribution even includes the Antarctic continent.

Transformation

Transformation of a pollutant within an ecosystem takes place in many ways. Harmful substances can be rendered innocuous or even helpful during the biodegradation process. But occasionally, a relatively harmless substance is transformed into a noxious form. A classic example is the transformation of metallic or inorganic mercury, which is relatively immobile, into methylmercury by microorganisms living in aquatic sediments.

Methylmercury is readily incorporated into detrital food chains, which may terminate with human consumption of contaminated fish and shellfish, producing the neurologic disorder known as Minamata disease. Nonbiogenic chemical transformations are more common in the environment (e.g., the conversion of sulfur dioxide and nitrous oxides in the atmosphere to form sulfuric and nitric acids and create acid rain).

Bioaccumulation

Bioaccumulation refers to the introduction of substances into ecologic food webs. Chemicals that behave in a manner similar to essential elements are most susceptible to rapid uptake and retention. Chiefly because of humans and their activities, the ecologist must now be concerned with the cycling of nonessential elements. For example, the radionuclides of strontium and cesium, whose chemical behavior is analogous to calcium and potassium, respectively, are introduced into the environment by nuclear reactors and represent a potential health hazard.

Biomagnification

Biomagnification results when the accumulation of a pollutant greatly exceeds the rate at which an organism eliminates it. The pollutant is concentrated in organisms at a low trophic level, where it is further concentrated and passed to the third level, and so on. For example, polychlorinated biphenyls (PCBs) are a large class of 209 separate chemical compounds that held many industrial applications before 1976, when they were banned in the United States. Each of these compounds has a different type and degree of toxicity, bioaccumulates at different rates, and behaves differently when free in the environment. In the 1970s, these PCB compounds were associated with adverse health effects in people eating fish from the Great Lakes. The PCBs were acquired by phytoplankton that innocuously acted as tiny scavengers of the pollutant, reaching levels of only 2.5 parts of PCB per billion parts of phytoplankton. These were then eaten by zooplankton, which, in turn, were eaten by larger zooplankton, in which PCB concentrations increased nearly 50-fold, reaching 123 parts per billion. The zooplankton were eaten by small fish, rainbow smelt, with PCBs increasing ninefold to 1 part per million (ppm). Next, the smelt were eaten by lake trout, which reached 5 ppm PCB, and finally consumed by humans (or other end-chain carnivores). At each step, the PCBs were sequestered in the fatty tissue of the carrier and stored. The final concentration of PCBs in herring gull eggs, which are rich in stored fat and sometimes consumed by humans, was 124 ppm, or 50,000 times greater than the original concentration in the phytoplankton.

Synergism

Synergism is the simultaneous action of separate substances or agencies that together produce a greater total effect than the sum of their individual effects. It is common to discover that a given substance behaves in one fashion in a controlled laboratory environment and in quite another when introduced into a natural ecosystem, where it interacts with a number of physical and chemical properties of the environment.

Toxic Substances

In recent years, toxic substances have received a great deal of attention in governmental regulations and the news media. Any chemical can be toxic, including table salt, sugar, and the chlorine in drinking water. Toxic substances are generally considered to be any chemicals or mixtures of chemicals, either synthetic or natural, that are poisonous to humans, plants, or animals under expected conditions of use and exposure. There are four major categories of toxic substances: pesticides, industrial chemicals, metals, and substances with radiation-emitting isotopes. Pesticides are lethal chemicals specifically designed to kill weeds, fungi, insects, mites, rodents, and other pests. Four pesticides have been banned from further use in the United States: DDT, aldrin, dieldrin, and chlordane. Industrial chemicals are particularly numerous, and a few have proven especially dangerous (e.g., asbestos, benzene, vinyl chloride, and PCBs). A number of metals, such as arsenic, lead, cadmium, and mercury, have also proven to be very toxic in the environment. The fourth category includes those substances with isotopes that emit various types of radiation, such as strontium, cesium, iodine.

Chemical toxicity occurs when a chemical agent produces detrimental effects in living organisms. The effects of a toxic substance can be immediate or long term and can harm selected tissues or the entire organism. Both the toxicity of the substance and the expected exposure to the organism must be considered to define the anticipated risk. Neurotoxins are likely the most significant toxic substances in both prevalence and severity that pose a risk to human health. Epidemiologically, a relatively small fraction of major neurologic disorders are inherited; most neurologic diseases appear to be associated with environmental factors. Many commercial chemicals used in very large amounts and known to persist in the environment have neurotoxic properties. In fact, insecticides, designed to have neurotoxic properties, are manufactured for deliberate release into the environment.

Ecologic Principles

Knowing how pollutants move in the environment and how they can be transported or transformed, how they accumulate or magnify to affect health, we need to review some basic ecologic principles.

Law of gravity. In recent history, the interdependency of the human species and the natural world has been too frequently overlooked or ignored. As we seek ways to alleviate problems associated with health, it is imperative to be cognizant of nature's operating principles. The "laws of nature" have not been repealed, and knowledge of these laws is vital to understanding the origin of health problems and in successfully designing strategies to reduce them. The law of gravity is particularly important to the ecologic system. Everything that goes up, including pollutants, must come down, and everything dumped on the surface of the earth must ultimately flow downhill. Water and even land masses, such as mountains, move slowly to the sea. It is imperative that we learn to design with nature, exploiting these principles to our advantage, rather than expending resources in a useless struggle, because nature always wins. It is important to remember three commonsense observations that are frequently overlooked because of their inherent simplicity.

Everything is connected to everything else, but some things are connected more tightly than others. This observation is the least obvious. As we go from a climate-controlled workplace to a correspondingly pleasant home, insulated from the vagaries of the weather even while en route, it is easy to forget that working in a climate-controlled environment is a very recent phenomenon, restricted to a minority of the world population. As we select foodstuffs from the bounty of 24-hour supermarkets, we seldom stop to wonder where a particular item came from; what chemical abuses it may have suffered during its growth, harvest, or transportation; or what unsuspected surprises may lurk beneath the protective cellophane.

Everything has to go somewhere. Although this observation is readily acknowledged, "somewhere" is generally considered synonymous with "away" and is not considered to be a problem until the "away" becomes your living space. This may produce the now-familiar "NIMBY" reaction (not in my backyard!). As human populations and industrial development grow, pollutants are produced in greater quantities and dispersed over longer distances. At the same time, unpopulated areas are diminishing. Some pollutants are conspicuous and readily detected. Others, perhaps more insidious, are detected only when sought; the search frequently requires elaborate instrumentation and methodology.

Everything is constantly changing. Although constant change is universally recognized, the nature and rate of change are generally unappreciated. The natural environment undergoes continual change. Some changes seem irreversible, permanent, or barely detectable from our perspective in time (e.g., geologic transformations and continental drift). Other changes are cyclic (such as the seasonal climate) or transient (floods or droughts). However, changes produced by the actions of human beings have become more prominent. Significant human-induced changes began with the domestication of animals and the development of agriculture. These led to the growth of large human settlements, soon followed by deforestation and the depletion of local resources. The rate of change increased greatly as muscle power was replaced by mechanical power and renewable energy resources (wood, wind, and water) were replaced by energy derived from fossil fuels. Today, human populations dominate the earth's ecosystems. Nearly one half of the earth's land surface has been modified by human activity. More than half of the accessible fresh water is used by humans for various purposes. Humans have become a global change agent.

Pollutants and Human Population Size

All of the environmental processes described so far can influence human health. Any pollutant or toxic substance introduced into the environment is subjected to these processes, many of which lead directly to human beings. Pollution of the environment occurs when these pollutants overwhelm the capacity of the environment to assimilate them without being thrown out of balance. Thus, pollution is a rate function involving a quantity of pollutant introduced over a period of time. This rate is directly correlated to population size.

It can be said that all pollution is the result of population growth. A single family, living on a subsistence level in the wild, burning wood as their fuel, and discarding rubbish and human wastes on the landscape, would seldom be a polluting factor in their environment. The population of a small village would denude the landscape of wood fuel, pollute the air with smoke from numerous wood fires, and litter the ground with rubbish and human wastes randomly dispersed. Cities, with more numerous inhabitants, totally overwhelm the environment with rubbish and human waste, necessitating the development of sewage and garbage disposal systems. Industrial development increases the number of pollutants and environmental insults. Our past practice of handling pollutants has been to just dump them, taking further action only when the natural systems have been overwhelmed. We need to reverse this practice and remove the bulk of pollutants before inflicting them on nature. Then the natural ecosystem can work for us by removing the final bit of pollution that always proves so difficult and expensive to neutralize.

Demographic changes can rapidly alter the stress inflicted on the environment. As population grows, the stress increases. If the population moves, both the nature and the intensity of an environmental problem can shift. For example, the recent decline of industrial productivity in the northeastern United States has resulted in a shift in the population caused by the exodus of workers (particularly young families) and an improvement in the surface water quality. The growth of population in the South, especially the arid Southwest, is increasing water pollution and straining the overall water supply.

The solution to one environmental problem may be the creation of another. Pollutants do not disappear. Sulfur that is scrubbed out of powerplant smokestack gases ends up as a sludge stored on the ground, where it may threaten water quality. Pollutants removed from wastewaters by precipitation end up in the bottom sludge, which also requires disposal. Unfortunately, if the sludge is burned, the pollutants may be released into the air to settle and become incorporated into the water or land once again. If the sludge is buried in a landfill, it may threaten surface water or groundwater supplies. Sewage treatment plants that aerate water as part of the process may discharge substantial amounts of volatile toxic substances to the air. Disposable plastic containers and bedpans used in the hospitals are often incinerated and go into the air. *Everything has to go somewhere.* What goes up, comes down and eventually enters the air, the water, and the ground.

In summary, virtually any pollutant that is introduced into the environment will subsequently be transported away from its point of entry. It may be transformed into another chemical form, either less or more hazardous. It will probably be accumulated by biologic organisms, possibly becoming magnified in its concentration. It is likely to react with other chemicals or physical processes and to produce unanticipated effects. Distinct and efficient chemical cycles and pathways that have evolved over millions of years ensure that toxicants will enter biologic systems and eventually reach humans or other organisms on which they depend. *Everything is connected to everything else, and everything has to go somewhere.* There is nowhere to hide. The only solution is to stop the pollution.

Interventions to Decrease Pollution

To decrease pollution, we must begin with our own lives and act to REDUCE, REUSE, and RECYCLE. Stop and make a list of ways you might:

- Use less resources
- Select products that are less toxic
- Reuse products
- Minimize use of disposable products
- Recycle
- Avoid incineration

How many strategies did you list for using fewer resources? Here are some examples of ways we can encourage communities to use less resources:

- Lobby manufacturers to use less packaging material
- Write to businesses, asking them to incorporate electronic communication systems, such as electronic mail
- Explain to consumers the "ecologic" benefit of purchasing concentrated bulk food and products
- Discuss with consumers the importance of buying products with less packaging material
- Encourage individuals and businesses to use ground cover that does not require irrigation or mowing

Reuse and recycling of products will reduce pollution and result in a healthier community. Local communities can encourage curbside recycling programs. One community established a program named "Pay-as-You-Throw" that charges rates based on how much a customer sends to a landfill. The result was a 23% reduction in the amount of solid waste discarded by residents.

After two homes were lost to the sea, a beachside community collected Christmas trees and placed the trees on the eroding shoreline. This small program has now developed into a major initiative that involves more than 10,000 residents along a 30-mile coastline. (Once a community comes together to tackle an environmental problem, such as an eroding shoreline, people will more quickly work together on other community health issues, such as crime reduction and prevention, after-school programs for children, and recreation programs for the elderly.)

Encourage community residents to establish individual and group compost areas, to bring reusable bags to the grocery store to pack groceries, and to buy reusable glass bottles. (Be an example at the health agency where you work and use beverage mugs instead of Styrofoam cups.) Encourage parents to use cloth diapers instead of disposable diapers. (You might offer statistics on how much money can be saved by using cloth instead of disposable diapers or glass baby bottles instead of bottles with disposable bags.) Increase awareness about the use of disposable items by having community groups, schools, and agencies lists the type and number of disposable items they use during one day.

Work with school systems to establish recycling programs. Many states offer assistance to public schools to establish recycling programs. How would you find out about such assistance for schools in your community?

Lobby for options that incorporate waste-to-energy management systems. For example, waste-to-energy incinerators can burn waste to create heat or electricity for nearby consumers. How many cities in your state have municipal solid waste-to-energy incinerators? Where would you go to find out this information? Writing an editorial for the local newspaper about the benefits of alternative energy sources is an excellent awareness-building strategy for community health.

Potentially recyclable materials include plastic, paper, glass, steel, aluminum, yard waste, used motor oil, and corrugated containers. When materials are recycled, energy is saved and pollutants reduced. What recycling programs exist in your community? Are the programs available to all residents? If not, why not? Is the community you are working in interested in a recycling program? If they are interested, which community agency(ies) would you go to for information about beginning a recycling program?

ENVIRONMENTAL ISSUES AFFECTING HEALTH

We are losing habitat that is the home to many plants and animals. The clearing of forests to create crop lands results in *deforestation*. This is most often done by cutting down and burning trees. Increasingly warm climates result in the disappearance of entire forest types and more frequent and intense forest fires. Deforestation contributes to soil erosion, a change in climatic conditions, and air pollution. Climate change results in increased *desertification*. Fertile land becomes desert due to hotter but not wetter conditions. Climatic change is achieved by altering the rain cycle by reducing forest area. Desertification also results from poor land management (i.e., an overgrowth of crops depletes essential nutrients from the soil). A loss of biodiversity results in the extinction of certain species of plants and animals and thus deforestation, desertification, and reproductive changes.

There has been an overall increase in temperatures throughout the world. The "greenhouse effect" is a contributing factor to this *global warming*. The greenhouse effect occurs from an increase in atmospheric carbon dioxide. The increase in atmospheric carbon dioxide is caused by burning fossil fuels and oil, which releases carbon dioxide into the atmosphere. This carbon dioxide allows sunlight to pass through the atmosphere to the earth to heat it, but also traps the heat that is reemitted by the earth. The increased temperature has contributed to an increase of certain vector-borne diseases, such as malaria and dengue fever. There is also an increase in heat-related mortalities and in premature labors. The community health nurse should help promote cost-effective strategies, such as a decrease in the use of fossil fuels for energy and an increase in the use of clean fuels such as sunlight and wind. Use of more efficient lights and appliances will also help to decrease the use of fossil fuels.

The protective atmospheric layer of ozone is gradually becoming depleted. This results from chemical interactions between air pollutants and ozone. The major source of air pollutants is chlorofluorocarbons (CFs). CFs are widely used in refrigeration, air conditioning, and aerosols. Ozone is a pollutant when found in ambient air, but it is not a pollutant in the stratosphere. Without an ozone layer in the atmosphere, it is estimated that skin cancer incidence rates would increase 60% and 20,000 more fatalities would occur in the United States every year due to the excess ultraviolet (UV) radiation penetration. UV light exposure contributes to cataracts and the depression of the immune system (there is a reduction of lymphocyte production and susceptibility to infectious diseases). It is estimated that two thirds of all cancers are caused by environmental factors (USDHHS, 2003).

An accumulation of a variety of wastes and their environmental effects results in planetary toxification. Contributing factors include air pollution, water pollution, acid rain, and accumulation of solid and hazardous wastes. Each household in the United States produces approximately 87 gallons of solid waste weekly. Thirty to forty percent of this waste comes from packaging materials. Health problems such as heavy metal poisoning and infectious disease can result from exposure to toxic wastes from illegal dumping.

Environmental Hazards Affecting Health

Physical Hazards

Physical hazards to health include radiation, lead, other heavy metals, and noise.

Ionizing radiation is found naturally in soil and rock. It can also be found in building materials such as granite. X-rays are a form of ionizing radiation. Radiation risks also include nuclear power emissions and nuclear weapons. Health hazards to humans from ionizing radiation include birth defects; increased rates of cancer, stroke, diabetes, cardiovascular, and renal disease; and immune system damage. *Nonionizing radiation* does not result in ionization when atoms are passed through the body. Sources of nonionizing radiation include electromagnetic fields, UV radiation, visible light, infrared light, and microwaves. Radiation leaks from microwave ovens that have improperly fitted seals can cause fatigue and headache.

Lead and other heavy metals are present in soil, water, and air. Lead is considered by the U.S. Environmental Protection Agency (EPA) as the greatest chemical risk to health. Sources of lead include vehicle emissions, burning coal, and decomposition of solid waste. Young children are at an increased risk of lead poisoning because of their propensity to put things into their mouths, such as lead paint chips. Exposure to lead is associated with learning disabilities in children. Mercury, a powerful neurotoxin, can be found in paint and some traditional medicinal remedies. Symptoms of mercury poisoning include listlessness and irritability. It concentrates in the kidneys, liver, and brain. Currently, some hospitals are trying to eliminate use of products containing mercury. Arsenic, which is found in pesticides, herbicides, and some over-the-counter poisons, causes nausea and vomiting, diarrhea, and abdominal pain in humans. Another heavy metal, cadmium, found in water supplies due to contamination from rechargeable batteries, causes nausea and vomiting, diarrhea, and prostration in humans. Exposure to small quantities causes kidney damage and bone demineralization.

Noise affects hearing, and prolonged exposure contributes to anxiety and emotional stress. It may cause insomnia, skin problems, swollen ankles, and heart disorders. Common sources of noise pollution are industries, vehicles, subways, and loud music. Hearing loss can occur from the excess noise produced by airplanes in neighborhoods that are near airports.

Biologic Hazards

Biologic hazards can be infectious agents, insects, animals, and plants. Common indoor biologic pollutants include animal dander, dust mites, cockroach parts, fungi/mold, bacteria, viruses, and pollen. Infectious agents are primarily transmitted by way of water or an infected person. Contamination of water supplies can occur from septic tanks and untreated sewage, rainwater flow, and medical waste. Air becomes polluted from improperly cleaned air-conditioning and heating systems. Biologic pollutants can be found in dirty air conditioners; humidifiers; bathrooms and kitchens without vents or windows; dirty refrigerator vent pans; laundry rooms with unvented dryers; unventilated attics; carpets; and water damage around windows, roofs, or in basements.

Humans are hosts to a number of disease-causing pathogens and parasites. Some act directly, transmitting from one human to another (e.g., smallpox, measles). Others require an intermediate vector, typically a biting insect or other arthropod (mosquitoes—malaria, yellow fever, dengue fever; biting flies—Leishmaniasis, trypanosomiasis, onchocerciasis; fleas—plague; ticks—Lyme disease, tickborne encephalitis; or snails—schistosomiasis). Each additional link in the transmission cycle allows for greater environmental influence, typically related to temperature or moisture. For example, the prevalence of malaria increases with higher temperatures and high amounts of rainfall.

Chemical Hazards

Chemical and gaseous hazards include poisons and air and water pollution. Poisoning occurs through cumulative exposure to insecticides, herbicides, fungicides, and rodenticides. Exposure can occur at work on farms and in industry, in the home through accidental ingestion, and from eating animals that have been exposed. Poisons cause sarcomas, lymphomas, myelomas, and respiratory and prostate cancers.

Air pollution, which occurs inside and outside, kills approximately 3 million people every year (outdoor 1 million and indoor 2.5 million). Contributing factors include automobiles, large industries, and small businesses, such as dry cleaners, household products, geography, and urbanization. Health effects from air pollution are many and include respiratory disorders, eye irritation, fatigue, and headaches. Indoor air pollution is most severe in buildings that are airtight and designed for energy conservation. Formaldehydes, carbon monoxide, nitrogen oxides, asbestos found in furniture and the structural compounds of buildings, aerosol deodorants, certain types of cooking and heating, and cigarette smoke are trapped inside buildings and cause nose and throat irritations, heart disease, central nervous system (CNS) damage, and certain cancers. Air pollution is linked to reduced lung function in children. Lung function growth in children who live in areas with increased air pollution in the form of acid vapor (found in smog) is decreased when compared to that in children who live in cleaner communities. Decreased lung function growth can lead to chronic respiratory problems in adulthood.

Water pollution is caused by acid rain, manufacturing, mining, septic tanks, salt and deicing chemicals on highways, sewage sludge, and certain chemicals. Less than 1% of the water on this earth is available for human consumption. Numerous health complaints are associated with water pollution, including bladder and colorectal cancers, CNS effects, skin irritation, alopecia, peripheral neuropathies, seizures, hepatitis and cirrhosis, infertility, congenital anomalies, developmental disabilities, anemia, renal failure, heart disease, and gastritis.

Global Climate Change and Human Health

Although change is a constant, the rate of climate change has quickened beyond doubt Warming of the earth's climate system is indisputable (IPCC, 2007). Global average air and ocean temperatures have increased. Glaciers and polar ice caps are melting and sea level is rising. Temperature increases have been greater at higher northern latitudes, and land regions have warmed faster than the oceans. Precipitation has increased in some parts of the globe but declined in others, characteristic of shifting weather patterns. Climate change has resulted from increases in the release of greenhouse gases (carbon dioxide, methane, nitrous oxide, and certain aerosols), changes in land cover due to human activity, and changes in solar radiance that have altered the energy balance of the climate system.

Climate change has concatenating consequences. For example, climate and soils determine the prevailing vegetation for any area. In turn, the vegetation ameliorates the microclimate of the ecoregion. Ecosystems influence climate by changing the energy, water, and greenhouse gas balance of the atmosphere (Chapin, Randerson, McGuire, Foley, & Field, 2008). Ecosystems both create and consume oxygen and carbon dioxide. They augment the water cycle through evapotranspiration, moving large quantities of water from below ground to the atmosphere. Ecosystems also affect the albedo, or reflectance, of the earth's surface, absorbing or reflecting various wavelengths of solar energy.

Climate change directly and indirectly impacts human health (Haines, Kovats, Campbell-Lendrum, & Corvalan, 2006). For example, climate change affects regional and local weather patterns. It can increase extreme weather events such as heat waves and cold spells, storms, floods, and droughts. Storms and flooding may cause direct mortality and injury, displace large numbers of people, disrupt transportation and rescue efforts, and despoil productive cropland, leading to crop failure and malnutrition. Standing water may increase water-related diseases such as cholera and malaria. Higher air temperature may lead to an increase in heat-related illnesses and deaths during summer but lower cold-related illness and death in winter. In urban areas, high temperatures can create air-inversion and stagnant air, decreasing the dispersal of air pollutants and increasing air pollution-related health effects.

Climate change affects both native vegetation and cultivated crops. Warming may lengthen the growing season, increasing crop yield but also augment pollen production of allergenic plants, increasing the incidence of allergic diseases. Precipitation may increase causing flooding or decrease leading to desertification, crop losses, malnutrition, and population migration.

In the human population globally, 335 infectious diseases emerged or increased in incidence between 1940 and 2004 (Jones et al., 2008). These diseases include newly evolved strains of established pathogens (e.g., multi-drug-resistant tuberculosis, chloroquine-resistant malaria), pathogens that have affected humans for the first time (e.g., HIV-1, severe acute respiratory syndrome [SARS] coronavirus), and human pathogens that have increased in incidence (e.g., Lyme disease). Sixty percent of these emerging infectious diseases have involved a nonhuman, animal source (e.g., SARS, Nipah virus). Further, 23% of these emerging infectious diseases involved an animal vector. It is hypothesized that climate change is driving the emergence of diseases with vectors sensitive to changes in rainfall and temperature.

All animals occupy specific geographic ranges that expand or contract over time, occasionally in response to changes in climate. Expansion may bring infected vectors into contact with host populations that lack prior exposure and have not developed immunity or resistance to the disease. Human population density has been a good predictor of these emergent disease events. Wildlife biologists have identified a dozen pathogens that may spread into new regions as a result of climate change: avian influenza, babesia, cholera, Ebola hemorrhagic fever virus, intestinal and external parasites, plague, Lyme disease, red tides, Rift Valley fever, sleeping sickness, bovine tuberculosis, and yellow fever. Wildlife diseases may enter domestic animal populations, where minor diseases may become major infectious agents due to high-density crowded conditions. Prominent diseases of domestic animals may affect wildlife populations, and both may cross over to humans when domestic and game animals are handled and consumed (Jones et al., 2008).

Nursing Interventions to Decrease Environmental Influences on Health

Primary Prevention

A nurse can use primary prevention to decrease pollution in a number of ways:

- Reduce/eliminate environmental hazards, such as with enforcement of legal codes and standards
- Educate community residents, business owners, and government officials on how to avoid environmental hazards, such as the routine application of sunscreen and use of ear plugs and safety glasses
- Become involved with political actions that provide strategies to minimize environmental exposure in populations
- Promote routine immunizations to minimize diseases caused by biologic agents

For example, an environmental community action group, in collaboration with citizens of its community, is conducting a public education project on pesticide use in their community. Their goals are to increase public awareness of pesticide use and their environmental and health impacts, provide the public's right to know about pesticide use, and take steps to reduce pesticide use and health risks, particularly to children. Strategies they use in their project are similar to conducting a community assessment. First, they collect information regarding pesticide use in the area; then, they seek changes in pest management practices to reduce chemical pesticide use, and they build support in the community for implementation of new policies. They utilize parent–teacher organizations to build support in the community and to support their pesticide reduction campaign's legislative agenda.

Secondary Prevention

The nurse can use many techniques involving secondary prevention:

- Monitor for signs of hazardous environmental conditions such as blood lead levels
- Assess for signs of illness related to environmental hazards in the community such as increased incidence of asthma and mental retardation
- Decrease environmental pollution (refer to the section earlier in this chapter)
- Treat and monitor disorders caused by environmental conditions such as asthma and blood lead levels in children

With funding from the U.S. EPA, state departments of health are working with local public health units to conduct lead screenings of children. Because most funding in the past has targeted children on Medicaid, the new program targets non-Medicaid children 1 to 6 years of age who have never been screened and who live in homes built before 1950. Lead poisoning in children affects growth and development and can cause nervous system and kidney damage, learning disabilities, attention deficit disorder, decreased intelligence, speech and language problems, poor muscle coordination, decreased muscle and bone growth, hearing damage, convulsions, coma, and even death. Screening is a first step to detecting problems associated with lead poisoning.

Tertiary Prevention

The following are some ways to use tertiary prevention to keep the environment clean:

- Eliminate environmental hazards to prevent re-exposure, such as removing asbestos, lead, and mold from buildings
- Help communities to manage the long-term effects of conditions that are caused by environmental hazards, such as the extra-care costs associated with mental retardation and asthma
- Participate in political activity that reduces environmental hazards including strict adherence to emission regulations and air and water quality standards

Here is what one community did at the tertiary prevention level. In 1999, it was learned that two public schools had been built on land contaminated with a variety of toxic industrial chemicals. Although some cleanup of the site had occurred, a variety of carcinogenic and other hazardous chemicals remained, and according to the state pollution control board, there was a potential health risk to people using the site. Although the control board's approval was not required for the site cleanup, parents learned that the site had never received a clean bill of health, despite the fact that it was used by over 800 school children. As a result, Citizens for a Better Environment, working with individuals, the state Environmental Protection Agency, and the state Pollution Control Board, proposed changes to the state Site Remediation Program that would ensure that site cleanups receive certification before schools are built and occupied by children, and that they remain safe after schools are occupied (Citizens for a Better Environment, 2002).

NURSING ACTION FOR HEALTHIER COMMUNITIES

Change begins at the community level by making residents aware of the environmental issues and hazards present in their community. The community health nurse focuses on the concerns of the community residents and targets the problems that the people choose to address. The responsibility of the community health nurse is to make the community aware of the environmental health risks and the actions necessary to reduce exposure and potential health problems. The community health nurse works with the community to develop strategies for change and reduce resistance to change. Development of coalitions is important. The community health nurse assists the community to contact and partner with environmental organizations for help in improving the community's health. The community health nurse encourages communities to become involved in political action required to eliminate, avoid, and reduce exposure to environmental hazards. Assisting a community group in drafting an editorial for the local newspaper or writing a letter to an agency or congressional representative is the first step toward political action. If asked to describe the specific health effects associated with environmental exposures, where can you find information regarding environmental exposures in your community?

In one community with heavy toxic air emissions from chemical plants, a librarian decided to make a difference. She offered classes for citizens on how to use the Internet to learn more about toxic air emissions. She taught residents how to study their potential health risks from exposures in their community. The citizens were exposed to various inhalant toxins such as benzene, 1,3-butadiene, and chloroform. The citizens learned that benzene can cause drowsiness, rapid heart rate, headaches, tremors, confusion, and unconsciousness. Long-term exposure (365 days or more) can cause leukemia and cancer of the blood-forming organs. 1,3-Butadiene is made from the processing of petroleum and is used to make synthetic rubber. Breathing small amounts for a short time can cause damage to the CNS, blurred vision, nausea, fatigue, headache, decreased blood pressure and pulse rate, and unconsciousness. Lower levels cause adverse effects such as eye, throat, and nose irritation. Chloroform is used to make other chemicals and can be formed when chlorine is added to water. Long-term inhalation exposure in high levels can damage the liver and kidneys. Both 1,3-butadiene and chloroform are considered possible carcinogens. In this community of 50,000 citizens, 61% of the population reported eye, nose, and throat irritation but only 50% perceived a negative impact on their health from air pollution. The informed citizens wanted to share the information about the harmful effects of toxic air pollutants with all the citizens in their community. What strategies would you recommend to the citizens for informing the community? To which community groups would you suggest the informed citizens ask to make a presentation? What role does the community health nurse have in promoting the efforts of these concerned citizens? In addition to the health effects of environmental toxins, what other important information can the community health nurse assist the citizens in retrieving?

Community Health Nursing Actions for Healthy Air

Air pollutants can make asthma symptoms worse and trigger attacks, especially in children. Air pollution makes it hard to breathe and causes symptoms such as coughing, wheezing, chest discomfort, and a burning feeling in the lungs. There are two pollutants in the air that affect asthma: ozone and particle pollution. Ozone, found in smog, is often worse on hot summer days in the afternoon and early evening. Particle pollution, found in haze, smoke, and dust increases when the weather is calm and pollutants are able to build up in the air. Particle levels are highest near busy roads, during rush hour traffic, near factories, and when there is smoke from wood fires in stoves or fireplaces and burning vegetation.

As a community health nurse, what interventions can you advise to citizens at risk for the adverse effects of air pollution? Where can citizens go to find up-to-date information about local air quality? People with asthma should exercise because regular exercise is important for health. Exercising in the early morning and away from busy roads or industrial areas should be recommended and so should exercising indoors when pollutants are especially high outdoors. Trying a less intense outdoor activity, such as walking instead of jogging, on high ozone level days will reduce the amount of pollution inhaled. The community health nurse can stress the importance of access to quick relief medication when active outdoors, especially for those beginning an activity program that is more intense than usual. Sources of information about air quality and asthma can be found on the websites listed in Box 4.1. Free EPA brochures on ozone, particle pollution, and air quality can be obtained by calling 1-800-490-9198.

BOX 4.1

WEB RESOURCES FOR INFORMATION ON AIR QUALITY AND ASTHMA

http://www.epa.gov/airnow
http://www.cdc.gov/asthma
http://www.epa.gov/asthma

Community Health Nursing Actions for Healthy Water

Water is essential for life. According to the World Health Organization (WHO, 2006), 1.8 million people die from diarrheal disease each year, and 88% of these deaths are linked to contaminated water. Annually in the United States there are 900,000 illnesses and 900 deaths linked to poor water quality (Chalupka, 2005).

Natural disasters such as the tsunami in Asia in 2004 and hurricanes Katrina and Rita in the United States in 2005 destroyed water and sanitation systems. Subsequently, diseases including cholera, typhoid, dysentery, and diarrhea may result. Provision of uninterrupted safe drinking water is one of the most important preventive measures toward which community health nurses can contribute following a natural disaster.

Even in nondisaster situations, local water supplies are threatened by organic and synthetic contaminants. Private wells are affected by runoff from herbicides sprayed on vegetation. Half of all Americans obtain their drinking water from surface water sources (lakes, rivers, streams), the other half from groundwater. Natural and synthetic hormones and pharmaceuticals often pollute surface waters. There are two sources of water pollution: point and nonpoint. Point sources are easily discernable sources that discharge chemicals into the environment (factories). Nonpoint sources are less discernable, carrying agricultural runoff or industrial runoff (melting snow, paved roads).

Community health nurses play key roles in assessing causes of illness from water contamination in any situation: disaster, local water supply, or private well system. Specific responsibilities for the community health nurse include education and advocacy to decrease the risk of waterborne illness in vulnerable populations and to improve the local drinking water supply. The nurse must become knowledgeable about the situation, counsel family members on how to protect their household water supply, consider the possibility of waterborne illness when encountering acute gastroenteritis of unknown etiology, and take steps to safeguard the community water supply. The following resources will assist you in assessing and working with communities toward healthy water.

- Local drinking water information: http://www.epa.gov/safewater/dwinfo/index.html
- Ground water and drinking water information: http://www.epa.gov/safewater/index.html
- Information on recognizing waterborne disease and the health effects of water pollution: http://www.waterhealthconnection.org

Excellent target objectives for promoting community health include the national health objectives related to environmental health in Healthy People 2020 available at http://www.healthypeople.gov/HP2020.

THE COMPLEX HUMAN ENVIRONMENT

The preceding sections described humans interacting with the physical world and other species in a simplistic fashion. The complete human environment is difficult to comprehend because of the multiplicity of interrelated elements. The delivery of health care sometimes goes awry because the influence of certain elements is underestimated or unappreciated. A conceptual model of the human environment from an ecologic viewpoint can often illuminate the problem and guide efficient intervention.

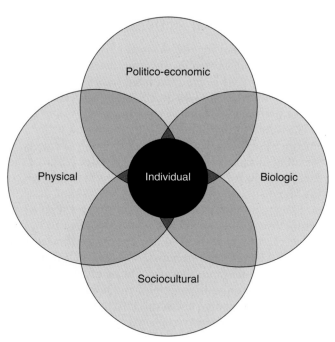

Figure 4.1   Model of the environmental systems that affect each individual.

An ecologic model (Fig. 4.1), like most models, proposes a framework from which to study and understand a phenomenon. The environment surrounds people wherever they go, whatever they do. An ecologic approach to the study of human health relates the biologic, physical, sociocultural, and politicoeconomic components of an individual's environment to any deviation from a state of health. The model can be applied to study the health of any defined subpopulation (e.g., infants, children, adolescents, and the elderly).

Environmental systems not only act on the individual person but also interact with one another, and a change occurring in one system will frequently affect others. Each system consists of components that act with and on other systems to bring about equilibrium or disequilibrium within the system.

Conceptually, both the subsystems and environmental systems are in a constant state of interaction (everything is connected to everything else and is constantly changing). Enumerating the variables within the systems and measuring the interaction among them are the keys to operating the model. In Figure 4.2, environmental systems and subsystems are displayed in a tabular arrangement, with variables boxed according to the systems most acutely affected by their interaction. Certain variables, such as migration and consumption of basic needs, equally interact with all systems as they affect the family and individual's functioning. Other variables, such as birth statistics (mother's age at birth, sex, birth order, and condition), are primarily within one system, affecting one developmental stage (the child) of one subsystem (the individual). Lines encasing variables are not set boundaries; rather, they serve as a guide to identify the system and subsystem most affected by variable manipulation.

The purpose of the conceptual model is to offer a framework from which to select significant variables related to the health status of a chosen individual. The variables that appear in Figure 4.2 are a synthesis of the epidemiologic, demographic, and

ENVIRONMENTAL SYSTEMS

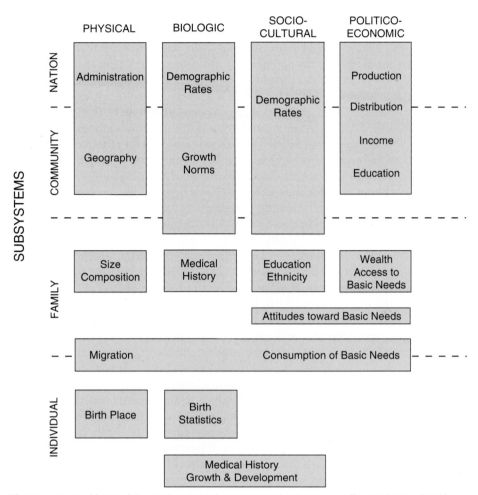

Figure 4.2 Model of the environmental systems and subsystems affecting human health.

social health indicators consistently proposed, tested, and recommended as valid and reliable indices of child health. Application of this model is described in the regional case history that follows.

Application: A Regional Case Study

The Problem

The following study concerns children with infection and their shared environmental variables. Much is known about the effects of infection; the morbidity and mortality statistics are salient testimony to the impact of infection on child growth, development, and survival. Surprisingly little is known, however, about the ecologic milieu that shrouds infected children or the causal paths by which the environmental variables interact to determine child health.

Epidemiologic studies of infection are plentiful, but their focus is usually on the incidence and seriousness of the problem, with little attention to the associated social or cultural forces. Similarly, sociologic analyses of infection focus on behaviors and attitudes, usually skirting the biologic as well as the economic and political factors. The objective of explaining this study is to demonstrate the usefulness of an ecologic model to identify and quantify the physical, biologic, sociocultural, and politicoeconomic variables related to infection among children.

Health statistics for children in rural communities, especially children of indigenous heritage, reveal that they have more problems than urban children. For example, in Chile, infant mortality rates in rural communities are more than twice those of urban communities. When risk is matched for ethnicity, indigenous children have a far higher risk, which is reduced somewhat if they live in urban areas but still remains substantially higher than that of nonindigenous children living in rural areas. The chance for indigenous children to attain the same mortality rate as nonindigenous children is directly correlated to years of maternal education.

In developing countries, income determines food consumption. With inadequate income, nutrient intake suffers. Malnutrition, defined as a deficiency of the essential nutrients required to support normal physiologic functions, has startling effects on health. The Pan American Health Organization found that a preexisting nutritional deficiency or immaturity (defined as a severe growth deficit) was the underlying or associated cause of death in 57% of deceased preschool children in the Americas. Infection was the leading (58%) cause of death, and 61% of those children who died of infection also had a nutritional deficiency (McFarlane, 1985). Malnutrition and infection demonstrate a synergistic and compounding relationship. Infection, a state in which microorganisms reproduce and cause damage to the host, is a radically different and more lethal process in a child than in an adult. Malnutrition and infection affect the vast majority of children in developing countries.

When a community seeks to maximize its resources of health personnel and capital goods to service the greatest number of children, it requires a tool that will (1) appraise the impingement of biopsychosocial variables that surround the child and (2) establish the relationships that link these variables to health status indicators such as the presence or absence of infection. Because infection is usually a short-term problem, whereas malnutrition is a chronic state of ill health, age-specific prevalence rates of infection are considered crucial indicators of health status and are used to measure health condition in this study.

Population and Methods

The Multinational Andean Genetic and Health Survey assessed the health status of the indigenous population living in Chile's northern province of Tarapacá. Northern Chile is geographically divided into three ecologic zones—the lowland coast, mountainous sierra, and highland altiplano—which differ radically in topography and climate. Associated with the differences are biotic changes that determine the type of agroeconomics, and thus lifestyle, that can be practiced. The health status of 988 children and 1,108 adults in 12 communities was determined; these people represented 70% to 90% of the people in any given village.

The International Classification of Diseases codes were used. Children with one or more diagnoses of infection were considered "infected," children with one or more noninfectious disorders were categorized as "noninfected," and children without coded diseases were considered "well" and "free of disease." In addition, family health variables were abstracted from census data collected concurrently.

Family wealth was scored according to the number of animals and amount of acreage owned. Four anthropometric measurements—weight, height, arm circumference, and subscapular skinfold—were used to study the relationship between growth and present health status. From known surnames, ethnicity was determined: non-Aymara (Spanish), Mestizo (mixed Spanish and indigenous), or Aymara (indigenous).

The people studied were primarily agriculturists who derived their livelihood from the land. Inhabitants of the highlands had little arable land, but large expanses of grazing pasture were available. They used their livestock (goats, llamas, and alpacas) to convert the inedible (to humans) natural vegetation into animal products (meat, milk, cheese, and fibers) suitable for human use. Conversely, residents of the sierra had more arable land, more irrigated fields, more diverse livestock (adding sheep and cattle) and agricultural crops, and thus more available foodstuffs. Coastal residents had the least arable land (desert stream floodplains) but benefited from a favorable climate and subsidized irrigation. Plant production was high and diverse on the coast, but animal products were restricted.

Population Characteristics

The physical examinations of children of all three ecologic zones revealed that 40% of them had one or more infections, 18% exhibited one or more noninfectious disorders, and 42% were well and free of disease. Infection did not decrease appreciably with age. Non-Aymara children living on the coast were most likely to be well and free of disease, whereas highland children had the highest rates of infection. The prevalence of noninfectious disorders showed little ethnic variability and no appreciable difference between coast and altiplano regions.

A complex clustering of interacting variables prevailed at the family level. Some, such as the number of people in the household, influenced child health directly (the larger the family, the more potential reservoirs for the incubation and transmission of infection). Other variables exerted their influence indirectly, acting through a web of interrelationships. A primary problem in understanding the ecologic determinants of child health is deciding how to assess the extent to which a given variable acts within the family's environment, directly or indirectly, to affect health status. Analysis of socioeconomic variables (maternal age, education, and health; paternal occupation and health; and family wealth) revealed that well children were likely to have a mother with secondary education and that infected children were likely to have a mother with no education.

Additionally, children with one or more infections were more likely to be cared for by a mother who was also infected, who was younger than 35 years, and who had minimal or no education. A large number of infected children in the altiplano resided in homes below the median wealth index, but neither wealth nor the father's occupation differentiated the health status of coastal or sierra children. Only among sierra children did the father's health correlate significantly to the child's health. Most early child and maternal health factors varied as a function of region but not of ethnicity.

When compared to well children, infected children consumed fewer foods and, regionally, altiplano children consumed the fewest foods. Region of residence with associated access to food, shelter, education, and health care proved more connected to child health than culture and associated lifestyle behaviors. Child health was determined by environmental factors operant at the individual, family, and community levels.

Model Application

Most children in developing nations (and some children in developed nations) reside in abject poverty, resulting in inadequate dietary intake and significant prevalence of infectious disease. The dilemma facing health workers and planners in all countries is how to use existing resources to the greatest benefit of the largest number of children. To promote child health, causal determinants of infection and malnutrition as well as cost-effective interventions must be identified. The problem is how to define and measure the crucial variables of child morbidity.

Most assessment models are linear, unidirectional, and not designed to look beyond the child or immediate family for health indicators. The ecologic determinants responsible for the prevalence, severity, and duration of the infection–malnutrition cycle are practically unknown. In developing countries, almost all pediatric morbidity data are obtained from hospital records; consequently, they offer uncertain direction for regional or community health planning, especially in rural areas where people have limited or no routine access to medical care.

The Chilean study used an ecologic model to sort physical, biologic, sociocultural, and politicoeconomic variables that impinged on child health. Descriptive and multivariate analyses were used to delineate the variables that exerted an appreciable effect on child health. Using ecologic concepts and the variables found to be important links to child health, a model of the ecologic chain of events has been constructed (Fig. 4.3). This "ecologic map" begins with the geographic region of residence—the community.

The region, or community, surrounds the child with a given set of physical forces, including climate, water supply, and topography. These forces interact with demographic structure and political and economic organization to determine the nutrient productivity of the land. Food production in any region is conditioned by economic forces (resources allocated to food production and food distribution); social forces

Figure 4.3　Model of the ecologic determinants of child health.

(land tenure); and political edicts (policy and legal implication of land ownership and use). These forces unite and determine the quantity and quality of land used for food production; the people and technology applied to the land to maximize production; and the diversity, nutritive value, and distribution of the produce. The physical, biologic, sociocultural, and politicoeconomic forces within each region determine the quantity and quality of nutrients available to the family for consumption.

The family consists of a clustering of interacting variables, many of which serve as gates, acting to impede or facilitate members' access to available nutrients. Simultaneously, infection risk factors abide within the household, variables that mitigate or accentuate the child's risk of illness. Both nutrient intake and infection risk concurrently determine health status, which is reflected in growth patterns.

The web of interconnection continues even further. Paternal health influences paternal occupation, which determines family wealth and, in turn, defines purchasing power and access to available nutrients. The number and age of siblings influence both access to food (through competition) and infection risk (through exposure). In addition, poor maternal health not only exposes the child to illness but also acts as a deterrent to adequate caregiving. Caregiving is also affected by maternal ethnicity, age, and education. Each factor determines the mother's knowledge and experience regarding basic health-promoting acts, such as hygiene practices, appropriate solid foods, and needed nutrients and physical care during illness. When the caregiver lacks knowledge or is ill, the child's risk of infection increases.

The child is a composite of risk factors that interact with familial and regional variables to set his or her health status and subsequent growth. The quantity and quality of nutrients consumed by the child determine weight gain and nutritional status. Weight gain is a product of both nutrient intake and a risk variable for infection. The malnourished child has impaired immunocompetence and is prey to infection. Also influencing a child's weight gain are weaning age and first solid foods; both affect the child's nutritive status and susceptibility to infection. Finally, the child's age and past medical history decrease or accentuate susceptibility to infection. In this study, it was the young, preschool children, ill within the last 2 weeks, who experienced the bulk of morbidity.

For most children, the interaction of nutritive intake and infection determines growth. Infection is wasteful and has a negative effect on nutrient absorption, metabolism, and use. As a result, the child loses weight, and growth is halted or retarded. Low nutrient intake equally retards growth. Children have greater nutritional needs relative to body mass: the younger the child, the more kilocalories per kilogram of body weight is needed for normal metabolism and growth. The risk of infection is high for all children, especially for infants and preschool-aged children, regardless of their nutritional status; however, when adverse infection–risk factors combine with marginal nutrient intake, the result is morbidity and delayed growth.

Policy Implication

Current assessment of world health indicates that lack of basic needs is the primary barrier to wellness. To provide basic needs and improve access to and availability of human services (e.g., education, health, sanitation), most countries have focused on providing selected basic needs to designated groups, such as school feeding programs or prenatal care. Unfortunately, regard for the environment, from which the needs arose, is usually omitted. To focus on selected needs without assessing the environment from which the needs arose ignores the complex interrelationships of the biopsychosocial system and negates the structure that created the health problems. Basic-needs intervention programs that do not address ecologic dynamics can create an illusion of success and allow continuation of social and political inequalities that are themselves major contributors to poor health.

Child health is ecologic and relates to the total environment that surrounds children and the physical ecosystem, as well as social, political, and economic organizations. Each system determines the production, availability, and distribution of resources and the eventual access of children to basic needs, which, in turn, dictates both health and growth. Children's health and nutrition problems will not be improved substantially until measures are instituted to eradicate poverty.

Using an ecologic model to identify and sort the determinants of infection among children in northern Chile, researchers found that the region of residence consistently emerged as a significant correlate of health. Region embraces politicoeconomic factors as well as a set climate and demographic state that determine nutrient productivity and access. Once the child acquires food, whether the nutrients are used to maintain and promote growth or are degraded by infection that retards growth and development depends on the family milieu, especially the mother's health, age, and education. Additional risk factors include family wealth, ethnicity, and paternal health. No one risk factor can be addressed independent of the others. Infection is promoted or hindered by a maze of intercorrelated variables, and to address only one or two does little more than vibrate the web of causation.

The root determinants of child health lie deep in the social, economic, and political fiber of the people. Child health cannot be improved independently of changes in the environment surrounding the child. To focus on selected prevention programs (such as improved nutrition or adequate housing) without simultaneously attending to the environment from which the deficits arise (such as existing political and economic policies) negates the determinant values of health and is an inappropriate use of time, money, and personnel.

Summary

Where does this knowledge of ecologic processes leave us? As practitioners of community health, how does this information aid us?

First, we must be aware that the health of any population can be affected by its surrounding environment. Next, be skeptical of any claims of perfect disposal schemes for pollutants; they do not exist. Remember that pollutants can travel long distances and remain undetected. Water treatment systems usually precipitate pollutants to a bottom sludge. Eventually, the sludge must be cleaned out. If it is burned, will the pollutants go back up the smokestack, only to settle into another watershed? If it is buried in a landfill, will the pollutants remain in place or seep into a groundwater reservoir, only to surface at your kitchen faucet? Everything—including pollutants— has to go somewhere, and it may be difficult to keep them in any one place.

Finally, as a consumer or a public advocate, do not demand perfect disposal schemes. Demand honest and realistic estimates of the risk that invariably accompanies any plan, no matter how appealing. Beware of flowcharts that indicate perfect control of pollutants at all stages of the cycle. Remember that it is people who handle pollutants, and the people factor can overwhelm every other part of any plan. It is people who load, transport, and dispose pollutants. It is people who operate and maintain pollution control systems. It is people who give illegal orders for "midnight dumping and roadside disposal." In some instances, particularly involving the ultimate disposal of nuclear wastes, we may be planning caretaking operations that exceed the realm of past human experience. Our oldest civilizations generally have not persisted for more than 5,000 years, and individual nations typically survive for far shorter periods. Can we honestly listen to glib talk of storing radioactive materials that will require maintenance for 10,000 years or longer—and take such plans seriously?

Critical Thinking Questions

1. Florence Nightingale recognized the connection of environmental conditions to human health. Based on what you have learned from this chapter, what are the major environmental conditions affecting the health of people in your community?

2. Exposure to lead and asbestos can happen at the worksite and then be transmitted on workers' clothing to the home, where it can affect family health. Think about the industries in your community, and identify potential sources of occupational exposure to substances that could be transmitted at home and affect family health.

3. Choose an environmental hazard, such as "ozone," and use the Internet Resources in this chapter to learn about the health effects of exposure to this hazard. What populations are at highest risk of health problems? What are the health problems? What can be done in the community to reduce exposure?

4. What information about health risks can you determine are present for a residential community near a chemical plant? What approaches can you take to obtain this information?

5. What can community members concerned about environmental toxins do to protect their health? What resources can you suggest to concerned citizens to assist them with a healthy action plan?

6. What are potential environmental health risks to patients, staff, and the citizens living and working near a large urban medical center? What are some specific strategies to decrease environmental health risks to these population groups?

7. How might a community health nurse respond to questions posed regarding the safety of well water versus public drinking water versus bottled water?

8. Choose an existing environmental health problem in your community, such as lead levels in old homes; poor air quality related to ozone or smog; or an environmental threat posed by the construction of or an existing landfill, airport, or housing development. (This is a good time to read the local newspaper and note the environmental issues.) Once you have chosen an environmental health problem, research the health effects and strategies to minimize the effects. Outline a 15-minute presentation, suitable for a group of parents of school-aged children, a group of seniors, or a group of pregnant women. (Of course, any interested group is just fine. The important point is to know your audience and tailor your presentation to the needs of the audience. Frequently faith communities and civic associations provide opportunities for interested citizens to gather.) Include references and sources for further information. Ask to make your presentation. Evaluate the responses of the audience. What questions were asked? What further information is needed? What action steps were discussed? What can be your continuing role in working with the group?

● R E F E R E N C E S

Chalupka, S. (2005). Tainted water on tap. *American Journal of Nursing*, 105(11), 40–52.

Chapin, F. S., III, Randerson, J. T., McGuire, A.D., Foley, J.A., & Field, C. B. (2008). Changing feedbacks in the climate-biosphere system. *Frontiers in Ecology and Environment*, 6, 313–320.

Citizens for a Better Environment. (2002). *Pesticide use reporting and reduction project*. Retrieved September 6, 2006, from http://www.wsn.org/pesticides.

Haines, A., Kovats, R. S., Campbell-Lendrum, D., & Corvalan, C. (2006). Climate change and human health: Impacts, vulnerability, and mitigation. *Lancet*, 367, 2301–2309.

IPCC (Intergovernmental Panel on Climate Change), (2007). Climate Change 2007: Synthesis Report, Summary for Policymakers. http://www.ipcc.ch/pdf/assessment-report/ar4/syr/ar4 _syr_spm.pdf. Accessed March 23, 2010.

Jones, K. E., Patel, N. G., Levy, M. A., Storeygard, A., Balk, D., Gittleman, et al. (2008) Global trends in emerging infectious diseases. *Nature*, 451, 990–994.

McFarlane, J. (1985). Use of an ecologic model to identify children at risk for infection and to quantify the expected impact of the risk factors. *Public Health Nursing*, 2, 12–22.

Nightingale, F. (1969). *Notes on nursing*. New York: Dover Publications.

U.S. Department of Health and Human Services (2003). Cancer and the Environment: What You Need to Know, What You Can Do. http://www.cancer.gov/images/Documents/5d17e03e-b39f-4b40-a214-e9e9099c4220/Cancer%20and%20the%20Environment.pdf. Accessed March 23, 2010.

World Health Organization (2006). Water, sanitation and hygiene links to health. Facts and figures updated November 2004. Retrieved December 29, 2005, from http://www.who.int/water_sanitation_health/publications/facts2004/en/print.html.

■ F U R T H E R   R E A D I N G S

ANA RN No Harm Training and Pollution Prevention Kit for Nurses: http://www.nursingworld.org

Collaborative for Health and the Environment: http://www.cheforhealth.org

Health Care Without Harm and the Nurses Work Group: http://www.noharm.org

University of Maryland School of Nursing's Environmental Health Education Center: http://www.enviRN.umaryland.edu

U.S. General Services Administration. (continually updated). Code of Federal Regulations. Title 40—Protection of the environment, part 50. National primary and secondary ambient air quality standards, part 129. Toxic pollutant effluent standards, part 141. National primary drinking water regulations, part 143. National secondary drinking water regulations. Washington, DC: U.S. Government Printing Office.

Internet Resources can be found on the**Point**, at http://thepoint.lww.com/Anderson6e.

Ethical Quandaries in Community Health Nursing

SUSAN SCOVILLE WALKER

LEARNING OBJECTIVES

Effective partnership with communities requires sensitivity to the tension between the beliefs, perceptions, and priorities of the community and those of the health care professional.

After studying this chapter, you should be able to:

1. Identify essential elements of health care ethics.
2. Describe ethical implications of the community-as-partner model.
3. Analyze community health proposals in consideration of ethical principles.
4. Formulate ethically sound decisions in partnership with communities.
5. Evaluate ethical decisions within the context of human needs.

Introduction

*T*his chapter reviews the general domain of ethics in health care to clarify the principles most often threatened or affirmed in health care decision making. Within the context of alternative approaches to ethical decision making and varying philosophical frameworks for defining the relationship between clients and health care providers, these principles are applied to the specific context of community health nursing. Finally, the concept of *community-as-partner* is reaffirmed as a guiding principle to unraveling the dilemmas encountered in the field of community health nursing.

WHAT IS ETHICS?

Ethics is a philosophical pursuit originating in an ancient discourse on the definition of "the good." To maintain a clear focus on ethics, it is helpful to contrast its domain to that of law, in order to avoid the tendency to confuse the two or to simplify the moral struggle to do the right thing by seeking a legal reason for action. The essential points of comparison are the following:

- Whereas ethics considers people as inherently good, law presumes them to be basically bad;
- Therefore, ethics proposes what a person *should* do, whereas law specifies what one *must* do;
- In fact, although one may be chastised if found in violation of ethical principles, there are no definite sanctions, whereas law imposes penalties in terms of fines and imprisonment.

Another point of confusion arises because the popular press often confuses the two terms or at least uses them interchangeably. Press coverage of the "ethics violations" of public officials actually deals with infractions of laws intended to bridge the gap between the two arenas and influence people to act in the "correct" way. The law is often seen as a way to enforce the current ethical values of a society because it responds more quickly to changing circumstances (O'Keefe, 2002).

Finally, ethics includes many levels of discourse, but the division of ethics most useful to health care decision making is that of applied ethics. The function of applied ethics is to provide a systematic, logical framework for analysis, discourse, and decision making that helps ensure that decisions are grounded in the philosophy of "good" actions.

APPROACHES TO ETHICAL DECISION MAKING

Although many philosophical approaches are discussed in the literature, two contrasting approaches are most helpful in applied ethics: deontology and teleology. Briefly, deontology is a rule-based approach, in which decisions are made by applying a set of rules of good conduct. Examples of such rules include personal moral codes and professional codes of ethics, such as the American Nurses Association (ANA, 2001) Code of Ethics for Nurses and the American Public Health Association (APHA, 2002) Public Health Code of Ethics. Deontology is grounded in the philosophy of Immanuel Kant and in the central precept of his teaching, that no person should be treated as the means to an end (Fry & Veatch, 2006; Petrini & Gainotti, 2008).

The contrasting approach is teleology, or outcome-based decision making, based on the philosophy of John Stuart Mill. Decisions are made on the basis of the greatest good for the greatest number (Fry & Veatch, 2006; Petrini & Gainotti, 2008). In actuality, the application of ethics to health care decision making usually involves a combination of these two approaches. Thus, the available options are evaluated first, to determine what option would be of greatest benefit to most of the parties involved and second, to ensure that the rights of all involved parties are respected.

The adequacy of either approach to health care ethics has come under scrutiny in recent years, however, as fundamental inequalities across geographical regions, strata of society, and age groups complicate the analysis (Daniels, 2006).

FRAMEWORKS FOR HEALTH CARE ROLES

Most people who enter the health care profession cite altruism as one of the reasons for their career choice. Given their desire to help others, the traditional framework of the relationship between health care professionals and the people they care for has been one of paternalism. In a traditional, literal rendition of this relationship, the physician holds the role of the father, the nurse is the mother, and the patient is the child. Indeed, this framework is inherently implied by those health care professionals whose chosen term for those in their care is "patient." Frequently, these health care professionals work in areas such as trauma, intensive care, and critical care, where they care for people who are often in acute distress and may not be able to be active participants in making decisions regarding their care.

In settings in which people can be active participants, a philosophy of contractualism applies. In these settings, the client and health care professional share in determining the options and selecting the best choice for that person.

Finally, in elective situations, such as plastic surgery, the balance of authority in decision making shifts away from the provider to the user of health care services, and the operative framework becomes one of consumerism, in which the consumer is clearly in control of choices among available options. Community health nursing is best understood within this framework, as exemplified in the model of community as partner. Effective, lasting community health nursing interventions depend on the ability of the community health nurse to relinquish decision-making control to the community and to trust its ability to make responsible decisions.

THE ROLE OF THE HEALTH CARE PROFESSIONAL

New roles of the health care professional within the framework of community as partner reflect an increasingly balanced participation between providers and recipients of health care. One role, developed and elaborated by nurse ethicist Sally Gadow, is that of advocacy. In her philosophical discourse, advocacy involves understanding the world view, life circumstances, and priorities of those requesting or receiving care and exploring the possible options with them in light of their preferences. In contrast to a strict contractualist or consumerist approach, however, the health care professional tries to imagine experiencing the situation of the person seeking care and offers an opinion of the best choice in full consideration of the other party's individuality (Gadow, 1990). The concept of advocacy has been refined by Racher (2007) to describe action within political, economic, and social systems on behalf of health interests of communities.

Another conception of the role of health care professional, particularly applicable to community health nursing, is that of catalyst. In this model, the community is seen to contain all the necessary qualities and resources for change, and the role of the health care professional is to provide the spark that will initiate change, as desired by the community and on its terms.

Both of these models clearly establish the primacy of the community and the fact that lasting change depends on the investment of the community. However, it is important to underscore that the health care professional is an active, concerned, supportive, sometimes challenging participant in the process. As an advocate or catalyst, the community health nurse can make the difference between success and failure of a community's efforts to improve the quality of life of its members.

SEVEN PRINCIPLES ESSENTIAL IN HEALTH CARE ETHICS

The process of ethical decision making involves analysis of alternative actions in light of moral and ethical principles. In health care ethics, seven pervasive principles are useful in making conscientious decisions. These are the principles of autonomy, respect

BOX 5.1

ETHICAL PRINCIPLES IN HEALTH CARE

1. Autonomy
2. Respect for persons
3. Beneficence
4. Nonmaleficence
5. Justice (distributive and retributive)
6. Veracity
7. Fidelity

for people, beneficence, nonmaleficence, justice, veracity, and fidelity (Box 5.1). In this section, each principle is defined and then applied to situations typical of those encountered in community health nursing.

Autonomy

The right of individuals to self-determination (autonomy) is the core value of western European and American law and ethics. In application to health care, it means that decisions should be made by those most affected, be they individuals, families, groups, or communities. Clearly, autonomy is the umbrella concept of the community-as-partner model. Many health care professionals will come and go, and any outside program, no matter how worthy, will endure only as long as those professionals remain active in the community, unless the community makes an autonomous investment to endorse and adopt the idea behind the program.

The altruistic nature of health care professionals presents a central challenge to the autonomy of those who receive their care. Often, the desire to care is so strong, and the appreciation of those who benefit from that caring so rewarding for the provider, that the result is a system of giving and taking that leads to increased dependency. It is striking to visit a remote community after a community assistance project of some kind has been operating there and be greeted with, "Who are you and what are you going to give us?" For some community health care providers, it seems that the urge to help is so strong that it can get in the way of empowering people to help themselves. The classical field of community development, as exemplified by the Peace Corps and other relief organizations, assists people to develop the skills needed to improve their own circumstances. Thus, in contrast to programs focused on providing goods or services, these programs operate at the grassroots level. Outside helpers work as catalysts with people in communities to discover their potential and as advocates to help the community learn how to access resources needed to move toward their goals.

Respect for People

The second essential ethical principle, respect for people, recognizes that every person and community has intrinsic value. Applying this principle to community health directs health care professionals to evaluate the effect of proposed initiatives in light of their implications for all who might be affected.

One example of applying the principle of respect for people might be to encourage a community to reevaluate its proposal to resolve its solid waste or toxic waste problem by transporting this waste to another community. The benefit to people in one community creates potential harm for those in another. Another example would be to give careful consideration before introducing western medical practices and ideals that might conflict with a community's cultural norms and folk-healing practices. Other examples will be discussed in more detail in the next sections in relation to justice issues and programs that are restricted to serve only a portion of the community in need.

Beneficence

The desire to act in the best interest of others, beneficence, is perhaps the strongest guiding ethical principle of health care professionals. Most people who enter the helping professions do so because of an altruistic desire to help others. Because of the desire to help people, to take care of them, and to alleviate their suffering, health care professionals often find themselves faced with conflicts between their desire to help (beneficence) and their respect for the other person's right to choose (autonomy). In fact, the principles of beneficence and autonomy are so often at odds that it is all but impossible to imagine an uncomplicated example of beneficence as applied to community health nursing. Even a community health initiative as apparently benign as an immunization campaign to protect community members from a communicable disease may conflict with the autonomy of people whose religious beliefs do not support the practice. The complexity of communities makes it unlikely that any community-wide activity will be uniformly beneficial to all sectors.

Nonmaleficence

Nonmaleficence, the avoidance of harm, is the silent partner of beneficence. Often, health care decisions may offer no really good option that will provide positive results, but at least there may be a choice that does not cause any outright harm. When proposals are considered for community health initiatives, it is important to evaluate not only what positive good (beneficence) may come from the activity, but also what harm might result, particularly if, as in the example above of solid waste and respect for people, the same initiative may well be beneficial for some community members and harmful to others. If a community attracts more industry to the area, the results may include increased job opportunities and better economic conditions for its residents, but there may be counterbalancing health risk factors such as environmental harm and decreased water and air quality.

Justice

The principle of justice has two aspects, both of them applicable to health care decision making. Most often, discussions of health-related justice center on *distributive justice*, the fair distribution of rights and resources. These discussions often center on allocation of scarce resources in ways that are fair and of greatest benefit to the most people. In this context, community health care providers and advocates argue for increased governmental support for preventive health programs that lead to better quality of life (beneficence) for the greatest number of people in the community (respect for people).

Well-meaning community programs designed to improve access to health services raise issues of distributive justice. In one example, a community coalition of diverse clinical providers and health care organizations developed a series of community health fairs in different neighborhoods in and near a small city. Initiated as a means of improving child immunization rates, in the early years the fairs were small and community oriented, combining health services and some aspects of a street fair, including games, food, raffles, and children's activities. Events were held three times a year, and the late summer fair was always the largest, because many children needed immunizations or athletic physicals before the start of school. Over time, civic groups joined in to provide school supplies for the back-to-school fair and other incentives for the other fairs. Incentives brought an ever-increasing number of people to the health fairs, including many people who came because of their need for the supplies (paper, pens, food, and blankets) rather than a need for health services. Because the intent of the organizers was to provide health services, there was often a requirement that participants receive a certain number of services to be eligible for the incentives. Service records from the fairs indicate that a number of participants traveled to health fairs in several communities and participated in repeated health screenings to receive the incentives.

Grant-funded community health research projects also raise issues of distributive justice when random houses in a particular neighborhood are selected for a project. A neighbor may be visiting on the porch at the time the field investigator visits and offers members of the selected household a stipend in return for participation. Culturally sensitive, caring field researchers who are invested in the community are known to dip into their own pockets and provide equal treatment to the neighbor even though the data will never be included as part of the study.

There is a second branch of the principle of justice, that of *retributive justice*, the arena of reward and punishment. Because of their generally altruistic nature, health care professionals may be reluctant to address this principle. However, the application of this darker side of justice is often tied closely to distributive justice. Allocation of resources is very often determined politically, and resources are awarded to those who have provided support to those in control of the resources. Thus, in poor communities everywhere, political candidates may provide transportation to the polls along with assurances of improved living conditions should they be elected. At the same time, grants and projects often come to communities that have demonstrated a strong voting record for those in power.

Many community health programs are funded by local, state, or federal government grants. Often, communities are selected to receive grant-funded services through the political and legislative process. Therefore, it is important for community health nurses to be active and to help community residents establish a voice within the local, state, and national political arena. Starting with knowing their own city, county, and state representatives, effective community health nurses can serve as a link between the community and its elected representatives and can facilitate interaction and support as a two-way process. If the community (including the nurse) can find ways to support politicians (photo opportunities, voting, attending rallies), it is more likely that politicians will reciprocate by funding needed programs.

Veracity

Veracity is the commitment to tell the truth. In community health nursing, veracity centers on honesty about who you are and what you bring to the community. In some communities, many programs and researchers have come, and gone and a cynical materialism has arisen in the community. Community health nurses may find themselves entering communities that have become accustomed to outsiders bringing in programs, goods, or services. It is difficult but necessary to be clear from the beginning that, in the spirit of community as partner, the only gift brought by the nurse is the gift of self, offering advocacy and energy to support the community.

Community health research raises issues of veracity. Many communities, particularly those with underrepresented population groups, are frequently visited by teams of researchers who screen residents for any number of health conditions or risk factors, including chronic illness and toxic exposure. Community health nurses, as community advocates, should help ensure that they and other researchers are honest with the community about exactly what is to be provided. All too often, residents do not understand that the only benefit from participation in a research study is the screening itself. Access to the results of health screening raises a separate issue of veracity, as well as issues of beneficence and nonmaleficence. It is of little benefit to know of a serious health condition if there is no access to treatment for it.

Fidelity

The last of the seven essential principles is fidelity, or faithfulness. To work with communities or individuals, the health care professional must be careful in making promises and steadfast in keeping them. This obligation may be embodied as simply as making and keeping appointments. It also may extend to keeping a pledge to report back to community leaders on the outcome of a project.

As discussed above in the section on veracity, community health research raises serious questions of fidelity as well as veracity in projects that involve health screening. To be effective on a long-term basis in a community, a community health nurse needs to network with health care providers in the community to obtain treatment for people made aware of serious health conditions by community health screenings. Much of the work of the community health nurse, then, involves building relationships to advocate effectively for treatment for community members diagnosed with serious health conditions. It is important to be aware of the reciprocal nature of this relationship and how it relates to issues of retributive justice and political involvement. Thus, if the community health nurse expects another health care professional to respond to a community and its needs, the time will come that the health care professional is entitled to ask for a favor in return. An effective approach is to consider what one's community, one's associates, or oneself might have to offer in advance of asking the favor. It is also good to know about tax incentives, public relations, referrals, and other nonaltruistic motives as well.

ETHICAL QUANDARIES IN COMMUNITY HEALTH

The diversity and complexity of communities inevitably lead to a plethora of conflicts between and among these principles. In this section, several examples will be discussed to illustrate some common quandaries that complicate community health partnerships.

Quandaries Regarding Autonomy and the Public Good

The potential conflict between autonomy and the public good (beneficence) is a prominent feature of many of the Healthy People 2010 National Health Goals. As delineated by the U.S. Department of Health and Human Services (2000), the health indicators used to measure progress toward reaching these goals include the following: physical activity, overweight and obesity, tobacco use, substance abuse, responsible sexual activity, and immunization. Clearly, with the exception of immunization and substance abuse, these indicators are health behaviors that carry no mandates. On the other hand, they represent expressions of personal freedom that are highly cherished and protected by a society that values individual freedom and respect for a person's right to choose. However, the purpose of the National Health Goals and the establishment of indicators that can be used to measure progress toward goal attainment is to reduce the human and economic cost of preventable, disabling health conditions prevalent in the United States today. The health effects of a fast-food diet and inactivity are well documented, yet it remains a matter of personal choice for individuals to change behaviors that harm only the individuals themselves and that can be modified only if the individual desires. Nevertheless, the community health nurse can act as an advocate and catalyst, by helping a community look at overall resources and alternatives that can promote health and a healthy lifestyle. Whether or not all individuals have free choice regarding health behavior decisions is open to discussion, considering the long-standing correlation of healthy behavior choices with socioeconomic status (Blacksher, 2008).

Quandaries Regarding Respect for People, Autonomy, Justice, and Beneficence

Although health care professionals desire to help improve people's lives and health status, they are often challenged to respect the rights of individuals or communities to choose other alternatives. For example, in many communities, a faltering economy has led to severe cuts in human services programs, often on the basis of perceived worth of the individuals. Among the first population groups to lose funding are the mentally ill and those with substance abuse disorders.

An example that illustrates the conflict between beneficence and respect for people concerns the activities of a group of community health nursing students who worked in a small, rural community on the Texas–Mexico border. The community is located on the Rio Grande River and has a population of around 3,000, including many migrant farm worker families. The community has an independent civic government but a very limited economic base and a weak infrastructure. On arrival in the community, the students conducted a detailed community assessment, in keeping with the community-as-partner model, using the community assessment wheel as a guide. As they discussed their findings, the students noted the young population of the community, with a preponderance of children and youth, the proximity to the river, and the safety issues inherent in children swimming and fishing in the polluted river. The students thought that a high priority for the community would be safety, and they were prepared to teach parents and children about the health risks of the river. However, as they got to know the community better and community members spoke up, it was clear that the community had much the same concern but a very different perspective on what to do about it. Although their primary concern also related to the children and youth, they focused on the need for recreation, in particular the need for an informal ballpark on the riverbank.

Another example of ethical issues of justice, beneficence, and respect for people focuses on the choice and condition of goods delivered to impoverished areas as part of public health relief efforts. Often, as winter approaches, appeals go out for blankets and warm clothing. Although the appeals specify that donated items should be new or in excellent condition, all too often organizers receive bags of clothing unfit for any use other than cleaning rags. Another notable example relates to food supplies sent to cultures with no appreciation for how to use them. Peanut butter was airlifted to Afghanistan to relieve hunger; it was unacceptable to the people, who did not have a taste for it, but who did find that some of their domestic animals were willing to eat it. In another instance, bulgur wheat, a Middle Eastern staple, was shipped to South America where it was unknown and went unused.

Quandaries Regarding Autonomy and Beneficence: The Case of Scarce Water

Probably the most frequent source of conflict faced by community health nurses is the desire to help people whose values are at odds with those of the person desiring to help them improve their health status. In an acute care setting, chronic tobacco smokers defy the best attempts to improve their health status unless they are invested in the process. In community health, a similar situation exists. Community health workers starting a new outreach program to identify people at risk for human immunodeficiency virus/acquired immunodeficiency syndrome (HIV/AIDS) found that they needed first to provide information and access to basic needs like housing and food. Community members were more concerned about immediate risks than the long-term possibility of AIDS.

Similarly, a group of community health nursing students was assigned to an isolated rural community near the Texas–Mexico border. The water supply of the community was known to contain a high level of naturally occurring arsenic. The students were eager to learn about the community's perception of their health risk and to help find ways to remediate the situation. Students were surprised by the results of their comprehensive community assessment. Community members acknowledged the natural presence of arsenic in their water and the potential for long-term undesirable health effects. However, they compared that unknown risk with the outright lack of an adequate water supply of any kind in a neighboring town. They weighed the risks and benefits and considered themselves fortunate to have water in an arid region. The health issue of highest importance identified by the community was the lack of accessible health services and the accompanying risks of traveling 50 miles each way on a dangerous highway to access services.

Quandaries Regarding Autonomy, Beneficence, and Justice: Access to Care

As the cost of health care increases, so does the population of uninsured and underinsured. Combined with the cost of litigation and extravagant settlements, open access to care is coming into question. When data showed a decrease in the number of eligible low-income families choosing to enroll their children in The Children's Health Insurance Program (CHIP), the low-cost, government-supported health insurance program, research revealed the most common explanation given by those who failed to reenroll was that they did not want to pay the $50 enrollment fee either because their children were not currently sick, or because they could go to the emergency room when a child was sick and receive free care. Emergency rooms, on the other hand, have started to look more critically at their role in the health care system and treat only those cases that qualify as emergencies; other cases are evaluated and offered a referral to a primary care clinic for a nominal fee.

Communities are also beginning to explore strategies to encourage or even to force families to participate in some form of health insurance or other payment plan.

As resources become scarcer and demand increases, these discussions are becoming more common and more frightening in their implications for other aspects of children's overall health when they include suggestions such as restricting access to recreational facilities or even public education.

Quandaries Regarding Autonomy, Beneficence, and Nonmaleficence: The Case of the Tarahumara

In northwestern Mexico, in the beautiful Sierra Madre mountain range, is the spectacular natural wonder called the Copper Canyon, home to one of the world's last remaining indigenous cultures, the Raramari, also known as the Tarahumara Indians. They live a simple life, based on a philosophy of harmony with nature. As civilization has taken over more and more of Mexico, the Tarahumara have moved into more and more rugged and inhospitable regions, and are now isolated deep in the canyons of the Sierra Madre. The Tarahumara prefer to sleep out under the stars, weather permitting, but they maintain small huts or cave dwellings both on the rim and at the base of the canyon. Due to the great variation in temperature from the rim to the base, they stay on the rim in summer to catch the cool breeze and move to the warmth of the canyon floor in the winter. The canyon is crisscrossed with paths used by the Indians to maintain communication with others in the community. The Tarahumara live in isolated family units and come together occasionally for special events. They are world-renowned long-distance runners, due to their dependence on foot travel on the steep mountain trails to maintain communication between families. They maintain a subsistence lifestyle, carving out steep fields on the mountainside in which they grow the corn that serves as the staple of their diet.

During the past 50 years, "progress" in the form of industrialization and modernization led to the development of one of the greatest engineering marvels of the world, the Chihuahua al Pacifico Railroad, running through the Copper Canyon on its way from Chihuahua, near the United States–Mexico border, to Los Mochis and Topolobampo, across the Gulf of California from Baja, California. With the railroad has come world accessibility to the natural wonder of the Copper Canyon and alternatives to the traditional subsistence farming lifestyle of the Tarahumara.

Scholars admire the beauty of this vanishing lifestyle and fear the effects of increasingly greater accessibility to the region and increased interest of outsiders in "improving" the lot of these people (Fontana, 1987; Gorney, 2008). Electricity has moved farther into the canyon, bringing with it washers, dryers, and television. Convenience foods have introduced hypertension, and increasing contact with outsiders has exposed the people to communicable diseases for which they have no immunity. One proposed development plan would bring commercial air travel into the area, while resort hotels would require as much water for one day as a Tarahumara family might use in a year.

Some say the world is entitled to be inspired by visiting one of the most beautiful unique regions on earth (autonomy) but also has an obligation to preserve a unique culture (respect for people). On the other hand, increased tourism has offered the Tarahumara an easier means to survive by surrounding the train and hawking their carvings and beautiful pine needle baskets to the tourists as they come through. The Tarahumara themselves express no qualms about enjoying some modern conveniences.

EVALUATION OF ETHICAL DECISIONS WITHIN A HUMAN NEEDS FRAMEWORK

Another interesting approach to examining ethical issues within the community-as-partner model is to use a human needs framework to evaluate the merit of a particular choice of action. In this context, the most basic (and perhaps, therefore, the highest priority) need would be physiological need, followed by safety, then belonging, self-esteem, and finally self-fulfillment (Maslow, 1970). It is arguable, however, whether this hierarchy also reflects a scale of priorities for any particular individual. The ethical dilemma may come down to valuing an individual's right to (autonomy) development of his or her fullest potential against the physiological or safety needs of the larger community. This dilemma is best illustrated in a discussion of access to and use of a scarce commodity: water.

Does an individual or group have the right to enjoy water for its beauty, while the community as a whole is in danger of running out of water for basic needs such as sanitation and drinking? The classic example is an upscale community in a desert region with a waterfall feature that loses substantial amounts of precious water through evaporation. Unrestricted home landscaping choices may also require excessive amounts of water; however, those plants may have particular significance and give a sense of well-being to people who have moved to a strange area. What responsibility does a developer have in terms of water infrastructure to ensure adequate water pressure to the adjoining community? How might water be fairly allocated if it is to be rationed—should each individual or each household be allowed a particular number of gallons? Should water conservation be required as a feature of all new construction?

Is access to water a right? Some unscrupulous developers have sold parcels of land with no infrastructure. Community activism has focused on bringing in water lines at no cost to the residents. But some residents do not want to pay for the hookups, nor for water usage at the going rate. Alternatives to sewer hookup include septic systems and solar composting toilets. However, well-meaning community development workers may run afoul of regulations, ordinances, and cultural preferences in trying to implement reasonable programs without sufficient research and background preparation.

Another example of conflict between individual self-fulfillment and community basic needs is the involvement of an increasing number of people in so-called extreme sports and other high-risk behaviors. For example, in addition to scuba diving, horseback riding, mountain climbing, ski jumping, and motorcycling, America's active, affluent adventurers are showing increased interest in personal light aircraft, mostly made at home and not inspected or requiring a pilot's license to operate. All these activities provide an outlet for self-actualization and stress relief. However, the costs to the emergency medical system are immense when the resources involved in a search-and-rescue mission are calculated, along with the costs of medical care. At what point does the individual assume the risk, and at what point do emergency medical services determine that the cost and risk are just too great to pursue a rescue? As the affluent population becomes greater and their leisure-time activities expand, this question will become ever more critical.

The second level of human need is security—one of the most common areas of concern identified by community residents on community assessment surveys. In the past, proposed interventions to improve public safety centered on close collaboration among law enforcement agencies in the community. However, as the level of violence has escalated, communities have started feeling less confident in the law enforcement's ability to manage the situation. One community reportedly passed an ordinance requiring all adult citizens to be armed. After publication of this ordinance, the crime rate markedly decreased.

Increased drug and migrant-related activities along the United States–Mexico border have left many residents disillusioned with the federal agencies charged with securing the border. Citizens complain about receiving no response when they call to report groups of individuals trespassing on private property. Concern for their personal and economic safety and security has led to the development of controversial groups of volunteer patrols that pledge to make the designated agencies respond by observing, notifying, and monitoring the response. The controversy centers on whether these groups actually are peaceful observers, as they claim, or vigilantes, and how they will be perceived by the federal agencies, the local landowners, and the persons they are seeking to apprehend. Some unfortunate incidents in the past have raised questions about how the groups will conduct themselves and how they will interface with the commuity and its law enforcement agencies.

Local residents also wonder about the motivation of people from other parts of the country who participate in this activity. Do they come as a patriotic gesture in the interest of homeland security, or as participants in a thrill-seeking extreme sport substitute? Are they prepared for the climate, terrain, and culture of the area? What sort of training do they have? How will they handle the boredom of watching and waiting and the frustration of observing and not taking action? What will be the demands on local resources for both infrastructure and emergency response?

Summary

Working in partnership with communities requires careful consideration of all seven primary ethical principles and the interplay among them. Autonomy, respect for people, and nonmaleficence are the principles most often threatened by the community health nurse's commitment to beneficence. Conscious awareness of this risk and application of the principles of justice, both retributive and distributive; veracity; and fidelity will assist community health nurses to analyze the ethical principles at stake at any given decision-making point in their work with communities. Their actions, then, will reflect the best possible application of the principle of community as partner and will promote the optimal overall health of a community within its own culture.

Critical Thinking Questions

1. As a nurse, how do *you* define the relationship between yourself and those for whom you care? What word do you use to describe the other(s) in that relationship? Why? Which ethical values are supported and which are threatened by your concept of this relationship?

2. Analyze the ethical implications of a community health initiative to decrease the rate of teenage pregnancy by means of health education in the public schools. Consider the following ethical principles in your analysis: autonomy, beneficence, nonmaleficence, and justice.

3. Imagine that you live in a community with a large number of homeless people. The climate is mild, and people live openly in the streets and parks. A proposal is to come before the city council to strengthen the vagrancy ordinance in

order to promote tourism. As a community health nurse working with the homeless, you have been asked to provide testimony. What will your position be and how will you defend it ethically? Prepare a 3-minute public testimony to address the issue.

4. What role might a community health nurse play in the community's deliberations regarding the presence of a volunteer security patrol group? How might you help the community prepare for likely sequelae?

● REFERENCES

American Nurses Association. (2001). *Code of ethics with interpretive statements.* Washington, DC: American Nurses Association.

American Public Health Association. (2002). *Public health code of ethics.* Washington, DC: American Public Health Association.

Blacksher, E. (2008). Carrots and sticks to promote healthy behaviors: A policy update [electronic version]. *Hastings Center Report*, 38(3), 13–16.

Daniels, N. (2006). Equity and population health: Toward a broader bioethics agenda [electronic version]. *Hastings Center Report*, 36(4), 22–35.

Fontana, B. (1987). *Tarahumara: Where night is the day of the moon.* Tucson, AZ: University of Arizona Press.

Fry, S. & Veatch, R. (2006). *Case studies in nursing ethics* (3rd ed.). Sudbury, MA: Jones & Bartlett.

Gadow, S. (1990). Existential advocacy: Philosophical foundations of nursing. In S. Spicker & S. Gadow (Eds.). *Nursing images and ideals* (pp. 79–101). New York: Springer.

Gorney, C. (2008). A people apart: Modernity looms for the Sierra Madre's Tarahumara. *National Geographic*, 214(5), 78–101.

Maslow, A. (1970). *Motivation and personality.* New York: Harper & Row.

O'Keefe, M. (2002). Ethics in nursing. In M. O'Keefe (Ed.). *Nursing practice and the law* (pp. 58–93). Philadelphia: F. A. Davis.

Petrini, C. & Gainotti, S. (2008). A personalist approach to public-health ethics [electronic version]. *Bulletin of the World Health Organization*, 86(8), 624–629.

Racher, F. (2007). The evolution of ethics for community practice [electronic version]. *Journal of Community Health Nursing*, 24(1), 65–76.

U.S. Department of Health and Human Services. (2000). *Healthy People 2010: Understanding and improving health* (2nd ed.). Washington, DC: U.S. Government Printing Office.

Internet Resources can be found on the Point at http://thepoint.lww.com/Anderson6e.

Empowerment and Healing

BRUCE LEONARD

LEARNING OBJECTIVES

Community empowerment and healing are concepts that provide the basis for community health nurses to build partnerships with communities. This chapter provides an overview of how community health nurses may apply the theoretical components of empowerment and healing in practice.

After studying this chapter, you should be able to:

1. Understand a framework for empowering communities through building healing relationships among community members.

2. Develop an understanding of healing as an important concept in the development of humanistic relationships and resolving barriers to promote community partnerships.

3. Apply a grassroots approach through participatory research as a pathway to community empowerment and healing for improved community health status.

Introduction

*P*artnerships between community members and health care professionals are critical for collaborative decisions that promote awareness and understanding of a community's health needs. Community health nursing has the potential to create relationships beyond the individual and develop program interventions that affect the community as a whole. Nurses have long been at the forefront of integrating health resources by forming partnerships with clients, families, and communities. Through the application and use of relationship-building concepts such as empowerment, we can influence and reshape the environment to address health disparities among those who are most vulnerable in our society. The process by which nurses develop healing or caring relationships in the community reflects interactions among the four major constructs of the nursing paradigm: health, environment, client, and nurse. Community health nurses have power to develop healing relationships or capacity-building activities that promote health and to empower others to engage community members in collaborative efforts, partnerships, and coalitions. Engaging community members in collaborative efforts that affect their well-being is integral to community health nurses' professional practice.

Community health nursing focuses on health, caring, and relationship building among community members. Community involvement is one of the critical elements of successful problem solving with communities. A basic tenet of community empowerment is that the community defines its own agenda. Community participation is a crucial element in engaging community members to develop agendas that serve as a cohesive force to mobilize community toward a process of change. For social change to be long term and relevant to the needs of a community, it must come from the community members themselves (Brown, 1991; Laverack, 2006). Community empowerment works like a catalyst in creating a sense of readiness to mobilize forces among community members or groups to engage in active community interventions to transform power relationships.

PERSPECTIVES ON COMMUNITY HEALTH PARTNERSHIPS

Community partnership programs have not always been equitably distributed or considered essential to community members. Many community health programs of the 1960s emphasized processes of community participation led by academic experts who were in control of health programs and who set the agenda for the types of programs offered within communities. These programs often failed because they lacked true community commitment and involvement. A major lesson learned from failures has been that effective partnerships require active community participation, community ownership and control of programs, and continual relationship building.

More recently, community health professionals have placed a new emphasis on having communities solve their own problems, with guidance from experts, by forming partnership alliances. The idea of community participation as a model for community health initiatives in the 1960s and 1970s has been supplanted by programs that focus on ideas of partnership, collaboration, community empowerment, and community capacity (Fraser, Dougill, Mabee, Reed, & McAlpine, 2006). Rather than allow self-interests of experts to guide a community, partnerships work by integrating the community's ideas, people, and resources in both the development and implementation processes. A community's level of commitment and involvement may be increased by capacity building in allowing them to gain knowledge, learn skills, and gain confidence to improve their health through partnerships (Raeburn, Akerman, Chuengsatiansup, Mejia, & Oladepo, 2007). The act of creating partnerships is a complex process of bringing together academics, community leaders, and health care providers to accomplish change. Effective partnerships require a sharing of power and decision making along with feedback mechanisms to assure understanding among all parties for successful implementation of community health promotion programs (Hanks, 2006). We will examine how nurses might use these concepts to expand their social consciousness.

Partnerships not only are important in implementing community-based programs, but also must be culturally sensitive to ensure success. When implementing a program, we need to assist communities in ways that match their perception of health problems. Partnership programs often fail if there is conflict between the health care provider's and the community's belief systems. We define our own health and illness beliefs based on our cultural and ethnic backgrounds, and on our own perceptions of how to be healthy or recognize illness (see Chapter 7).

Historically, nurses have had a rich practice in the community transforming both individual and public health for the poor and disenfranchised through political advocacy. Lillian Wald (1915), who coined the term *public health nurse* in 1893, provides probably our prime example of working with communities to improve health. Our historical focus of nursing in the community has been replaced by "site managed care systems," such as hospitals and primary care clinics that require the client to come to a facility rather than the nurse providing care within the community. Although many nurses today are employed by organizations that provide home health care, community health nursing is more than just providing health care to an individual; it focuses on the aggregate population in providing *primary health care* as opposed to primary care. The concept of *primary health care* embraces the ideals of the World Health Organization's Alma Ata declaration (World Health Organization Primary Health for All, 1978) of providing essential health care based on the needs of the community, emphasizing health and well-being as a fundamental right for all.

Modern health care emphasizes individualized medical care as opposed to providing aggregate community-based health care. Our present "system" of health care has not served our profession well and has resulted in fragmented programs and limited return on improving the overall health in communities. In many respects, modern-day nurses who work for large hospital-based institutions whose focus of care has been on the individual have lost their unique voice, innovation, and drive to be proactive in community affairs. Nurses frequently remain blind or silent to what is going on around them in the community; however, what goes on in the community is really the pulse that drives our health care needs. Our challenge as community health nurses is to transform our health care system into one that reflects the values and needs of our communities based on the concepts of *primary health care.*

Community nurses may transform our fragmented system of individualized health care by reformulating a vision for the future. We must look beyond our past and explore new avenues aimed at improvement of health for all. Rather than focusing on disease-specific problems, we should explore developing new programs with a community focus on providing primary health care. People in communities deserve comprehensive nursing care aimed at improvement of health and quality of life. Health in this country cannot be improved just by providing health services, but needs to be based on principles of equity, participation, and involvement of communities in making decisions about health care. Successful participation implies negotiation without manipulation and equity in relationships between community members and health care workers who embrace common goals in providing health care with accessible programs and service for all.

EMPOWERMENT THROUGH COMMUNITY PARTICIPATION

Community participation is a social process involving people from specific geographic localities who share common values in identifying their needs (Rifkin, 1986). Participation in formulating the framework for primary health care in a community may lead not only to better services but also to services based on existing socioeconomic conditions. Rifkin (1986) describes three approaches to community participation in health programs commonly used by different countries (Fig. 6.1). One is the medical approach, which is focused on curing diseases and is controlled by the medical profession. The second is a health services approach, which mobilizes people to take an active role in the delivery of services based on modifying unhealthy behaviors. The third is a community development approach in which people are involved in the decision-making process to improve health. The first two approaches to health care are called "top-down" approaches, in which experts

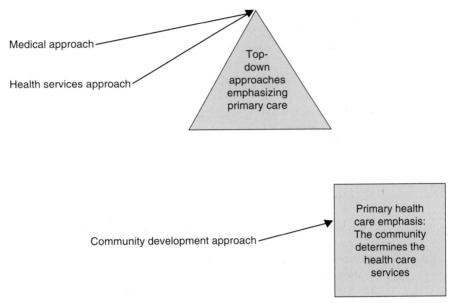

Figure 6.1 Three approaches to community participation in health care (Rifkin, 1986).

prescribe their values of health care for the public. The third approach is at grass-roots level in which members within the community determine what health care services should be provided. It is more consistent with the principles of primary health care.

Essential components for community participation include the following: (1) a framework to define the community; (2) shared awareness by members of the community; and (3) mechanisms to mobilize the community to recognize its needs and develop a culture of participation (Meleis, 1992). Through empowerment, community health nurses can enable people to make decisions and to act on issues they believe are essential to their health or well-being.

Empowerment through participation has three essential components to which nurses must be sensitive in order for community transformations to occur (Box 6.1). First, participation is an active process, not a process in which one group or organization imposes its values on the community, but a process of mutuality, in which all have voice. Second, participation involves choice, implying people have the right and the power to make decisions that affect their lives. Third, the decisions made through participation must have the potential to be effective, and there must be social systems to allow decisions to be implemented. Community participation, according to Rifkin, Muller, and Bichmann (1988), "is a social process whereby specific groups with shared needs living in a defined geographical area actively

BOX 6.1

ESSENTIAL ELEMENTS OF COMMUNITY EMPOWERMENT

- Active process (one that is nonjudgmental and characterized by mutuality)
- Choice (right to make decisions)
- Effective participation (decisions are implemented)

pursue identification of their needs, make decisions and establish mechanisms to meet these needs" (p. 933).

The role of the nurse in community empowerment is to build effective partnerships through community participation. Only our imagination, vision, and moral or ethical values limit the climate of empowerment we create. The holistic model of nursing provides one vision based on principles of healing that integrate all human potentials in formulating client-based partnerships. Nursing is about building moral, healing relationships that address the human response to illness and health-seeking behaviors of those who live within the communities around us (Watson, 1999, 2006).

HEALING IN THE COMMUNITY

In the history of humankind, both Western and Eastern philosophies have illustrated healing not only in the context of the physical body, but also through more abstract descriptions related to cognitive processes of the mind; magical, mythical, or spiritual components; along with an innate universal energy force occurring within or around the nature of all things (Newman, 1986; Quinn, 1992; Quinn, Smith, Ritenbaugh, Swanson, & Watson, 2003; Rogers, 1970; Watson, 1995, 2006). Healing within the context of community empowerment is a bonding or bridging process that enables community members to work together effectively to achieve common goals such as improved quality of life and community health. The process is similar to that described by Putnam (1995) in the development of "social capital." Putnam describes two types of social capital: bonding capital and bridging capital. Bonding capital is the relationship-building process among people or groups who already know each other. Bridging capital brings together people who don't know each other. Putnam's theory of social capital is that the more people connect with each other, the more they will trust each other, and the better off they will be collectively. Healing within the framework of empowerment involves developing a series of norms that enable people to connect and develop trust with each other.

The concept of healing in nursing relates closely to the theoretical underpinnings of holism (Quinn, 1989, 1992, 1997; Quinn et al., 2003; Scandrett-Hibdon & Freel, 1989; Watson, 1995; Wendler, 1996). Holism is based on a theory introduced by Smuts (1926) that reflects nature's tendency to synthesize units into wholes. The work of nurse theorists such as Rogers (1970) and Newman (1986) reflects many of the philosophical underpinnings of holism, in which humans are depicted as constantly interacting with their environment in multiple rhythmic patterns. Healing within the context of community empowerment is seen as a dynamic process involving the interplay of human energies that transforms people toward wholeness in understanding their connectedness among themselves, others, and the environment.

The process of healing is both physical and mental. It allows persons or communities to resolve emotional wounds and enjoy their full potential as human beings. Healing is more than just the physical, biologic healing of a wound. Although the physical wound may heal completely without leaving a scar, the mental wound from the experience may not. Healing, when applied to nursing in the community, is a process of moving the community toward wholeness or a state of health or well-being (Chinn, 1989; Quinn, 1992; Watson, 1999). Nurses facilitate healing through their interactions with clients based on moral agency of nonjudgmental caring (Hemsley, Glass, & Watson, 2006; Watson, 1999). For healing to occur, then, there must be unconditional acceptance between the nurse and the client (community, family, or individual) (Erickson, Tomlin, & Swain, 1983; Parse, 1981; Quinn, 1992; Watson, 1990). Hall (2005) asserts, "We become nurse healers when we follow a personal and spiritual path that helps us strive to be the very best we can" (p. 4).

Community problems, such as inequities in health care or disenfranchisement from society of persons who are at risk due to poor physical, psychological or social health, may create chaotic energy patterns between communities, families, and individuals. Resolving community problems through community-based partnerships may facilitate healing as community members are empowered to search for ways to resolve issues to attain harmony within the community and the environment.

DEVELOPING RIGHT-RELATIONSHIPS

Nurses relate to clients, communities, and families on many psychosocial levels. In the development of a nurse–client relationship, nurses may facilitate healing through interactions with clients and communities. For healing to occur, there must be a balance of unconditional acceptance between the nurse and the client as a whole person. The transformation of becoming whole is what Quinn (1997) identifies as the right-relationship among one or more levels of the human system. Right-relationship is defined "as any pattern of organization within the system that supports, encourages, allows, or generates actualization and self-transcendence—at any and all levels" (Quinn, 1997, pp. 2, 3). Nurses play a critical role in assisting communities, families, and individuals in the process of becoming whole as they facilitate right-relationships. The development of the right-relationship is not an ethical or moral judgment, but a pattern of organization that generates self-transcendence or self-actualization.

The ability to heal may be expanded to communities as a whole. If you imagine communities made of systems connected to form a natural healing web, nurses could create synergistic healing partnerships among individuals, families, and communities similar to energy flowing through electrical wires. Environmental energy fields are integral parts of human life patterns. In a healing web, nurses could integrate different worldviews to create a holistic perspective, one that values diversity of culture and humanness in forming partnerships with multiple community systems. A nurse working in a healing environment would want to look at what is creating disharmony within a community and pattern the environment to promote health and community well-being. Through communication and by formulating partnerships among community systems, nurses may pattern the environment to develop healing partnerships or right-relationships. Relationships created within a natural healing web would allow for the development of extraordinary states of consciousness for true community healing to take place.

Community health nurses have the potential to transform community systems into healing–caring environments. Figure 6.2 displays a model of the concepts of healing and the interactions between the nurse and community. Communities are composed of many core groups and subsystems in the community-as-partner model. Community health nurses assist community members in the healing process by transforming relationships. If relationships are limited or confined to the elements where "academic experts" maintain control of the health care resources—through either medical or health care services approaches as identified earlier by Rifkin (1986) that emphasize primary care—communities may not be able to maximize their human potentials to become proactive for healing processes and outcomes to occur. Although the "primary care model" of health care strives for predictable outcomes

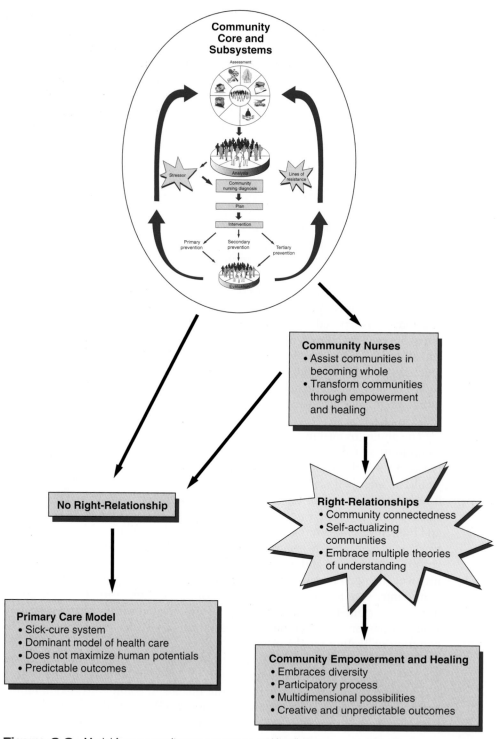

Figure 6.2 Model for community empowerment and healing.

in curing disease, people may not be healed in the process. If nurses do not develop right-relationships with communities, community members may not be able to maximize their potential to become empowered. Community health nurses who practice in a healing framework strive to develop a sense of connectedness or right-relationships with community members. Nurses who practice in a healing environment embrace multiple theories of knowing or understanding. Relationships built on the healing model embrace diversity: outcomes may be creative or unpredictable but are right for the community as a whole. These outcomes are congruent with primary health care.

In the traditional "primary care" approach to health care, community health care workers viewed community members as sources for data gathering or recipients of care. The conventional approach to health care has been paternalistic, resulting in fragmented or unwanted programs with community members as passive recipients. Community health partnerships, by contrast, emphasize active participation by community members and health care workers not only from a variety of disciplines but also from every relevant segment of society. The goal for community health care workers, then, should be to empower community members to visualize their needs and actively participate in planning and implementing needed change—the tenets of primary health care.

TRANSFORMING COMMUNITIES THROUGH EMPOWERMENT

How can nurses assist communities to expand their healing resources? Empowerment means different things to different people and depends on the context. Community participation exists on many levels that may range from passive compliance by acceptance of the status quo to true shared decision-making (Schwab & Syme, 1997). Empowerment is an avenue for communities to gain control of resources and transform inequities of power through social change. Only through the ability to organize and mobilize community forces can individuals, groups, and communities achieve social and political change necessary to rectify their powerlessness (Laverack & Wallerstein, 2001). Empowerment enables people to take control of their lives and community resources. Nurses work to empower communities not for domination or control of people, but rather to facilitate the development of others to promote change.

Dialogue is a critical element for community transformations to occur. All voices in a community are important. Paulo Freire (1997), a Brazilian educator, contributed philosophic and theoretical writings on empowering people through education to reverse the dehumanization and objectification of oppressed people. His concerns deal primarily with class oppression, but his philosophies have been applied to empowerment of professions such as nursing, feminist theory, and vulnerable populations among communities at risk for poor health.

Community partnerships develop through a process of empowerment. Four characteristics of an empowered community (conceptualized from Paulo Freire's [1997] *Pedagogy of the Oppressed*) follow:

- Faith in people
- Trust established through dialogue
- Hope in positive transformations benefiting the community as a whole
- Discussions grounded in critical thinking without fear of repercussions by those who are in power

Freire (1997) hypothesizes that dialogue or communication between people is the key to empowerment. Each of the empowerment characteristics is discussed below.

Faith in people implies that all people have the *potential* to provide a voice in community affairs. Faith in humanity encourages a commitment between community members to create and transform the bonds of human communities and interconnect those who live on the fringes or are the most vulnerable to the whole of society. Vulnerability includes individuals or communities who are camouflaged in our society, such as the homeless, chronically disabled, immigrants, or low-income single parents. Vulnerable populations are at great risk for harm in society and are often those with the least social capital. Risk encountered by the vulnerable are generally not voluntary or under their control. The more risk encountered, the more vulnerable the person or population becomes. Vulnerability leads to symptoms of victimization, alienation, helplessness, or powerlessness, all opposite approaches to empowerment.

Freire (1997) believes that dialogue is a primary component in transforming those who are most vulnerable to be empowered, but we cannot have dialogue without *trust*. Trust in people is founded on the principles of truth and integrity in our words. Many well-intentioned community projects have failed through false leadership of people saying one thing and doing another or designing projects for their own personal reality, ignoring those the project is intended to serve. Trust occurs when people cooperate to transform ideas into a reality and are committed to making a difference or create change.

Hope is another vital component of empowerment (Freire, 1997). Hope engenders a sense of inner strength that propels people to act, mobilize forces, and envision a better tomorrow. Hope is all encompassing in providing people protection against despair and giving them strength and determination to live when misfortunes in life occur. Empowerment through hope inspires an ability to move beyond the present difficulties and see a future with possibilities. Empowerment through hope is not an entity of imagination acquired while sitting still, but rather a transformational process fought for with conviction. Empowerment is not an instant transformation, but rather a slow process of weaving thin threads of society together through dialogue, like a spider weaves a web.

Trust, faith, and hope are significant concepts that relate closely to developing healing relationships, but it is through the process of critical thinking and evaluation that people are ultimately empowered. For empowerment and communication to be successful, people must engage in critical thinking, continually evaluating and re-evaluating the premises behind their thoughts (Freire, 1997). People need to be free to exchange ideas, weighing the positive and negative impacts of change on themselves or their communities. As new realities emerge, people must evaluate their world critically and not remain naive or blind to those who are most vulnerable in communities. Naive thinking justifies maintaining the status quo or the continual oppression of those who are at the greatest risk for harm. For social inequalities to change, we must develop through education new abilities to influence others and transform our communities.

Empowerment is gained through critical dialogue and reflection of critical thought, not necessarily from what is known. It is a process of going from the known to the unknown and reflecting on the possible, with hope for a better tomorrow. Without critical dialogue, true learning ceases to exist and only knowledge—not wisdom—is passed between the empowered and the oppressed. Critical thinking encourages the transformation of knowledge into wisdom for those who are most vulnerable. The wisdom gained through critical thought, faith, trust, and hope in humanity may transform oppressive social structures into powerful communities with a voice (Fig. 6.3).

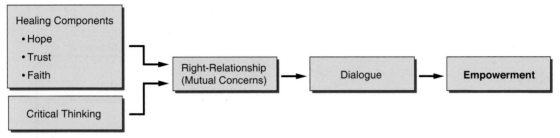

Figure 6.3   Key components for social transformation.

EMPOWERING COMMUNITIES THROUGH HEALING

Empowerment and healing involve synergistic processes and outcomes. Community health nurses are responsible for caring for and supporting communities, families, and individuals as they respond to ill health, violence, or dissonance within society. Nurses are skilled in compassionate caring and the application of scientific knowledge and technology. We are also skillful at humanistic universal–psychosocial–spiritual interactions that support our clients and empower them in the change process. The nurse's role as a healer does not directly create change in others but creates the processes or conditions for change to occur. For compassion and healing care to be sustained, the communities we work with must be willing and able to care for themselves. Communities must be willing to awaken their healing capacity from within. The capacity for healing a community faced with a horrific act of violence and senseless loss of life by extremists on the fringes of society, for instance, may stimulate but not necessarily *cause* healing. The psychological scars communities face as the result of sudden acts of violence may persist unless the causes of the social imbalances are resolved. Healing is an intrinsic capacity of the community, and, as health care professionals, nurses have the potential to facilitate the healing process to balance the inequities faced by those with the greatest risk for social harm.

Nurses need to awaken the healing capacity within themselves to facilitate the process of healing others. "Awakening the healer within, however," as Wells-Federman (1996) states, "requires us to face both the limitations and the miracles of our humanness and our work with balanced perspective" (pp. 14, 15). We need to care for ourselves as human beings, balancing our commitment to practice with the need to heal others. Effective healing can transpire only through our own self-awareness to take responsibility for making change in our lives that will contribute to the well-being of others. Nurses, as universal–psychosocial–spiritual beings, have the unique capacity to understand healing interventions as well as the ability to look beyond the symptomatic causes of disharmony in our communities, placing nursing in a unique position to empower communities to change through healing interactions.

A Healing Consciousness

The emergence of a healing consciousness in which communities envision a mind–body–spirit connection with humanity can only occur through dialogue. Dialogue provides the critical mass for community transformations to take place. Dialogue enables communities to see their inequities and transform their environment through healing interventions.

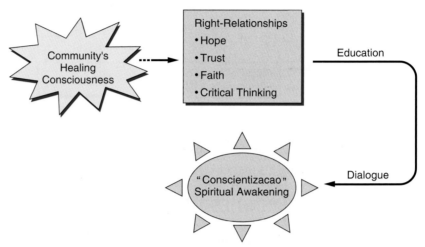

Figure 6.4   Promoting a healing consciousness in communities.

"The spirit of dialogue involves an openness to new ideas" (Koerner & Bunkers, 1994, p. 51). This spirit of openness implies people are willing to listen to others and negotiate with an understanding of opposing viewpoints. Empowerment is a process of hope, trust, faith, and critical thinking based on mutual concerns and love for other human beings. Empowerment is a dualistic interactive process involving investment in understanding yourself and others and a willingness to impact change for the betterment of humanity.

The process of promoting a healing consciousness in communities parallels Freire's (1997) process of human liberation of oppression through education. Education, according to Freire, should provide a human awakening of consciousness or what he calls "*conscientizacao*." The awakening of the spirit develops through processes of reflection and critical thinking between the teacher and the students (Fig. 6.4). The open exchange of ideas through dialogue does more than just pass old knowledge in justifying the inequities in communities; it provides new insight to the understanding of political, social, and economic forces of oppression.

In the modern Western paradigm of the world, "a person is merely in the world, not with the world or with others; the individual is spectator, not re-creator" (Freire, 1997, p. 56). In the postmodern paradigm of a healing consciousness as a model for nursing, only our imaginations and our own fears limit reality. Empowerment and healing are touchstones essential to the nursing process. Nursing is a profession based on mutual understanding of clients, families, and communities. Healing provides the force of liberation to empower communities to reconcile forces of oppression and transform the human consciousness to awaken our capacities for humility, love, and reciprocal cooperation. For healing and empowerment to emerge as a new consciousness, community health nurses must engage in active, critical dialogue that promotes understanding, mutual cooperation, and critical reflection of community aspirations. Nurses may institute global change through the application of the concepts of healing and empowerment and help our communities achieve their hopes and dreams.

Transformation of Global Community

The transformation process of empowering a community through the integration of healing relationships by community health nurses has the potential to change the global environment of health care and promote healthy environments for all. The community development approach to health care involves empowerment participation with the application of healing practices by all members of society regardless of culture, social status, gender, or ethnicity. As the world shrinks through global electronic communication, we are exposed daily, through the news media, to inequities in our global environment. We are able to witness first hand the adversities of famine, drug abuse, unemployment, genocide, murder, and lack of health care worldwide. Community health nurses must not remain blind to these inequities, but advocate transforming our societies into healing communities based on principles of trust, hope, love, and faith in humanity.

Our unique vantage point as nurses is our ability to communicate, dialogue, and form partnerships with clients, families, and communities. Nurses are in a prime position to chart a new course for the delivery of health care and resolve many of the social injustices for the world's disenfranchised using the principles of empowerment and healing.

EMPOWERING A COMMUNITY THROUGH PARTICIPATORY ACTION RESEARCH

One method community health nurses may employ in empowering a community to focus on health problems is participatory research. This is performed through collaboration between health professionals and community members. Participatory research is problem-focused or context-specific research centered on a particular problem involving all participants. Participatory research is similar to action research, in which each person or group engaged in the process is committed to improvement through continuous interaction among dialogue, research, action, reflection, and evaluation (Hart, 1996). Individuals are active participants in change and are not passive objects. Through participatory research, community members can gain skills to think critically and analyze the health concerns of their community.

Participatory research is a form of emancipatory inquiry that addresses inequities and injustices in health and society (Aston & Meagher-Stewart, 2009; Fraser et al., 2006). It incorporates conversations that produce both collaboration and self-awareness between nurses and their community. The methods of participatory research incorporate scientific research, education, and political action developed primarily out of the works of Freire (1997). The emancipatory process of participatory research also employs both critical and feminist theories. Critical theory emphasizes a critical analytic approach to discussing social problems by active reflection and synthesis through continuous dialogue. Behaviors may be changed through questioning the learner and providing feedback. In understanding the social and political patterns of oppression, community members may be able to emancipate themselves from oppressive power structures (Corbett, Francis, & Chapman, 2007). Feminist theory shares many of the humanistic values of nursing based on concepts of caring, intuitiveness, and valuing others' worldviews and experiences (Meleis, 1997). A feminist perspective provides a powerful language to enhance our understanding or to provide insights for social change.

Wallerstein (1999) identifies six core principles of participatory and action research. These include (1) the participants in the research project determine the research agenda; (2) the research project should benefit the community as a whole, and allows community members to make informed decisions and act collectively; (3) the relationship between health care experts and community members should be a collaborative effort based on the principles of shared dialogue (Freire, 1997); (4) community members should have access to all information and knowledge from which they might normally be excluded; (5) the process should be democratic and empower the participation of a wide range of community members; and (6) community members and the researchers should strive to achieve mutual goals.

The goal of participatory research is social change, not just the advancement of new scientific knowledge. Emancipatory inquiry is designed to have a direct effect on the lives of all participants in the research process, not just the life of the researcher. Individuals involved in participatory nursing research are able to explore how inequities in society are linked to their own health and, therefore, are enabled to act on this knowledge through empowerment (Henderson, 1995).

The Nurse's Role in Participatory Research Programs

In instituting participatory research programs, nurses help communities identify, understand, find solutions, and determine common goals in resolving community problems. The problems examined through emancipatory inquiry are those that community members believe are important and not necessarily those identified by health professionals in the community. Nurses are challenged to awaken the spirit of social change among those who are most vulnerable in our communities. Emancipatory inquiry provides a framework to expand the political consciousness of the disenfranchised in a community. As Henderson (1995) reminds us, "The goal of emancipatory inquiry is neither prediction nor understanding, but emancipation, both within the research process and within society" (p. 64).

Community health nurses can be the eyes and ears of a community. We have considerable credibility in the community as health professionals. Our clinical and educational experiences guide us in assessing the pulse of our surroundings. We have numerous tools for implementing change in the community environment based on theory and experience. Nurses have strong interpersonal communication skills, understand the importance of client–nurse relationships, are willing to learn from others, and know how to maximize the health resources of a community. Through our professional encounters with clients, we learn to solve problems almost intuitively and attempt to fix them before harm occurs. Our solutions are not always the right answer, however, if the end result is not congruent with the views or beliefs of those affected. A better solution is to empower the community to resolve its problems while at the same time expanding their healing resources. Participatory research is an excellent method for nurses to implement change, even on a small scale.

Developing a Participatory Research Program

An example of participatory research by the community health nurse might be your recognition of the importance of informing clients of influenza vaccines for seniors during the flu season while working at a senior center checking blood pressures in a low-income, African-American neighborhood. In talking with clients, you may find that very few in this community have had flu shots, but many have friends who died last year or were seriously ill from influenza. The seniors seem very concerned by news broadcasts predicting a major flu epidemic. You assess that this may be an important health issue to bring up at the monthly senior center board of directors meeting next week.

On the way back to the local public health department, you decide to stop by the epidemiology department to examine the community statistics related to influenza over the past few years. In analyzing the data, it is evident that low-income seniors in the county had a death rate 50% higher than those with higher income. The death rate for seniors living near the senior center where you were taking blood pressures was significantly higher than the rest of the city. The data also indicate that there is an overall higher death rate for senior African Americans within the county. You feel compelled to act because this is a significant health problem where nursing might make a difference.

Over the next week, you do a literature search and put together a proposal to present to the senior center's executive board members to develop a participatory research influenza immunization program with the support of the public health department. You reflect on how to make your proposal successful, knowing there are several barriers. A potential barrier identified is the need to make the program culturally sensitive to the African-American community. Many seniors around this senior center have limited access to health care, lack transportation, and have minimal understanding of the importance of influenza vaccinations. Your literature search, as well as the experience of your practice, reveals some key issues related to the African-American communities. Religion is central in their lives; cultural beliefs and health practices are often underutilized, regardless of their impact on well-being; and family support networks and informal health care systems play important roles in maintaining health during periods of stress or crises (Russell & Jewell, 1992). The community health diagnosis for this proposal might be: decreased influenza immunization rate of senior African Americans living in this community related to (1) cultural barriers, (2) low socioeconomic status, (3) attitudes, and (4) lack of resources for health promotion and disease prevention, as manifested by statistical evidence of high mortality rates and low immunization rates.

Your proposal includes a conceptual framework for increasing the effectiveness of an immunization program for the senior center based on the components of the community-as-partner model. The plan incorporates African-American cultural values relating to health and illness practices. The strategies include three main components: increasing the active participation of community members from the senior center in the program design, implementation, and evaluation process; tapping into the established formal and informal community networks; and structuring the plan to be culturally sensitive with the assistance of the executive board of the senior center and the religious leaders in the community.

A fundamental component of your proposal is empowering senior African Americans to receive their flu immunizations through health promotion. Health promotion entails motivating the community, families, and individuals toward obtaining their optimum state of well-being, health, or happiness. The strategies should encourage the best quality of life with goals toward continuous improvement in the overall health of the community. The health status of a community is directly related to the individual health-related behaviors and environmental conditions and is indirectly affected by environmental factors, which influence health behaviors (Brown, 1991). Communities can directly influence their health status by targeting individual health-related behaviors and can change health-damaging environments to health-promoting environments. Brown states, "The ultimate objective of community action for health promotion must be to empower people to improve their individual and collective health" (p. 455).

Three essential elements of health promotion identified by Brown (1991) involve (1) encouraging individuals to change and sustain personal behaviors that prevent disease and promote healthy lifestyles; (2) encouraging health-promoting behaviors that discourage health-damaging behaviors of individuals; and (3) creating an environment that promotes health by eliminating health hazards from the physical environment. According to Brown, most health promotion programs focus on encouraging individuals to change their health behaviors, but seldom look at empowering people to change the lifestyle or environment that shapes their behavior and influences their lifestyle. The goal is to increase the number of seniors immunized against the flu, and the objectives are to assist seniors to overcome their fears of immunizations, increase seniors' knowledge about the flu, increase their political power, and improve their physical health. The community-as-partner model, the concepts outlined for developing a participatory action research plan, and Brown's theory of health promotion are several tools community health nurses can use to promote change.

With the approval of the executive board of the senior center, the nursing interventions to meet the objectives of the immunization project focus on participatory research, emphasizing education and focus group community interaction. The focus group addresses strategies to make the program successful, including clarification of information on flu immunizations, stressing healthy outcomes, keeping the message culturally sensitive, and decreasing fears of the vaccine.

The missing component in our discussion on developing a participatory research program for our immunization project is the ethic of connectedness or developing the right-relationship with the senior African-American community members. We have mentioned the critical component of cultural sensitivity, but we need to focus our energies on building healing relationships in the process of participatory research. The relationships nurses develop in the processes of human interactions are crucial to the success of all community programs. We cannot ignore the political, social, environmental, cultural, and economic relationships among all community members. How we interact with communities on all social levels has an impact on our ability to provide a voice to those who are most vulnerable in our society. Community health nurses are morally responsible for providing a voice that maintains a dialogue of healing or caring and builds a dynamic of empowered connectedness within the community-as-partner model.

Summary

Community nurses can provide the critical conscience of health in a community. As a group, nurses can provide the bonding capital and bridging capital for community members to work together effectively to achieve common goals for improved community health and quality of life. Empowerment and healing are processes that require active community participation by community members and formal organizations to work together to achieve mutually agreed on outcomes based on trust. Empowerment is not just a program nurses create, but a process enabled by community health nurses to transform thinking through dialogue in reconstructing a healing environment for all. Only through continued activism can nurses expose the social injustices that continue to contribute to powerless communities. Through community empowerment and healing, nurses can provide a moral voice to inspire change to regain our historical roots as vanguards of the community.

Critical Thinking Questions

1. How might empowerment be applied in community nursing practice?

2. What are the essential processes for empowerment and healing to occur within a community?

3. As a nurse, how might you describe empowerment as a transformational process?

● REFERENCES

Aston, M., & Meagher-Stewart, D. (2009). Public health nurses' primary health care practice: Strategies for fostering citizen participation. *Journal of Community Health Nursing*, 26, 24–34.

Brown, R. E. (1991). Community action for health promotion: A strategy to empower individuals and communities. *International Journal of Health Services*, 21(3), 441–456.

Chinn, P. L. (1989). Nursing patterns of knowing and feminist thought. *Nursing and Health Care*, 10(2), 71–75.

Corbett, A. M., Francis, K., & Chapman, Y. (2007). Feminist-informed participatory action research: A methodology of choice for examining critical nursing issues. *International Journal of Nursing Practice*, 13, 81–88.

Erickson, H. C., Tomlin, E. M., & Swain, M. A. (1983). *Modeling and role-modeling a theory and paradigm for nursing*. Englewood Cliffs, NJ: Prentice-Hall.

Fraser, E. D. G., Dougill, A. J., Mabee, W. E., Reed, M., & McAlpine, P. (2006). Bottom up and top down: Analysis of participatory process for sustainability indicator identification as a pathway to community empowerment and sustainable environmental management. *Journal of Environmental Management*, 78, 114–127.

Freire, P. (1997). *Pedagogy of the oppressed* (New Revised 20th-Anniversary Edition ed.). New York, NY: Continuum.

Hall, B. A. (2005). *The art of becoming a nurse healer*. Orlando, FL: Bandido Books.

Hanks, C. A. (2006). Community empowerment: A partnership approach to public health program implementation. *Policy, Politics, and Nursing Practice*, 7(4), 297–306.

Hart, E. A., C. (1996). Action research as a professionalizing strategy: Issues and dilemmas. *Journal of Advanced Nursing*, 23(3), 454–461.

Hemsley, M. S., Glass, N., & Watson, J. (2006). Using Watson's conceptual model to investigate the extraordinary and transformative experiences of nurse healers. *Holistic Nursing Practice*, 20(2), 85–94.

Henderson, D. J. (1995). Consciousness raising in participatory research: Method and methodology for emancipatory nursing inquiry. *Advances in Nursing Science*, 17(3), 58–69.

Koerner, J. G., & Bunkers, S. S. (1994). The healing web an expansion of consciousness. *Journal of Holistic Nursing*, 12(1), 51–63.

Laverack, G. (2006). Improving health outcomes through community empowerment: A review of the literature. *Journal of Health Population and Nutrition*, 24(1), 113–120.

Laverack, G., & Wallerstein, N. (2001). Measuring community empowerment: A fresh look at organizational domains. *Health Promotion International*, 16(2), 179–185.

Meleis, A. I. (1992). Community participation and involvement, theoretical and emperical issues. *Health Services Management*, 5(1), 5–6.

Meleis, A. I. (1997). *Theoretical nursing development and progress*. Philadelphia: Lippincott.

Newman, M. A. (1986). *Health as expanding consciousness*. St. Louis, MO: Mosby.

Parse, R. R. (1981). *Man-living-health: A theory of nursing*. New York, NY: John Wiley & Sons.

Putnam, R. D. (1995). Bowling alone: America's declining social capital. *Journal of Democracy*, 6, 65–78.

Quinn, J. F. (1989). On healing, wholeness, and the haelan effect. *Nursing and Health Care*, 10(10), 553–556.

Quinn, J. F. (1992). Holding sacred space: The nurse as healing environment. *Holistic Nursing Practice*, 6(4), 26–36.

Quinn, J. F. (1997). Healing: A model for an integrative health care system. *Advanced Practice Nursing Quarterly*, 3(1), 1–6.

Quinn, J. F., Smith, M., Ritenbaugh, C., Swanson, K., & Watson, J. (2003). Research guidelines for assessing the impact of the healing relationship in clinical nursing. *Alternative Therapies in Health and Medicine*, 9(3), 65–79.

Raeburn, J., Akerman, M., Chuengsatiansup, K., Mejia, F., & Oladepo, O. (2007). Community capacity building and health promotion in a globalized world. *Health Promotion International*, 21(S1), 84–90.

Rifkin, S. B. (1986). Lessons from community participation programs. *Health Policy and Planning,* 1, 240–209.

Rifkin, S. B., Muller, F., & Bichmann, W. (1988). Primary health care: On measuring participation. *Social Science and Medicine an International Journal,* 26(9), 931–940.

Rogers, M. E. (1970). *An introduction to the theoretical basis of nursing.* Philadelphia, PA: F.A. Davis.

Russell, K. J., & Jewell, N. (1992). Cultural impact of health-care access: Changes for improving the health of African Americans. *Journal of Community Health Nursing,* 9(3), 161–169.

Scandrett-Hibdon, S., & Freel, M. I. (1989). The endogenous healing process: Concept analysis. *Journal of Holistic Nursing,* 7(1), 66–70.

Schwab, M., & Syme, L. (1997). On paradigms, community participation, and the future of public health. American *Journal of Public Health,* 87, 2049–2052.

Smuts, J. C. (1926). *Holism and evolution.* New York, NY: Macmillan.

Wald, L. (1915). *The house on Henry Street.* New York, NY: Henry Holt.

Wallerstein, N. (1999). Power between evaluator and community: Research relationships within New Mexico's healthier communities. *Social Science & Medicine,* 49(1), 39–53.

Watson, J. (1990). Caring knowledge and informed moral person. *Advances in Nursing Science,* 13(1), 15–24.

Watson, J. (1995). Nursing's caring-healing paradigm as exemplar for alternative medicine? *Alternative Therapies,* 1(3), 64–69.

Watson, J. (1999). *Postmodern nursing and beyond.* New York, NY: Churchill Livingstone.

Watson, J. (2006). Caring theory as an ethical guide to administrative clinical practices. *Nursing Administration Quarterly,* 30(1), 48–55.

Wells-Federman, C. L. (1996). Awakening the nurse healer within. *Holistic Nursing Practice,* 10(2), 13–29.

Wendler, M. C. (1996). Understanding healing: A conceptual analysis. *Journal of Advanced Nursing,* 24, 836–842.

World Health Organization Primary Health for All. (1978). *World health organization primary health care. Report of the international conference of primary health care.* (No. 1). Alma Alta, USSR: World Health Organization.

Internet Resources can be found on the**Point** at http://thepoint.lww.com/Anderson6e.

Cultural Competence: Common Ground for Partnerships in Health Care

JUDITH C. DREW

LEARNING OBJECTIVES

This chapter discusses the concept of cultural competence as a primary factor in improving access to quality health care for all Americans, regardless of their ethnic and cultural backgrounds. Brief theoretical perspectives on diversity, ethnicity, culture, and cultural health care systems are presented to provide the tools needed to assess and improve your own cultural competence as well as participate in building common ground for health care partnerships between individuals, health services agencies, and communities.

After studying this chapter, you should be able to:

1. Describe the characteristics of cultural competence as manifested by individuals, health services agencies, and communities.
2. Discuss the role cultural competence plays in meeting the Healthy People 2010 goals and objectives.
3. Acknowledge the influence of diversity, ethnicity, and culture on perceptions and expressions of health and illness beliefs and behaviors and on the development of health care partnerships.
4. Rediscover your own cultural identity and its role in shaping who you are.
5. Recommend specific approaches and strategies that you, your employer, and the larger community can use in the delivery of culturally competent health care to at-risk populations identified in Healthy People 2010.

Introduction

*C*ultural competence begins with an awareness of our own cultural beliefs and practices but is arguably more than a state of awareness. Being culturally competent means that we understand how cultural beliefs and practices influence our daily lives and recognize that people with cultural backgrounds different from our own have unique values, life ways, health practices, and interpersonal styles (Administration on Aging [AOA], 2009; Drew, 1996). Several experts describe cultural competence as a set of characteristics, grounded in respect for others, that enables persons from diverse backgrounds to live and work together effectively (Alexander, 2008; Campinha-Bacote, 2002; Gustafson, 2005; Katz, 2005; Kleinman, Eisenberg, & Good, 2006; Leonard & Plotnikoff, 2000; Smith, 2002). The ability to live and work together effectively means setting aside prejudices and biases we might have about other people's cultural beliefs and being open to understanding others. Although some individuals may feel threatened by or defensive about cultural differences, the skills and understandings that prevail in a state of cultural competence can guide us confidently through the processes of abandoning our "ethnocentric" views and experiencing growth and richness in our lives as we learn more about other people (AOA, 2009; GUCCHD, 2009).

As health care providers, we must make the commitment to learn actively and use the knowledge and skills needed to work competently with culturally diverse clients, their families, and communities. Such imperatives are consistent with the goals and objectives of Healthy People 2010 (HP 2010), our nation's health promotion and disease prevention agenda. Comprising 10 leading health indicators and hundreds of objectives, HP 2010 initiatives are guided by two overarching goals: (1) to increase length and improve quality of healthy life; and (2) to eliminate disparities among subgroups of the population (USDHHS, 2009). Instrumental to the success of HP 2010 is the cultural competence of individuals, agencies, and communities that can significantly improve access to quality care and reduce disparities by designing health promotion programs and illness intervention services that are available, acceptable, and appropriate to the cultures they seek to serve (Drew, 1997; Smith, 2002).

A growing body of evidence indicates that one of the major reasons that health services remain inaccessible and underutilized by some ethnic and cultural group members is because the services are not responsive to the needs of those they need to serve. The health services are not culturally competent (AOA, 2009). Clearly, health disparities exist and are due, at least in part, to problems experienced in accessing and effectively utilizing health services (Betancourt, Green, Carrillo, & Ananeh-Firempong,, 2003; Tervalon, 2003; Zuvekas & Taliaferro, 2003). Reducing and eventually eliminating disparities depends on building common ground among clients, providers, agencies, and communities so that culturally competent health care partnerships can grow in number and quality of services. Efforts to develop these competencies and partnerships must accelerate if we are to meet the health challenges of our ever-changing population demographics.

The demographic composition of the United States population will continue to change dramatically for the next several decades. Experts suggest that growth in racial and ethnic group diversity will continue at a rapid rate throughout the 21st century (Zoucha, 2000), causing descendants of European whites to become the *new minority*. As a result of these trends, health care providers will interact more frequently with clients of diverse ethnic and cultural backgrounds whose health beliefs, languages, and life experiences differ greatly from their own. Therefore, to help us prepare to meet the health needs of our ever-changing population, this chapter offers descriptions of concepts and strategies that will assist you in building cultural competence, beginning with an enlightened awareness of diversity, ethnicity, and culture, and illustrating their influence on individuals' and communities' health and illness beliefs and practices. Self-assessment and an analysis of client–provider interactions are presented as learning experiences with implications for practice. After all, successful health promotion and illness intervention outcomes depend on our abilities to competently reach and work effectively with the diverse individuals and communities we serve. The Internet resources listed at the end of the chapter offer access to educational materials and service-oriented programs about cultural competence that reach beyond the scope of this chapter.

DIVERSITY, ETHNICITY, AND CULTURE

Derived from the Latin *divertere*, meaning *to turn in opposite directions*, diversity is the condition of being different or having differences. No attempt is made here to imply a ranking, ordering, or prioritizing of differences; they simply exist. How we look at and deal with differences in human attributes can either build bridges or construct barriers with individuals in and across groups and communities. Rather than considering differences as sources of conflict, we should view them as part of the whole of social and individual identity. A celebration of differences can become commonplace when we understand that the principal strengths on which our country is built suggest a tolerance for individual uniqueness and a collective creativity.

Recognizing that each of us differs in what we consider functional in our lives, we must understand that those who act differently from the mainstream are not deficient in something or "disadvantaged;" they are rich in a different culture and are "other-advantaged" (Madrid, 1988). In daily practice, nurses provide care to patients and families who represent our global communities. Yet, we know little about the basic cultures, beliefs, and values that shape our clients' health and healing beliefs and behaviors. As our clients and our health care settings become increasingly multicultural, care providers across all disciplines must understand the role culture plays in determining health and illness needs and behaviors and strive to become culturally competent (Dreher & MacNaughton, 2002; Katz, 2005).

Asking clients to teach us about themselves will extend to others our sensitivities about being different and will empower others to share their own awareness. Taking the time to value both the differences and commonalities across ethnic and cultural groups will provide us with valuable insights into the human experience and enable us to build bridges between providers and the growing numbers of diverse clients.

Based on the population trends discussed earlier (U.S. Census Bureau, 2005), a *new minority* is emerging. For the first time in American history, descendants of European whites will assume minority status by mid-century. In its purest form, the term minority implies a condition of difference based on enumerating an identifiable characteristic. Wirth (1945) has suggested that a minority is "a group of people who, because of their physical or cultural characteristics, are singled out from others in the society in which they live, for differential and unequal treatment, and who therefore regard themselves as objects of collective discrimination" (p. 347). Health care providers need to make several important adjustments in response to this population shift while continuing to appreciate the special histories of all minority group members, past, present, and future. Regardless of how group memberships are described, all people want to have their ancestries and identities preserved and respected. All want to tell their stories about their unique struggles as well as their successes at overcoming barriers presented by change, exploitation, and prejudice (Taylor, 2005). Despite the fact that for many centuries European Americans comprised the majority population in the United States of America, little is known about the individual struggles they and their ancestors faced when prejudice and persecution drove them from their homelands. Some stories are surprisingly similar to those shared by persons of current minority status. In addition, we cannot lose sight of the fact that members of the new majority will carry with them their experiences of being minority. We still have a long way to go to improve the delivery of health promotion and illness intervention services to all groups of Americans who are at great risk, whether they are members of our new or former minorities or majorities. To do this, we must understand that differences in health and healing beliefs between individuals, care providers, and care recipients are rooted in heritage, ethnicity, and culture (Stryer, Weinick, & Clancy, 2002). This understanding is the basis for building common ground on which partnerships for positive health outcomes are constructed.

Whether ethnicity is associated with minority or majority populations, ethnic groups are composed of people who share a unique cultural background and social heritage that is passed from one generation to another. Ethnicity should be understood as a social differentiation that engenders in us a sense of self-awareness and exclusivity, a sense of belonging. Our ethnicity gives us membership in a distinct group and differentiates us from those in other groups. Our distinction is often based on such cultural criteria as a common ancestry; shared history; a commonplace of origin; language; dress; food preferences; and participation in rituals, networks, clubs, or activities (Holzberg, 1982). For example, when members of an Italian-American family gather at a wedding, the nature of the celebration expresses the ethnic culture in many ways. The ceremony and the formalities of receiving witnesses and guests are unique to each group and are representative of "the way things are done." At the celebration that follows the exchanging of vows, the guests may feast on antipasto, linguini, chicken marsala, and cappuccino. Soon after, the accordion player might strike up the tarantella, an Italian folk song. Young and old alike may grasp hands and promenade as they laugh and sing. Late in the evening, the elders may share stories about "the old country" with excitement and pride. Although members of this group may have emigrated at different times and may have been born in America, they share common bonds based on native language, history, and values. The passing of these beliefs, values, knowledge, and practices takes place through the rituals of sharing and participating in cultural events and celebrations.

It may be helpful to think of your own ethnic culture and ponder the following questions as you proceed through this chapter. With what group(s) do you identify and why? What are your common bonds? What cultural rituals do you celebrate and with whom? What are the purposes and meanings of your gatherings and celebrations? What types of things are shared and learned when people get together? What types of foods are prepared for the event? Are there dances, special rites, or ceremonies? Each of us can probably identify several shared beliefs, values, and practices that make us members of unique collectives, and many of us strive to preserve our rich cultures and histories by passing them on to each successive generation. Foods, languages, and other bonds of common ancestry are the cultural aspects of ethnicity that serve to offer consistency and structure to life, and provide individuals with abilities to interpret life events as significant and meaningful (Ford & Kelly, 2005; Kim-ju & Liem, 2003).

In health and illness, an ethnic group's shared beliefs, symbols, and customs serve as common reference points that members use to judge the appropriateness of their decisions and actions (Kleinman, 1978). However, attention must be given to variations within and between generations that are sometimes attributed to acculturation, socioeconomic status, and education (Congress, 2004). All health care providers should take care not to generalize beliefs and practices to every member of an ethnic group or culture (Campinha-Bacote, 2003). Although ethnicity captures the larger cultural component of human experiences, we must not permit our awareness of a culture to erode its members' individual identities and dignity.

CULTURE, HEALTH AND ILLNESS, AND NURSING

Ethnic culture is the medium through which a person's beliefs, standards, and norms for health and illness behaviors are structured, learned, shared, practiced, and judged. Cultural beliefs give meaning to health and illness experiences by providing the individual with culturally acceptable causes for illness, rules for symptom expression, interactional norms, help-seeking strategies, and determining desired outcomes (Kleinman, 1980). For example, when you awake before school with dryness in your throat and cramps in your stomach, several beliefs about what could be wrong and how you should act in response to what is wrong are set into action. What is causing this to happen to me? What can I do about it? Should I stay home from school? Whom should I call to help me? What will people think if I stay home today? The answers to these questions and the actions you take are learned and are influenced by the experiences you have had with your family and the larger ethnic aggregate. In some cultures, a special home remedy tea can be taken for specific complaints of dry throat and cramps, and going to work or school is an expectation. Other cultural groups may expect you to be visited by a healer, stay home from work or school, and tell no one else about your problem.

Noted psychiatrist and anthropologist Arthur Kleinman studied members of many diverse ethnic groups to gain an understanding of the links between cultural beliefs and health and illness behaviors and actions (Kleinman, 1980; Kleinman et al., 2006). The findings of his studies are especially helpful in guiding community practitioners who interact with clients in their homes and various types of community institutions. Like other researchers, he found that cultural beliefs based in shared meanings, values, and norms are the basic guidelines people use for recognizing that something is wrong, interpreting what it might be, and organizing a plan of appropriate actions (Kleinman, 1986). For example, before action is taken in response to a problem, individuals and family members must first agree that the symptoms represent a problem. Next, there is an examination of all possible and probable causes, which may range from behaviors and foods to violations of cultural norms. Once a cause has been identified, a plan of action is made and appropriate treatment is determined. In addition, how we act when we are "ill" is determined by our ethnic culture. Some cultures have specific norms for sick role behavior, whereas other cultures suggest that you continue to carry out your everyday role to the best of your abilities. In this overall illness recognition and management process, cultural beliefs influence the reasons the client formulates to explain the illness, the language and terms used for communicating the health problem, the choice of whom one talks to about the problem, the range of acceptable healing alternatives, how choices are made, and expectations for treatment outcomes (Drew, 1996, 1997; Helman, 2000; Kleinman, 1980).

For those of us in the nursing profession, culturally sensitive health care continues to be a central focus of a holistic and humanistic philosophy that guides our practice (Campinha-Bacote, 2002; Dreher & MacNaughton, 2002; Gustafson, 2005; Zoucha, 2000). Because nursing is defined as the diagnosis and treatment of human responses to actual or potential health problems (American Nurses Association, 2003), the role of cultural beliefs in guiding a client's health practices and responses to illness episodes is an important nursing concern (Gustafson, 2005).

The healing goals of culturally sensitive care can only be achieved through conscious efforts at gaining knowledge of different groups' ways of explaining, understanding, and treating health problems. Certainly gaining this knowledge and putting it to use will take some time, but it is important for practitioners to learn the strategies presented in this chapter for eliciting from clients their cultural models for health, illness, help seeking, and healing.

CULTURAL HEALTH CARE SYSTEMS

Basic to successful interactions between clients and providers is the understanding that we are all different from one another, with different ethnic and cultural backgrounds, and, therefore, different health and illness beliefs and practices. There's that word again: "different." But despite our differences, we come together at a mutually agreed on place to achieve a common goal: to maintain or regain health. The dilemma presented here is that health means different things to each of us; we recognize it and measure changes in it differently, act in diverse ways when faced with these changes, and seek different methods for achieving healing outcomes. The settings where we meet and interact with each other may take on different veneers and titles, but they are all what Kleinman (1980) calls *cultural health care systems*. The simple fact that culture influences health and illness beliefs and behaviors serves as a constant reminder to us that wherever clients and providers interact, there is a system, and it is influenced by the beliefs, values, norms, and standards that each of us brings to it. Cultural health care systems are made up of individuals experiencing and treating illness and the social institutions where interactions between clients and providers take place (Kleinman, 1980, 1986).

Sectors of Cultural Health Care Systems

Each cultural health care system can have several recognized sectors. The three sectors Kleinman's model addresses are referred to as popular, folk, and professional. Typically, the popular sector is composed of ordinary people, families, groups, social networks, and communities. The lay practitioners and healers comprise the folk sector, whereas the professional sector is composed of the licensed health professionals (Kleinman, 1980). Let us look at these sectors in some detail.

Popular

The popular sector of cultural health care systems is made up of informal healing relationships that occur within one's own social network. Although the family is at the nucleus of this sector, health care can take place between people linked by kinship, friendship, residence, occupation, or religion (Helman, 2000). In the United States, there are as many versions of the popular sector as there are ethnic cultures. In neighborhoods where many ethnic groups have settled, popular sectors of health care systems are found to have several different ways of managing health, illness, and healing.

In the popular sector, the process of defining oneself as ill begins with a self-diagnosis confirmed by significant others based on the implicit standards of what it means to be well (Angel & Thiots, 1987; Helman, 2000). Consequently, a person is defined as ill when there is agreement between self-perceptions of impairment and the perceptions of those around him (Weiss, 1988). The social, ethnic, and cultural values, on which the illness judgment is based, focus on the experience of discomfort, failure to function as expected, and a change in physical appearance. Whether a symptom is recognized as significant or normal is also influenced by the occurrence, persistence, and prevalence of the symptoms among group members (Angel & Thiots, 1987; Drew, 1997; Helman, 2000).

Once a symptom has been recognized as significant, decisions about appropriate healing actions must be made. These decisions are also usually based on beliefs, standards, and norms passed along from previous generations. For example, the affected individual makes decisions about seeing a physician for a health problem, as opposed to taking care of the symptoms at home, in collaboration with family and the social network. If the symptom is commonly observed in other members of the family or community and home remedies have successfully treated the problem, then going to the physician is not a priority. Within this sector, both the care recipient and the network counselors share similar assumptions about the observed symptoms and recommended healing strategies. Therefore, misunderstandings are rare, and the healer's credentials are based on experience rather than professional education and licensure (Fortin, 2002; Fox, 2005; Kleinman, 1980).

Folk

The folk sector of cultural health care systems includes the interaction between a client and sacred and secular healers. Most healers share the same basic cultural values and beliefs as their constituents. In many cases, family members and others in the social network work alongside the client and the healer to discover and treat the problem. Sources of holistic health problems are believed to include relationships the client has with other people, with the natural environment, and with supernatural forces (Helman, 2000).

Treatment rituals and strategies are prescribed to correct disequilibrium and to promote healing. Healers have little formal training, although some have served an apprenticeship with another, more accomplished healer. Most are believed to receive healing powers through family position, inheritance, signs, revelations, or gifts (Lewis, 1988).

Within the folk sector, illnesses are defined as syndromes from which members of a group suffer and for which their culture provides a cause, a diagnosis, preventive measures, and regimens of healing (Weller et al., 2002). It is very important that beliefs about causes of illnesses be compatible with selected treatments. In some cases, family and folk healers may be the only people who can effectively recommend or perform healing rituals. For example, some Hispanics believe that *susto* results from a traumatic experience or that sickness is a punishment from God. *Susto*, or fright, is an emotional response to a traumatic experience and is recognized as an illness that involves the loss of one's spirit from the body. Symptoms include crying, loss of appetite, listlessness, insomnia, nightmares, and withdrawal. *Susto* requires treatment by a *curandero* whose healing rituals attempt to get the individual's spirit back into the body. Sometimes complementary and supportive treatment from a psychiatrist is sought (Leonard & Plotnikoff, 2000; Ruiz, 1985; Trotter, 2001). Working with clients and families to learn acceptable forms of healing for these problems is imperative.

Professional

The professional sector of cultural health care systems is made up of organized health professionals who are formally educated and legally sanctioned (Kleinman, 1980). Unlike in the popular and folk sectors, the clients and the providers in the professional sector typically differ in their social and cultural values, beliefs, and assumptions. Based on these differences, and taking into account the unfamiliar surroundings and rules of the institutions where care is given in the professional sector, the client–provider relationship may be one of mistrust, suspicion, and conflict.

Although many collaborative, complementary, and alternative models of healing are gaining popularity, practices in the professional sector remain dominated by a biomedical disease and treatment orientation. A biomedical orientation suggests that disease is a physiologic and psychological abnormality. This view is exclusive of and counter to the popular, holistic view of illness as a meaningful experience perceived and constructed in sociocultural context (Angel & Thiots, 1987; Saha, Arbelaez, & Cooper, 2003). Some of us have prepared a home remedy for a sore throat or have applied a poultice to relieve a headache or a persistent cough. These are examples of actions taken, in the popular sector, in response to symptoms that are interpreted as part of a meaningful illness experience. In the professional sector, these same symptoms may be viewed as significant threats to health.

Decision Making Within the Sectors

People who become ill make choices about whom to consult in the popular, professional, or folk sectors of the cultural health care system. Overwhelming evidence suggests that those choices are influenced by the individual's subjective definition of the illness, its meaning, and its expected course (Fabrega, 1974). Attitudes toward different types of providers and decisions about whom one should seek for help vary according to how the symptom is interpreted and what it means to that person as a significant life event.

Forming these decisions is also a function of shared, family, and culture-based learning (Mechanic, 1992). Remember back to your childhood and a significant episode of not feeling well.

- Who decided what was wrong with you?
- What were the interpretations of your symptoms?
- Who made the decision about what to do for you?
- With whom did this person consult?
- Did the meanings of your symptoms and who was consulted have anything to do with the selected treatments?
- What were the expected outcomes from your treatments?
- How were those outcomes evaluated?

Just as important as examining your own health, illness, and healing beliefs and practices is investigating the significance of these factors and processes in your clients' illnesses.

In developing a help-seeking pattern, most people establish a therapeutic network, which may include informal relationships with people and providers from some or all of the three sectors of cultural health care systems. Different types of providers, including family members and folk healers, may be used concurrently or in sequence, depending on the client's perception of the cause of the problem, course of the illness event, and desired healing outcomes (Angel & Thiots, 1987; Helman, 2000; Kleinman, 1980; Mechanic, 1992). Typically, people make their help-seeking choices based on prior learning, symptom significance, compatibility between the philosophies of the sectors, and evaluation of the treatment outcome (Genao, Bussey-Jones, Brady, Branch, & Corbie-Smith, 2003). It seems logical that clients, in the process of seeking help, may involve a network of potential consultants ranging from informal structures in the nuclear family to select laypeople and professionals.

Conflict among Sectors

Given our diverse cultural backgrounds, we should not be surprised to find that research across many health-related disciplines provides evidence that barriers, conflicts, and misunderstandings among the system's sectors are, in part, related to the differences in cultural beliefs about illness causation and management. Although we may never have viewed conflicts through Kleinman's (1980) perspective before, we have all encountered conflicts between providers and clients. We may have even been the clients! Have you ever gone to the physician only to find that he or she recommended a treatment that was not what you expected? Have you ever found that a medication prescribed by the physician is something that you would rather not take? None of us is a stranger to these types of conflicts. Even after students in undergraduate and graduate nursing programs are offered a greater knowledge of ethnicity and culture, the conflicts in beliefs and practices between sectors and resultant barriers to effective health care remain unresolved. The lack of progress in reducing barriers can be linked to professional providers' relative inattention to the popular sector of cultural health care systems. Have you ever heard a professional provider say, "This client is difficult" or "This client is noncompliant with his medicines and he won't follow his diet?" Perhaps you have made such comments yourself without thinking that what has been prescribed or recommended may not be compatible with the client's beliefs about treatment and healing. The problem could be more basic than a mere treatment conflict; perhaps the client and provider have incongruent beliefs about what is wrong and what caused the symptom of illness. In the popular or folk sector, illness is sometimes thought to be a somatization of a client's uneasiness with a stressful relationship, the natural environment, or supernatural forces. This is an example of how cultural beliefs about the cause and management of an illness provide the client with a foundation for interpreting the illness experience as meaningful.

Because belief systems in the popular and folk sectors have often been termed as "unorthodox," "lay," "subjective," or "nonscientific" (Kleinman, 1980), and have been associated with non-Western societies, a client's preference for such healing practices may have been dismissed by some professional health care professionals. This dismissal is problematic because if recommended treatments do not fit the perceived cause, then the client may not follow suggested protocols.

If these problems are to be resolved, we need to understand and accommodate the ideologies and practices of diverse individuals. Professional providers must consider the significance of the illness interpretations and meanings for clients, thus facilitating a more comfortable and secure client–provider relationship. We must focus on the popular sector if working relationships are to have successful outcomes. Conflicts, misunderstandings, and barriers to effective health care will be reduced only by commitment to gain knowledge about the popular sector, where health beliefs and health practices are activated (Kleinman, 1980) and where 70% to 90% of all illness episodes are recognized and treated (Zola, 1972). The nursing profession's commitment to health and holism and its capacity to understand complex sociocultural responses to real and potential health problems make it the most logical choice for a professional segment to act as a client advocate in facilitating interactions between the sectors. Appropriate advocacy must be based on the ability to understand the popular sector's realities and to translate and negotiate between the system's sectors with the goal of reducing barriers to culturally sensitive care. In doing so, nursing will lead the charge for cultural competence among providers and will model the application of those attributes for health care institutions.

Without a doubt, differences are sources of conflict and misunderstanding in client–provider relationships (Angel & Thiots, 1987; Balsa & McGuire, 2003). A detailed understanding of cultural health care systems will provide us with many reasons for the existence and resolution of real and potential barriers between providers and laypeople in the caregiving process. Beyond a basic understanding of the ingredients for conflict, this paradigm of differences should be used by providers, partners, and communities as a guide for becoming culturally competent.

THE CULTURALLY COMPETENT PROVIDER

Cultural competence implies an awareness of, sensitivity to, and knowledge of the meaning of culture and its role in shaping human behavior (Campinha-Bacote, 2003; Malina, 2005). If culture, broadly defined, is socially transmitted beliefs, values, ways of knowing, and patterns of behavior characteristic of a designated population group (Fortin, 2002; Kleinman, 1980), then cultural competence is the ability to express an awareness of one's own culture, to recognize the differences between oneself and others, and to adapt behaviors to appreciate and accommodate those differences (Alexander, 2008; Smith, 2001). Culture includes more than race and ethnicity and may include a person's gender, religion, socioeconomic status, sexual orientation, age, environment, family background, and life experiences.

Cultural competence depends on the development of an attitude of acceptance of others among health care providers. It is a process that begins with one's willingness to learn about cultural issues, proceeds with the commitment to incorporate the importance of culture at all levels of care, and is put into operation by making adaptations in services to meet culturally unique needs. Although some practitioners may have specific knowledge of the languages, values, and customs of other cultures, the most challenging tasks are understanding the dynamics of difference in the helping process and adapting practice skills to fit the client's cultural context.

Developing an awareness and acceptance of cultural differences is required as a first step in the process of becoming a culturally competent individual (Campinha-Bacote, 2002; Zoucha, 2000). Many ethnic minorities have beliefs and practices about health, illness, and treatment that differ significantly from the Western, scientific medical paradigm around which the U.S. health care delivery system is structured (Good & Good, 1981; Kirmayer, Groleau, Looper, & Dao, 2004; Fox, 2005). However, negatively labeling people because the provider believes them to differ from him or her and the mainstream is unacceptable. Differences must be explored and understood so barriers to seeking health care can be reduced. Understanding differences begins with an awareness that they exist and continues with a willingness to accept them. In the sections that follow, there are suggestions for exercises to enhance your awareness of your own culture.

Assessing Our Cultural Awareness

A major component of cultural competence is an acknowledgment and awareness of one's own culture and a willingness to explore one's own feelings and biases. Each person is responsible for building an awareness of how culture influences his or her own ways of thinking and making decisions. Included in this awareness must be an acknowledgment of how day-to-day behaviors reflect cultural norms and values perpetuated by our families and larger social networks. To develop this awareness, several experts (Alexander, 2008; Campinha-Bacote, 2002; Hutchinson, 1989; Leonard & Plotnikoff, 2000) suggest that we ask ourselves questions that will direct our exploration of our cultural heritage and how our daily interactions are influenced by that culture. Sample questions include the following:

- To what ethnic group, socioeconomic class, religion, age group, and community do I belong?
- What about my ethnic group, socioeconomic class, religion, age, or community do I wish I could change and why?
- What experiences have I had with people different from me? What were those experiences like and how did I feel about them?

- What is there about me that may cause me to be rejected by members of other cultures or ethnic groups?
- What qualities do I have that will help me establish positive interpersonal interactions with people from other cultural groups?

One strategy used in teaching diversity awareness to health professions students is a cultural assessment project that serves as a purposeful self-examination and an exercise in appreciating differences. The project asks you to begin by identifying your own cultural beliefs and values about health and illness, education and vocation, foods, religion, and role expectations. (You can do this now as you read this section.) Once identified, think through your responses and make notes about how you remember being taught about some of those values, practices, expectations, habits, and traditions. Ask yourself:

- Where and how was knowledge about my heritage passed on to me?
- Who are the people in my network responsible for influencing and shaping the lives of the young people?

Proceed with this project by seeking out someone known to you but who has a background, heritage, or ethnicity different from your own. Ask that person's permission for an interview and ask them the same things you asked yourself in establishing your basic cultural richness. When you have the data you set out to compare with your own, sit down, and analyze what sociocultural similarities and differences the two of you have.

This exercise is particularly beneficial to the beginner who has not ventured into self-awareness projects from a cultural beliefs and values perspective. Having analyzed similarities and differences, proceed with your analysis and focus on predicting potential areas of conflict between the two views as well as the positive, congruent strengths. These may be as simple as food preferences and celebrated holidays or as complex as preferred vocations, generational hierarchies, and healing rituals. You may complete the practice assignment by asking the following question: *What potential strengths in similarities between us should I build on to begin interactions with this client?*

As this cultural assessment project points out, all interacting parties bring with them unique histories, communication styles, and learned expectations. Together, these contribute to potential misunderstandings and misinterpretations that manifest the dynamics of difference. Therefore, strategies of relating with clients must include eliciting information about their health and illness practices, as well as basic ethnic and cultural norms. Specific knowledge about the culture is necessary for the relationship to be structured within the helping framework. Bringing down barriers and facilitating the negotiation of individualized plans of care will support positive health outcomes for all clients. The ultimate goal in planning collaborative approaches to illness treatment and healing is to preserve the dignity of the client and to foster health promotion and healing programs that are likely to meet with adherence because they support rather than offend the client.

Eliciting Health and Illness Beliefs

We have explored the idea that cultural health beliefs are the major determinants of a person's recognition and management of an illness experience. Although these beliefs exist independently of and prior to a given episode of illness, they are activated when one has to cope with and explain a particular experience or situation (Kleinman, 1980). Therefore, as practitioners, we should expect that it is appropriate to elicit cultural health beliefs when (and not before) an illness experience becomes a reality.

According to several researchers, time and experience with an illness are necessary for the client to work the set of beliefs into a functioning set of reasons for the illness, directions for sick role behavior, and options for achieving healing (Good & Good, 1981; Kirmayer et al, 2004). Understanding ethnic interpretations of health and illness enables the practitioner to further clarify the sources of beliefs from which clients formulate their illness realities.

This process begins with eliciting the client's subjective explanations for the cause, duration, and characteristics of symptoms. Further discussion with the client should include exploring the client's expectations for acceptable treatments, outcomes of the treatment, and the substance of the client–provider interaction (Fortin, 2002; Fox, 2005). Kleinman's (1980) original set of questions can be adapted to ask clients about their perspectives on health and illness experiences. Attention to the answers to these questions increases the cultural competence of the provider:

- What do you think caused your problem?
- Why do you think it started when it did?
- How long do you think it will last?
- What have you done about your problem?
- With whom did you discuss your problem?
- What kind of help and from whom would you like to receive help for your problem?
- How will you know when your problem is getting better?

Additional questions formulated by this author for purposes of conducting explanatory model research include:

- What do you call your problem?
- What worries you most about having this problem?
- How did you come to know that you were having a problem?

Finding answers to these questions may take time and will take a conscious effort to collect and use. However, the process is well worth the time and commitment as we gain a greater understanding and respect for all clients' health beliefs and practices. This understanding can lead to both improved client–provider relationships and treatment outcomes. An analysis of the answers to these questions and much introspection will enable health care providers to understand the complexities of cross-cultural interactions.

Adapting Skills

Providers must develop critical skills so that cultural assessments can be elicted and appropriate sociocultural care can be delivered in conjunction with prescribed treatment interventions. Delivering culturally competent care implies a contextual understanding that treating the illness and understanding what it means to the individual are as important as working to resolve the disease process (Kleinman, 1988). Although nurses study communication strategies as part of their educational preparation, the cognitive skills necessary to understand another's cultural beliefs and backgrounds need cultivation, refinement, and practice.

Sound physical and psychosocial assessment skills, sensitive interviewing skills, active listening, neutral body language, and self-awareness are the basic attributes required of culturally competent providers. Several of these attributes can be built using the contents of this chapter, but it is expected that the practitioner will seek out continuing education that will expand the skills necessary for thorough data collection. For example, physical assessment of people of a different race may be a learning need for some, whereas spending more time in cultural self-assessment and analysis of potential conflicts between providers and their clients may be a priority for others.

Active listening, which is a learned skill that requires a lot of practice, is a necessary component of sensitive interviewing. It is helpful if you can audiotape a "client" interview that employs role-playing so you and a colleague can critique your style. Use the following questions to evaluate your progress toward becoming a skilled interviewer:

- Am I using slang or jargon that is only understood by other professionals?
- Are the questions I ask presented so rapidly in sequence that the client has no time to think and organize a response?
- Do I paraphrase a question so many times that it has lost its original intent?
- Are the questions I ask so long that the focus is diluted beyond recognition?

Sometimes the reasons questions seem to go unanswered are related to interviewing skills, styles, and competencies. For example, are you comfortable with pauses, or do you have the need to always hear a speaking voice, even if it is your own? Are you asking appropriate follow-up questions that will probe a client's response to an earlier question? It is important for you to demonstrate that you value what the client is saying. Active listening and planning appropriate responses are a sure way of accomplishing the task.

You must also learn how to present yourself with neutral body language during interactions with clients. Not everyone likes being touched or having someone else in their personal space. Although we may think touch is important in healing, remember it may not be culturally appropriate to the clients we serve.

In addition to physical assessment data, eliciting patient and family explanations of health status and illness realities helps providers take the patient's perspective seriously in organizing clinical care strategies. In turn, the provider's effective communication style assists patients and families in making more useful judgments about when to enter into treatment, with which practitioners, for what treatments, and at what ratio of cost and benefit (Kleinman, 1988). It is imperative to approach health teaching and self-care training with the attitude that providers and patients are collaborators and are working toward the same goals of positive outcomes for the patient and the family. Negotiation among patients and providers over conflicts in explanation, interpretation, and understanding can reduce barriers to effective care and instill in the patient the provider's respect for alternative viewpoints and preferences. These strategies work together to close the gap between the patient and the provider (Kleinman, 1988; Tervalon, 2003) and are necessary to increase access to care and improve health for our entire nation.

THE CULTURALLY COMPETENT AGENCY

Cultural awareness, sensitivity, and competence are necessary attributes for all health care providers and for the delivery systems of which they are a part. It makes no sense to have culturally competent practitioners in settings that are culturally ignorant. In services to individuals, families, and communities, culturally competent systems of care must acknowledge and incorporate the importance of culture, appreciate the dynamics of difference, and make a commitment to adapt services to meet unique needs (AOA, 2001). Culturally competent programs and services respect their clients' and staff members' cultural beliefs and include in their mission statements goals to maintain and improve the self-esteem and the cultural identity of employees and clients. The driving forces behind culturally competent service delivery are knowing and understanding the people that you serve. It means appreciating the importance of culture and avoiding prejudices and biases. It also means that you and your organization understand and work to change the sociopolitical influences that create barriers to quality care.

Several types of movements toward agency-level cultural competence have been reported in the literature. When success is measured by community acceptance and use, some agencies are recognized as more successful than others (AOA, 2001). Generic outreach models may be rejected by ethnic minority groups because the services are often the same ones offered to mainstream groups. This approach is perceived by many to maintain rather than remove barriers (Betancourt et al., 2003; Smith, 2002; Stryer et al., 2002). A more meaningful and successful approach to agency cultural competence is mainstream support of local programs and services that employ and use staff who have similar cultural backgrounds to those for whom the services are intended (Zuvekas & Taliaferro, 2003). This approach means that multilingual and multicultural services should be offered in some neighborhoods and communities. A needs assessment must be employed to identify the types of services and the systems of service delivery that are most acceptable and efficient (AOA, 2001).

For many existing agencies and delivery systems, structures, services, and competencies must be modified or created to be consistent and compatible with the cultures they encounter in their client populations. Culturally competent services, systems, agencies, and practitioners possess the capacity to respond to the unique needs of populations whose cultures differ from dominant or mainstream America.

Awareness that racial, ethnic, and minority groups have different needs, have been underserved, or have underutilized available services has created an interest in agency cultural competence. Assessing the types of services identified as wanted and needed by target populations is crucial to the reception and use of services by people with culturally diverse backgrounds. Agencies striving for cultural competence must be able to accept the values of the community's ethnic cultures, and develop and refine services and skills for working with the local population (Zoucha, 2000).

Summary

Educators and providers must remember that ethnicity provides a sense of belonging to people in a pluralistic society—a celebration of differences in identity, strength, and survival. An understanding of ethnic culture is necessary for coping with and appreciating differences. Research supports the roles of heritage and identity in influencing people's behaviors and attitudes and the perpetuation of ethnicity throughout generations. Rather than eradication of differences, stimulation of conflict, and goals for sameness, cooperation with and respect for others with different heritages must be the focus of future practice and research. Cultural competence is an imperative for meeting HP 2010 goals for health promotion and improving access to quality care. It empowers individuals and providers alike to develop and nurture healing partnerships in health care that are aimed at successful health outcomes for all Americans. Many of the skills providers' need are in place and available for enrichment through awareness, specialty and continuing education, and careful listening to what our clients teach us. For more information, explore the references listed at the end of the chapter and the Internet Resources that can be found on thePoint (http://thepoint.lww.com/Anderson6e).

Critical Thinking Questions

1. The clinical director of the outpatient clinic where you work is often heard complaining about the unit secretary "who just doesn't seem to understand or speak English very well." Sometimes you notice other nurses laughing at the secretary's accent and native dress. You want to help others change their behaviors. What will you do? Be specific and use the hints in this chapter to make and carry out a plan.

2. You are invited to the wedding of a very close friend whom you have not seen in many years. He is marrying the love of his life, a Japanese woman he met while working in Project Hope. He calls you a few weeks before the wedding and asks you to escort the parents of his bride-to-be so they will feel "at home." He tells you that this is their first trip to the United States and they do not speak English. How will you prepare for this special assignment?

● REFERENCES

Administration on Aging (AOA). (2009). *Achieving cultural competence: A guidebook for providers of services to older Americans and their families.* Retrieved February 3, 2009, from http://www.aoa.gov/prof/adddiv/cultural/CC-guidebook.pdf

Alexander, R. G. (2008). Cultural competence models in nursing. *Critical Care Clinics of North America,* 20(4), 415–421.

American Nurses Association. (2003). *Nursing's social policy statement* (2nd ed.). Washington, DC: Author.

Angel, R., & Thiots, P. (1987). The impact of culture on the cognitive structure of illness. *Culture, Medicine, and Psychiatry,* 2, 465–494.

Balsa, A. I., & McGuire, T. G. (2003). Prejudice, clinical uncertainty and stereotyping as sources of health disparities. *Journal of Health Economics,* 22(1), 89–116.

Betancourt, J. R., Green, A. R., Carrillo, J. E., & Ananeh-Firempong, O. (2003). Defining cultural competence: A practical framework for addressing racial/ethnic disparities in health and health care. *Public Health Reports,* 118(4), 293–302.

Campinha-Bacote, J. (2002). The process of cultural competence in the delivery of healthcare services: A model of care. *Journal of Transcultural Nursing,* 13(3), 181–184.

Campinha-Bacote, J., (2003). Many faces: Addressing diversity in health care. *Online Journal of Issues in Nursing,* 8(1). Retrieved September 30, 2005, from http://nursingworld.org/ojin/topic20/tpc20_2.htm

Congress, E. P. (2004). Cultural and ethical issues in working with culturally diverse patients and their families: The use of the culturagram to promote cultural competent practice in health care settings. *Social Work in Health Care,* 39(3–4), 249–262.

Dreher, M., & MacNaughton, N. (2002). Cultural competence in nursing: Foundation or fallacy? *Nursing Outlook,* 50, 181–186.

Drew, J. C. (1997). The ethnocultural context of healing. In P. Kritek (Ed.). *Reflections in healing.* New York, NY: National League for Nursing.

Drew. (Summer, 1996). Culture as medium in health and illness [Feature article]. *Nurse Investigator.* New York, NY: MD Anderson/Sloan Kettering Publications.

Fabrega, H. (1974). *Disease and social behavior: An interdisciplinary perspective.* Cambridge, MA: MIT Press.

Ford, M. E., & Kelly, P. A. (2005). Conceptualizing and categorizing race and ethnicity in health services research. *Health Services Research,* 40, 1658–1675.

Fortin, A. H. (2002). Communication skills to improve patient satisfaction and quality of care. *Ethnicity & Disease,* 12(4), S3-58–S3-61.

Fox, R. C. (2005). Becoming a physician: Cultural competence and the culture of medicine. *New England Journal of Medicine,* 353(13), 1316–1319.

Genao, I., Bussey-Jones, J., Brady, D., Branch, W. T., & Corbie-Smith, G. (2003). Building the case for cultural competence. *American Journal of the Medical Sciences,* 326(3), 136–140.

Good, B., & Good, M. J. (1981). The meaning of symptoms: A cultural hermeneutic model for cultural practice. In L. Eisenberg & A. Kleinman (Eds.). *The relevance of social science for medicine.* Boston: Reidel.

GUCCHD, (2009). The Georgetown University's National Center for Cultural Competence. Retrieved February 18, 2009, from http://www11.georgetown.edu/research/gucchd/nccc/resources/index.html.

Gustafson, D. L. (2005). Transcultural nursing theory from a critical cultural perspective. *Advances in Nursing Science,* 28(1), 2–16.

Helman, C. (2000). *Culture, health, and illness: An introduction for health professionals.* (4th ed.). Oxford: Butterworth-Heinemann.

Holzberg, C. S. (1982). Ethnicity and aging: Anthropological perspectives on more than just the minority elderly. *The Gerontologist*, 22(3), 249–257.

Hutchinson, I. (1989). *Strategies for working with culturally diverse communities and clients.* Bethesda, MD: The Association for the Care of Children's Health, Maternal and Child Health Bureau.

Katz, A. (2005). Caregiving is culture. *Journal of Professional Nursing*, 21(3), 139–140.

Kim-ju, G. M., & Liem, R. (2003). Ethnic self-awareness as a function of ethnic group status, group composition, and ethnic identity orientation. *Cultural Diversity & Ethnic Minority Psychology*, 9(3), 289–302.

Kirmayer, L. J., Groleau, D., Looper, K. J., & Dao, M. D. (2004). Explaining medically unexplained symptoms. *Canadian Journal of Psychiatry*, 49, 663–672.

Kleinman, A. (1978). Clinical relevance of anthropological and cross-cultural research: Concepts and strategies. *American Journal of Psychiatry*, 135(4), 427–431.

Kleinman, A. (1980). *Patients and healers in the context of culture.* Berkeley, CA: University of California Press.

Kleinman, A. (1986). Concepts and a model for the comparison of medical systems as cultural systems. In C. Currer & M. Stacy (Eds.). *Concepts of health, illness, & disease: A comparative perspective.* New York, NY: Berg.

Kleinman, A. (1988). *The illness narratives: Suffering, healing, and the human condition.* New York, NY: Basic Books.

Kleinman, A., Eisenberg, L., & Good, B. (2006). Culture, illness, and care: Clinical lessons from anthropologic and cross-cultural research. *Focus*, 4(1), 140–149.

Leonard, B., & Plotnikoff, G. A. (2000). Awareness: The heart of cultural competence. *AACN Clinical Issues: Advanced Practice in Acute Critical Care*, 11(1), 51–59.

Lewis, M. C. (1988). Attribution and illness. *Journal of Psychosocial Nursing*, 26(4), 14–21.

Malina, D. (2005). Compliance, caricature, and culturally aware care. *New England Journal of Medicine*, 353(13), 1316–1319.

Madrid, A. (1988). Diversity and its discontents. *Black Issues in Higher Education*, 5(4), 10–18.

Mechanic, D. (1992). Health and illness behavior and patient-practitioner relationships. *Social Science & Medicine*, 34(12), 1345–1350.

Ruiz, P. (1985). Cultural barriers to effective medical care among Hispanic-American patients. *Annual Review of Medicine*, 36, 63–71.

Saha, S., Arbelaez, J. J., & Cooper, L. A. (2003). Patient-physician relationships and racial disparities in the quality of health care. *American Journal of Public Health*, 93(10), 1713–1719.

Smith, D. B. (2002). Eliminating the disparities in treatment: The link to healing a nation. *Journal of Healthcare Management*, 47(3), 156–160.

Smith, L. S. (2001). Evaluation of an educational intervention to increase cultural competence among registered nurses. *Journal of Cultural Diversity*, 8(2), 50–63.

Stryer, D. B., Weinick, R. M., & Clancy, C. M. (2002). Reducing racial and ethnic disparities in health care. *Health Services Research*, 37(5), xv–xxvi.

Taylor, R. (2005). Addressing barriers to cultural competence. *Journal for Nurses in Staff Development*, 21(4), 135–142.

Tervalon, M. (2003). Community-physician education partnerships: One strategy to eliminate racial/ethnic health disparities. Commentary on "Teaching physicians-in-training to address racial disparities in health: A hospital-community partnership." *Public Health Reports*, 118(4), 357.

Trotter, R. T. (2001). Curanderismo: A picture of Mexican-American folk healing. *Journal of Alternative & Complementary Medicine*, 7(2), 129–131.

U.S. Census Bureau, Population Division (2005). Population estimates (revised). Retrieved October 24, 2005, from http://www.census.gov/popest/estimates.php

U.S. Department of Health and Human Services. (USDHHS). (2009). *Healthy People 2010* (2nd ed.). *With understanding and improving health and objectives for improving health.* Washington, DC: U.S. Government Printing Office. Retrieved February 3, 2009, from http://www.health.gov/healthypeople

Weiss, M. G. (1988). Cultural models of diarrheal illness: Conceptual framework and review. *Social Science & Medicine*, 27(1), 5–16.

Weller, S. C., Baer, R. D., de Alba Garcia, J. G., Glazer, M., Trotter, R., Pachter, L., et al. (2002). Regional variation in Latino descriptions of *susto*. *Culture, Medicine & Psychiatry*, 26(4), 449–472.

Wirth, L. (1945). The problem of minority groups. In R. Linton (Ed.). *The science of man in the world crisis.* New York, NY: Columbia University Press.

Zola, I. K. (1972). Culture and symptoms: An analysis of patients' presenting complaints. *American Sociological Review*, 5, 141–155.

Zoucha, R. (2000). The keys to culturally sensitive care. *American Journal of Nursing*, 100(2), 24GG–24II.

Zuvekas, S. H., & Taliaferro, G. S. (2003). Pathways to access: Health insurance, the health care delivery system, and racial/ethnic disparities, 1996–1999. *Health Affairs*, 22(2), 139–153.

Internet Resources can be found on thePoint at http://thepoint.lww.com/Anderson6e.

Partnering With Communities for Healthy Public Policy

JULIA HENDERSON GIST

LEARNING OBJECTIVES

This chapter focuses on the importance of healthy public policies for healthy communities.

After studying this chapter, you should be able to:

1. Discuss the different types of policy.
2. Describe the process of health policy development and the interface of politics.
3. Explain how community health nurses can contribute to health policy.
4. Apply the steps of policy development.
5. Partner with community groups to form healthy public policy.

Introduction

*N*urses work with communities to promote population health. To promote the health of the community, health policy development is required. This chapter discusses the process of health policy development and why policy development is a part of the role of a community health nurse. Examples of nurses who have worked with communities to influence and develop policy are reviewed. Additionally, information is given on how to become part of the policy development process in a community and how politics is part of the policy development process. Finally, we use concepts of health policy development to analyze community health issues and derive an action plan.

POLICY COMES IN DIFFERENT FORMS

Policy is defined as a plan or course of action, as of a government, political party, or business, intended to influence and determine decisions, actions, and other matters (*American Heritage Dictionary*, 2000). Other authors describe policy as "the principles that govern action directed towards given ends" (Titmus, 1974, p. 23) and "a consciously chosen course of action (or inaction) directed toward some end" (Kalisch

& Kalisch, 1982, p. 61). The development of policy includes the choices that a society, organization, or group makes regarding their goals and priorities, including how they will allocate their resources. The development and use of policies gives the entity a goal or a plan of action. The policy formed should reflect the values, beliefs, and attitudes of those who are designing the policy.

Policy is often explained further by describing its various types. The types we describe in this chapter are public policy, social policy, institutional policy, organizational policy, and health policy. When describing the different types of policy, often we find that a policy may fit several different types depending on the perspective of the person describing it. For example, public policy regarding assault laws may become part of health policy as we make laws for victims' rights to health care compensation following intentional injury.

Public policy applies to all members of a society and includes prescribed sanctions for failure to comply, such as fines for driving while intoxicated or fines for factories that do not comply with emission regulations. Public policy is formulated by governmental bodies and frequently restricts personal choice to improve public welfare, such as fines for unsafe driving. Additional examples of public policy include seat belt laws for both children and adults and legislation that regulates where and to whom tobacco products may be sold and the fines or penalties that apply with failure to comply.

Policy that promotes the welfare of the public is termed *social welfare policy*. Examples of social welfare policy include child labor laws and income assistance, such as Social Security. Social welfare policy tends to focus on the nation's minorities and vulnerable populations. Aid to Families with Dependent Children (AFDC) as well as Temporary Assistance for Needy Families (TANF) and Supplemental Security Income (SSI) are examples of public welfare programs. Further information is offered about TANF in Table 8.1.

TABLE 8.1

Examples of Legislated Health Services

Programs	Benefits	Eligibility
Medicare	Health insurance program	65 years or older Disabled people <65 End stage renal disease or Lou Gehrig disease
Medicaid	Health care Insurance assistance Nursing home coverage	Low-income residents and also pregnant women, a parent or relative caretaker of a dependent child under age 19, the blind, people with a disability or with a family member in their household with a disability, or people aged 65 years or older
State Children's Health Insurance Program (SCHIP)	Doctor visits Immunizations Hospitalizations Emergency room visits	Children <19 years of age from families who earn too much to qualify for Medicaid but who meet SCHIP eligibility
Temporary Assistance to Needy Families (TANF)	Financial and medical assistance to needy dependent children and parents or relatives with whom they are living	People who are pregnant or responsible for a child <19 years of age, have a low or very low income, and are either underemployed, unemployed, or about to become unemployed
Women, Infants, & Children (WIC)	Supplemental foods, nutrition education, and referrals to health care	Pregnant, breastfeeding, and postpartum women; infants; and children up to age 5 who meet a low-income standard

U.S. Department of Labor (2005). Your Benefits Connection. Retrieved November 7, 2005 from http//www.govbenefits.gov

Institutional policy governs work sites. Institutional policies are based on the institution's mission and goals, and they determine how the institution will function and relate to employees. Institutional policies state when the work shifts begin and end, the location and rules of smoking environments for employees and clients, and criteria for paid sick leave and vacation time.

Organizational policy is formed and applies to groups who have similar interests or special interests, such as professional associations. An example of organizational policy is a state nurses' association or a specialty nursing organization that determines governing rules for membership, such as designated credentialing or registration.

Health policy includes the laws to promote the health of citizens. Often health policy is considered a part of public policy when it is directly related to legislated health care services and reimbursement (Mason, Leavitt, & Chaffee, 2007), such as Medicare and Medicaid. Health policy is established in many ways including legislation, rules and regulations, and institutional mission and goals. Health policies determine what services are paid for and by whom, who is eligible to receive care, and who qualifies for financial assistance. Examples of health programs that are guided by health policy are described in Table 8.1.

Policy can be made in any organizational system and at many levels including community agencies, state organizations, and national and international groups. Health policy may also be characterized by the level (i.e., community, state, national, or international) at which the policy development occurs. For example, health care policy decisions made on a community level, such as a new health clinic for low-income families, is funded with budget allocations from local city and county governments. State funding for health care policies may also focus on the provision of health care as well as policies related to the licensure of health care professionals and the regulation of health care institutions. At both state and local levels, policies may be formulated in legislation or emanate from regulations that control health-related behavior by citizens, such as state laws and local ordinances that limit smoking in public places. National health policy focuses on issues of concern to all citizens, such as legislation and regulations that focus on patient safety in hospitals and ensure access to public health care.

If policy reflects the needs of the public, then the public must assist in the development of the policy. How can community health nurses assist citizens to be part of health policy formulation? Community health nurses who work with community residents have a unique perspective for health policy decision making because of their nursing knowledge, their role as an advocate for community health, and their understanding of the political process. We begin with a brief historical overview of how nurses have partnered with communities and populations of need to form healthy public policy.

NURSES INVOLVED WITH POLICY: SOME EXEMPLARS

Florence Nightingale was active in setting policy to implement organizational changes including hand washing and cleanliness procedures in the military hospitals in which she practiced during the Crimean War (Palmer, 1977). Nightingale believed that once she determined a course of action to be beneficial to the patients, it was then her responsibility to make sure that the policy continued to be followed. Even after Nightingale's health declined and she could not practice nursing, she worked from her bed to see that health care policies were implemented throughout the United Kingdom. Nightingale (1873) wrote, "Every great reformer began by being a solitary dissenter . . . But in every case it was a positive dissent; ending not in a protest, but in a great reform" (p. 26). Nightingale believed not only in being a part of the policy process, but also in being a participant in a positive process.

Another pioneer nurse in public health policy-making was Lillian Wald, who practiced in the early 20th century in the tenements of New York City. She worked tirelessly to improve the health of some of the poorest residents who were often immigrants. She created cooperative relationships with organizations to provide her clients with needed items and services. Wald kept track of various incidents in her community and would relate the incidents when they were needed to influence and educate the public to understand their responsibility to the underserved community (Buhler-Wilkerson, 1993). Working with government and health officials, Wald led policy reform to improve living conditions, form child labor laws, and establish clinics for the residents. These reforms led to the establishment of the Henry Street Nurses' Settlement, for which Wald sought and received financing from private individuals. Various services were provided by the Settlement, including a milk station, a convalescent center, county homes, first aid stations, maternity services, home visits, kindergartens, job training, and recreational activities. This establishment was the beginning of what is now known as public health nursing.

Margaret Sanger was another nurse who saw policies that needed to be changed and worked to improve the life of her community residents. Sanger sought to increase the use and availability of birth control measures, such as condoms and spermicides. Sanger's dedication to changing contraception policies began when she connected her mother's premature death to having experienced 18 pregnancies. Sanger helped to change laws that prohibited education about, use of, and sending information through the mail about contraception (Wardell, 1980).

Today, community health nursing is guided by the American Nurses Association (ANA) Code of Ethics with Interpretive Statements (2005) and the ANA Social Policy Statement (2003). Both of these documents include sections on nurses' responsibility to the public and threats to the health and safety of the community. The ANA Code of Ethics also specifically states that nurses "participate in institutional and legislative efforts to promote health and meet national health objectives . . . support initiatives that address barriers to health such as poverty, homelessness, unsafe living conditions, abuse and violence, and lack of access to health services" (ANA Code of Ethics, 2005, 8.2).

More recently, Healthy People 2020 directs providers of care, including community health nurses, to work toward the achievement of four overarching goals: to eliminate preventable disease, disability, injury, and premature death; to achieve health equity, eliminate disparities, and improve the health of all groups; to create social and physical environments that promote good health for all; and to promote healthy development and healthy behaviors across every stage of life (U.S. Department of Health and Human Services, 2009). Health care providers are encouraged to work with communities to implement health programs to further the health of the community and to use the Healthy People goals to set an agenda for community health improvements. Setting an agenda for health improvements involves using knowledge, expertise, and experience to work with local organizations and officials to enact health policies and set goals for the individual communities.

Florence Nightingale, Lillian Wald, and Margaret Sanger addressed community issues for community health. Today, our challenge is to work with community residents to identify the health issues of concern and collaborate to form an action plan.

POLICY OR POLITICS?

How is policy affected by politics? How does politics shape policy? *Politics* is defined as "the process of influencing the allocation of scarce resources" (Mason et al., 2007, p. 5). However, politics is a word that has assumed a meaning much broader and much less neutral than the definition. When a discussion of politics occurs, often the context determines the meaning. A person's perception of politics will depend on his or her experiences and knowledge of politics. Politics occur within all organizations whether they are for-profit businesses, not-for-profit service agencies, social gatherings, faith communities, health care settings, or governmental agencies. The manner in which politics operate, positively or negatively, in an organization will depend on the rules that have been established as acceptable within that organization, whether the goals are important to the participants, and whether one person is in a position to change the rules of the organization (Mason et al., 2007).

The community health nurse lobbies for the allocation of resources and shapes policies by analyzing the impact of the policy on community health. Lobbying for resources and analyzing the impact of policy on health defines politics. The community health nurse is a politician for health. Politics is sometimes portrayed negatively when it appears that the politicians will do whatever is necessary to achieve their goals. Now is a good time to review Chapter 5 and consider the connection between politics and ethical quandaries. Consider the following potential ethical quandary. Schools in a geographic area with a high tax base fund a full-time school nurse for each public school. Schools in the same geographic area with a low tax base cannot afford a nurse for any of the schools. Should the taxpayers living in the geographic area with school nurses share their revenue to budget school nurses for schools without a nurse? Defend your answer. Describe how you could bring citizens together to discuss the issue. What health data would you want to gather about the students (in both the schools with and without a nurse) before the meeting? What would be the goal of the meeting?

POLICY-MAKING IN ACTION

Policy-making occurs in many settings and among many people. Any system involving people will necessitate policy-making. Policy-making systems include governmental organizations, such as state, county, and city public health departments; federal and state legislatures; offices of the governor and mayor; as well as local and state regulatory agencies, such as public utilities, housing, and zoning. Additionally, private, not-for-profit organizations, such as faith communities, the American Red Cross, the Shriners, United Way, and the Lion's Club also are policy-making systems.

The Process

The basic building blocks of nursing, the steps of the nursing process, are similar to the process used in policy-making. Please refer to Table 8.2 as we discuss this process.

Step 1: Problem Recognition and Definition

Policy-making begins with recognizing and defining the problem of interest to the policy makers. We can use as an example a frequently encountered problem in urban community health—paved walkways (i.e., sidewalks) in disrepair. Broken or uneven paved walkways are a danger to all pedestrians. For example, pedestrians may be forced to walk around broken paved walkways and into the street, putting them at increased risk for a motor vehicle accident. The community health nurse may

TABLE 8.2

Steps of the Nursing Process and Policy-Making Process

	The Nursing Process	The Policy-Making Process
Step 1	Assessment	Problem recognition and definition
Step 2	Diagnosis	Policy formation
Step 3	Planning	Policy adoption
Step 4	Implementation	Budgeting and policy implementation
Step 5	Evaluation	Policy evaluation

become aware of the problem of inadequate paved walkways through observation; conversations with community members and business owners; and reports from local police, hospital, or emergency aid workers who file accident reports. The community health nurse would confirm the problem by gathering information on the number of accidents that have occurred to different age groups. Next, the community health nurse would compare the number of accidents on inadequately paved walkways to the number of accidents on adequately paved walkways.

Step 2: Policy Formulation

Once the problem has been clearly defined, the policy maker (i.e., the community health nurse) determines what type of policy is required and who has jurisdiction over the problem. A policy would be proposed to maintain safe paved walkways. Or in nursing process terms, a diagnosis is made. Returning to the example of the paved walkways, the community health nurse would determine which agency and persons were responsible for the construction and maintenance of the paved walkways. Paved walkways on public property are usually the responsibility of public (i.e., city) government. Therefore, the appropriate place to begin a discussion about the need for safe paved walkways is city government, often city council members. Now is a good time to stop and learn who the city government representatives are where you live. What are their names? When were they elected? Where are their offices? How can you contact government representatives to discuss community problems affecting health and public safety, such as paved walkways in disrepair and the related information on accidents?

Continuing with Step 2, policy formulation, a group of concerned community members, including the community health nurse, must write a proposal to be presented to the responsible city government officials. The proposal is usually a brief statement about the problem and the need for action (i.e., a policy) to correct the problem. The goal of the proposal is to have the walkway issue placed on the agenda for consideration by city government policy makers when a meeting is convened. In order to bring the issue of inadequately maintained paved walkways to the attention of the authorities, increased public awareness is necessary. The community health nurse and interested citizens can increase public awareness by writing letters to the editor of the local newspaper regarding the lack of safe walkways and associated accidents. Detailing incidents of persons injured as a result of the walkway condition and presenting the information to local faith-based, service, and civic organizations as well as at public forums is an excellent way to inform the public about the problem.

Now is a good time to take a break, get a beverage, and review today's newspaper. What issues affecting the public's health are discussed in the newspaper? What further information would you need to gather to document the extent of this problem? How would you identify the responsible agency? What strategies do you suggest to increase public awareness about the problem?

Step 3: Adoption of the Policy

The third step of the policy-making process, which coincides with planning in the nursing process, is the adoption of the policy by the appropriate agency. Once a policy proposal has been presented to responsible officials and the policy has been adopted, governing rules and regulations are formulated to administer it. For example, the department responsible for paved walkways will be specified, along with a schedule for routinely assessing the condition of walkways and completing necessary maintenance. It is important for the community health nurse and interested community residents to be present during the discussion of the policy proposal by the public officials. The nurse and citizens must always request an opportunity to testify as to the importance of safe walkways and be prepared to offer the names of specific walkways needing immediate repair. Finances will need to be allocated to begin the fourth step, the process of implementation.

Step 4: Implementation

Following approval from the appropriate agency and allocation of a budget, the policy can be implemented. For the paved walkway example, implementation is the completion of paved walkway repairs. Frequently during Step 4, public education programs are necessary to increase awareness of the new policy, especially if the new policy requires a change in citizen behavior, such as seat belt use or no smoking in public places.

Step 5: Evaluation

After the policy had been implemented, the final step is evaluation of the new policy of paved walkway repair and maintenance. When the goals of the policy—routine walkway maintenance and repair—are being met, then the policy for safe walkways is effective. However, if the evaluation determines that paved walkway maintenance and repair is not completed, then the public policy process would begin again. The community health nurse must continue to collect data on the occurrence of accidents on pedestrian walkways. Accident data can help determine the efficacy of the new walkway policy. If accidents and injuries continue to occur at paved walkways, then the community nurse would collect data to determine the association of the injury to the condition of the walkway. The data may indicate that the cause of the pedestrian accidents is not associated with the condition of the walkway but rather with the lack of paved walkways. If the problem is lack of paved walkways as opposed to our first problem of paved walkways in disrepair, then the community health nurse begins the policy-making process anew with the goal being a policy for the construction of new paved walkways.

Policy versus Program

You may be asking, "What is the difference between a 'program,' funded by local government, to repair paved walkways and a 'policy,' formed and funded by local government, to repair walkways?" Programs are usually a set of actions to achieve a goal, such as a program to build paved walkways around all schools in an area. In contrast, policy is a set of principles, frequently formally agreed on, such as those that govern the construction and routine maintenance of walkways. Frequently, paved walkways are required to be built for all new construction as part of a city building code; however, the maintenance and repair of the walkways is not formulated into a policy or code. Therefore, a community may confront the need for additional public policy regarding the maintenance of paved walkways. Let's discuss another public policy action that began with community action.

An additional policy that has followed the policy-making process and has impacted the health and well-being of children is that of mandatory child safety seat laws. The first step of the policy-making process, problem recognition, began when the incidence of children being killed or severely injured in motor vehicle accidents was associated with the injured or deceased children being unrestrained on vehicle impact. Citizens (i.e., policy makers) gathered data, consulted experts, and formulated a policy to address the issue. The policy was then presented to the appropriate governing body, which in this case was the state legislature. The requirement of child safety seats was discussed, debated, and approved by majority vote. A date for implementation was determined. Once the policy was implemented, the policy makers continued to measure the effectiveness of the policy and determine if fewer deaths and injuries to children occurred following the policy. The answer has been yes, but the policy makers continue to adjust the policy to make children safer, such as increasing the age of children that are included in the child restraint law.

IMPORTANT HEALTH POLICY ISSUES FOR ALL COMMUNITIES

Over the past several decades, three areas of greatest concern in health care have been (1) access to care; (2) cost of care; and (3) quality of care. These concerns have taken center stage in national health care and are issues of great concern on the community level. There has been much debate over the financing of health care and the health care delivery system in the United States. Some Americans contend they have the right (access) to the best care (quality) at the lowest cost (cost) regardless of their level of income. These issues continue to be at the forefront of nursing and health care policy discussions.

In 2007, the ANA legislative initiatives included the issues of access, cost, and quality at a level at which action can be implemented. For instance, access to care now includes access to health coverage, health plans, and Medicare reform. Cost of care includes advanced practice nurse coverage, health plans, Medicaid cost containment, medical errors, medical malpractice liability/tort reform, and Medicare reform/prescription drugs. Finally, quality of care now includes adequate and appropriate nurse staffing, mandatory overtime, safe health care reporting, "whistle-blowing" protection for nurses, and safe patient handling. It is now the role of the community health nurse to be aware of these issues, to learn how they affect the community, and to partner with the community to become a united voice for the citizens. Health care reform continues to be debated as this book goes to press. It is the responsibility of every nurse to understand the current legislation, be active in forming legislation and always advocate for health promotion and disease prevention.

HOW CAN A NURSE AFFECT HEALTHY PUBLIC POLICY?

Nurses can and do influence health policy. Box 8.1 lists steps a community health nurse can take to advance policy-making, and each action is discussed below.

- **Learn the legislative process.** To influence and initiate changes in the health care system, the nurse needs to know about the legislative process. Nurses can learn about the legislative process by visiting websites of local, state, and federal governments. Many of these websites exist to educate the public on the legislative process and to inform constituents on how to be more involved. Information may also be obtained from government Internet sites which inform and educate citizens on how to participate in local/city government by serving on boards or committees.

BOX 8.1

WHAT CAN A NURSE DO TO INFLUENCE HEALTH POLICY?

1. Learn the legislative process
2. Stay informed on current issues
3. Identify government representatives
4. Be an active constituent
5. Speak out

- **Stay informed on current issues.** It is important that community health nurses stay informed on issues that are important to the profession of nursing, to the community members we serve, and to the community at large. Without remaining current on the issues, it is impossible to know what information to collect, with whom to share the information, and when to speak out. Reading the local newspaper with attention to local community issues is an excellent way to stay informed.
- **Identify government representatives.** Most government websites have links to enable constituents to identify their representatives and provide addresses and phone numbers for contacting representatives.
- **Be an active constituent.** Nurses can be active members of a constituency by writing letters, making visits, or calling representatives. Nurses as professionals may also choose to provide nursing expertise as policies and programs are being designed and to work with coalitions who have similar interests in the issues.
- **Speak out.** Community health nurses can also be advocates for the people with whom they work. Being an advocate involves speaking for those who cannot speak for themselves. An additional role of a community health nurse is to be knowledgeable of new programs, evaluate whether targeted groups are being served as proposed, and keep policy makers aware of progress or lack of progress toward goals.

Finally, remember that successful policy-making depends on you. To be a part of a successful policy-making process and healthy policy formation, stay focused on the needs of the citizens. Listen attentively. Personal relationships are the currency by which things happen. Be persistent. Show that you are concerned and will remain involved. Be prepared with data to demonstrate the effect of the problem on community health. Be positive. People are drawn to positive people. Positivity is a low-cost investment that has a high return. Be patient with the policy-making process, whether it occurs through a legislative body or a smaller organization. Time to reflect on the policy is part of the process, so patience is vital. Exhibit passion for the health issue. Your commitment will make a memorable impression on the community and policy makers. Lastly, be professional in every way and in everything you do. A lack of professionalism will always be remembered long after the issue is forgotten.

APPLYING YOUR NEW KNOWLEDGE IN HEALTHY PUBLIC POLICY

To apply your new knowledge in forming healthy public policy, please complete the following scenario. You read and hear news reports documenting an increase in the number of children drowning in your city. You ask, "What can I do?"

Remembering the steps of the policy-making process, you begin with data collection. You need to know the actual number of children drowned this year compared to previous years. Has the number of deaths increased or decreased? Learn what the death rate from drowning is for children younger than 5 years this year compared to the last five years. Establish the death rate from drowning for children older than 5 years and younger than 18 years this year compared to previous years. (Now is a good time to review the calculation of rates and age-specific rates in Chapter 3.) What are the circumstances surrounding the deaths, such as time of day, day of the week? What are the specific ages and genders of the children who drown? Were the children unattended at the time of drowning? How many children drown in public pools? How many in private pools? What type of policy regulates pools in your city? Is there a policy for fences around pools? If yes, how high must the fence be? Must the fence be locked? Are lifeguards required at public pools? What about alarms for trespassers after pool operation hours? Are there regulations about having private pools in your city? Are there penalties for not complying with the policy? How often are the policies reviewed?

The next step would be to decide if there is a problem and if a new or revised policy is needed. If a problem exists, then it would be necessary to determine who has jurisdiction for the problem. Is it a local issue or a state issue? This distinction may depend on the location of the drownings and who has the authorization to implement and enforce the policies.

After determining that there are an increased number of children drowning or being injured at pools, and determining who has jurisdiction for the problem, then a policy would be formulated to address the identified issue. To address the problem, the policy might institute regulations on fencing of pools, minimum height of fences, closure and locking of gates, penalties for noncompliance, and determination of who monitors compliance. Included in the policy proposal might also be a request for funding to educate the public on the dangers associated with pools and pool safety. Public awareness could be increased through school education, workplace meetings, highway billboards, or mailings. The policy proposal would then be presented to the appropriate legislative group. When a policy proposal is presented to a governing council, a presentation by the community health nurse and citizens in support of the policy is very helpful. Personal accounts of a family that lost a child to drowning are powerful testimony. You may also solicit support from other health care providers and request they offer expert testimony on the issue of pool safety and child drowning. If the policy is approved, then financial resources must be allocated for the implementation of the policy. Setting a date for implementation is the next step. Included in the policy is the importance of public education on the health problem of children drowning and the new policy. After the policy has been implemented, the community health nurse needs to review the statistics on child drowning at pools each year to compare with previous years and to learn if the new pool policy is effective in decreasing the number of children drowning. This example is intended to encourage you to examine your local newspaper frequently and consider opportunities for you to act to form healthy public policy.

Summary

We have discussed the different types of policy and spent considerable time describing the process of healthy policy development, including the role of politics. We have stressed the importance of the community health nurse and community residents forming a partnership to enact healthy public policy, and we have described the specific steps of the policy development process. You are now ready to begin the dynamic process of partnering with community groups for healthy public policy.

Critical Thinking Questions

1. Discuss the different types of policy, offering examples of each.

2. Describe the personal attributes that contribute to successful policy-making and explain how a community health nurse could use each attribute toward improving health care for a community.

3. What actions can you as a community health nurse take to enact healthy public policy for each of the problems listed below? For each problem, list a plan of action according to the five steps in the policy-making process.

   a. No potable water supply in a segment of your rural county.

   b. No emergency plan for the evacuation of older community residents during an anticipated weather disaster, such as flooding.

   c. No paved bike paths in your community.

● REFERENCES

The American Heritage® Dictionary of the English Language (4th ed.). (2000). Boston, MA: Houghton Mifflin.

American Nurses Association. (2003). *Social policy statement* (2nd ed.). Silver Spring, MD: American Nurses Publishing.

American Nurses Association. (2005). *Code of ethics for nurses with interpretive statements*. Retrieved April 10, 2010, from http://nursingworld.org/ethics/code/protected_nwcoe813.htm

American Nurses Association. (2007). Nursing's legislative and regulatory initiatives for the 110th Congress. Silver Spring, MD: American Nurses Association, Department of Government Affairs.

Buhler-Wilkerson, K. (1993). Bringing care to the people: Lillian Wald's legacy to public health nursing. *American Journal of Public Health*, 83(12), 1778–1786.

Kalisch, B. J. & Kalisch, P. A. (1982). *Politics of nursing*. Philadelphia, PA: J.B. Lippincott.

Mason, D. J., Leavitt, J. K., & Chaffee, M. W. (2007). *Policy & politics in nursing and health care* (5th ed.). St. Louis, MO: Saunders.

Nightingale, F. (1873). A sub-note of interrogation; What will our religion be in 1999? *Fraser's Mag*, July, 25–36.

Palmer, I. S. (1977). Florence Nightingale: Reformer, reactionary, researcher. *Nursing Research*, 26(2), 84–89.

Titmus, R. M. (1974). *Social policy: An introduction*. New York, NY: Pantheon.

U.S. Department of Health and Human Services. (2009). *Healthy People 2020: The road ahead*. Retrieved April 10, 2010, from http://www.healthypeople.gov/hp2020/

U.S. Department of Labor. (2005). Your Benefits Connection. Retrieved November 7, 2005 from http//www.govbenefits.gov

Wardell, D. (1980). Margaret Sanger: Birth control's successful revolutionary. *American Journal of Public Health*, 70(7), 736–742.

■ FURTHER READINGS

Bell, J. & Standish, M. (2005). Communities and health policy: A pathway for change. *Health Affairs*, 24(2), 339–342.

Thomas, S., Billington, A., & Getliffe, K. (2004). Improving continence services—A case study in policy influence. *Journal of Nursing Management*, 12, 252–257.

Toofany, S. (2005). Nurses and health policy. *Nursing Management*, 12(3), 26–30.

Internet Resources can be found on the**Point**. at http://thepoint.lww.com/Anderson6e.

Informatics and Community Health Nursing

TERESA J. WALSH

LEARNING OBJECTIVES

This chapter introduces you to the process of using and applying electronic information resources to promote the practice of community health nursing.

After studying this chapter, you should be able to:

1. Explain the process of using and applying electronic resources.
2. Locate, evaluate, and use electronic sources of health information.
3. Apply various search strategies to locate and retrieve electronic information.

Introduction

*I*nformatics describes the science of information. Community health nurses use a variety of information to make health decisions and are expected to use informatics in practice to reduce errors; to obtain, evaluate, and manage information; in decision making; and in communication (Institute of Medicine [IOM], 2003). However, before we can use information we must decide what information we need; obtain and evaluate the information; and then organize, synthesize, and communicate the information. Nurses who use informatics can better implement changes in health care. For example, new ways of retrieving, tracking, and storing patient information using computer technology demonstrate how informatics can support practice. Community health nurses focus on identifying sources of information on which to base health care decisions to improve the health status of aggregates and the community as a whole. The process of gathering information electronically to apply to community health nursing practice is the focus of this chapter.

Before we begin you will need to familiarize yourself with commonly used terms associated with electronic information. Please refer to Box 9.1 for commonly used words and abbreviations. We begin with a historical overview of health information retrieval.

Selected Vocabulary of Electronic Information

Bibliographic database: An electronic database available on the Internet that organizes a collection of publications providing information about the title, author, source of the data, and a brief summary (i.e., abstract) of the document. Most bibliographic databases offer limited or full text of documents. These databases are often focused on one type of information such as health care and medical research or publications from the social sciences.

Blog: This term is a combination of two terms, web and log, thus blog. A blog is like an online diary, offering chronological sharing opportunities, usually on a specific subject.

Boolean searching: Using terms AND, OR, and NOT in the search string. These terms assist the user in increasing the precision of the search.

Directory: A list of websites found on the Internet that have been organized by a hierarchy determined by the author of the directory.

FAQ: Frequently asked questions, a list often compiled as a help feature on websites or search engines to assist the new user.

Favorites: Similar to bookmarking in Netscape, this is a feature used in Internet Explorer to create a list of websites you can return to later for further review.

Home page: The first screen or view of a website. The home page may have a welcome and links to more information about the site and Help pages to assist the new user.

HTML: Hypertext markup language is a format for creating documents for browser viewing. Text in the document is formatted with specific coding called "tags" to communicate with the browser program.

Hyperlink: Also known as a link, a hyperlink is a word or phrase or even icon or picture that the browser reads and uses to access another resource. The link may take the user to another website or another part of the website. You will know you have accessed a link when your cursor changes from a pointer to a hand when it is moved over the link.

Internet: A worldwide collection of networks in communication using special protocols.

ISP: Internet Service Providers (ISPs) provide access to the Internet for a fee. You may access your ISP by using a telephone dial-up service, a cable network, or a wireless service provider.

Keyword: A descriptive term that can be used to search documents. When you use basic keyword searching, you are commanding the program to identify every document that has the word (your keyword) anywhere in the document. Keyword searching is useful to identify large amounts of information on a topic.

Mashup: When two or more sources of data are combined to create an online tool, often using mapping features.

Menu bar: Located at the top of your computer screen when you access your browser, the menu bar has a series of pull-down menus with commands to allow you to navigate your computer, the Internet, or a website.

Search engine: A tool that uses computer programs to search the Internet for websites and indexes those sites by keywords. You can access the search engine and search the indexed sites using keywords to describe your needed information. Each search engine uses a specific type of indexing, so different information sources could be produced searching different search engines with the same keyword.

Search string: The words and commands you enter into a search box to identify your desired information. Single word searching is keyword searching; adding Boolean terms or quotes around a phrase can increase the precision of the information yielded from the search engine.

URL: Uniform resource locator is the term for an Internet address and is shown on your browser in the locator bar. The URL provides clues about the origin of the website, whether a commercial (.com) or an educational (.edu) site.

box continues on page 132

BOX 9.1 (continued)

Web browser: Specific programs are needed to view websites on the Internet. Your Internet Service Provider (ISP) will have a browser for you to view the Internet. Most common browsers are Internet Explorer (IE), Opera, or Netscape.

Wiki: An online collaborative writing opportunity often used in learning environments to allow multiple users to add to a growing document or site. Community agencies might use such a tool to develop a member site.

World Wide Web: The World Wide Web (WWW) is part of the Internet supporting use of information exchange including pictures, sounds, and movies using what is known as Graphical User Interface (GUI).

Ackermann and Hartman (2003), Dee (2005), National League for Nursing (2005) and Skiba (2007).

EVOLUTION OF HEALTH INFORMATION RETRIEVAL

Resources for use in community health nursing practice have evolved appreciably since Lemuel Shattuck first recommended the collection of vital statistics on community members in his 1850 report on public health in Boston (The Public Health Museum in Massachusetts, 2005), or when Florence Nightingale first published *Notes on nursing: What it is and what it is not* in 1860 (Nightingale, 1860). These early publications stated the need for exact observation and recording of information such as the age, gender, cause of death, and number of infections experienced by a community over a period of time. Florence Nightingale stressed the importance of collecting and organizing health data. For example, her charts showed the decreased mortality in the military hospital at Scutari during the Crimean War following nursing interventions to improve hygiene.

Now is a great time to get a beverage and look at some electronic information. A chart showing decreasing military deaths as a result of nursing interventions is available at http://www.florence-nightingale-avenging-angel.co.uk/Coxcomb.htm from the British website *Florence Nightingale: Avenging Angel*.

FORMAL ACCESS TO ELECTRONIC LITERATURE ON HEALTH

In America, the first collection of regularly published medical and health information was available in *Index Medicus*, first published in 1879 by the forerunner of the National Library of Medicine (Miles, 1982). As the National Library of Medicine grew during the 1900s, formal cataloging of information led to publication of a list of titles owned and published for the medical community. In 1964, this computerized list became known as *Medical Literature and Analysis Retrieval Systems* or MEDLARS (National Library of Medicine). In 1971, MEDLARS was computerized to provide access to medical literature. In 1997, MEDLARS Online (MEDLINE©) became available on the World Wide Web (WWW) (National Library of Medicine, 2005). Today MEDLINE is available electronically at the National Library of Medicine website http://www.ncbi.nlm.nih.gov/sites/entrez offering access to over 11 million documents, including articles with publication dates from 1965 to the present. This database is available at no charge and can be accessed online. A tutorial to help you learn to use MEDLINE can be accessed at the following site: http://www.nlm.nih.gov/bsd/disted/pubmedtutorial/.

Another important electronic database available to support informed community health nursing decisions is the Cumulative Index for Nursing and Allied Health

Literature (CINAHL©). CINAHL was initiated by a group of hospital librarians keeping index cards of articles helpful for the hospital's nurses. Today, CINAHL is a bibliographic electronic database offering some full text access, usually available through medical or academic libraries. The most recent nursing and health care literature published is indexed in CINAHL, which is a valid and reliable source of information for community health nurses planning programming for aggregates in their community practice.

CINAHL is keyword searchable, meaning you can list primary words describing your topic of interest, such as "pregnancy" or "asthma." You can also search CINAHL using specific author names. Abstracts—short, descriptive paragraphs that provide summaries of articles—can assist you in choosing which full-text articles will be most helpful. Full-text publications and conference materials are also available in CINAHL, and you may limit your search to only those articles available in full text. However, for thorough searching, limiting a search to full-text articles is not an effective approach as it eliminates many valid publications not available electronically as full text.

Additional electronic databases of interest to community health nurses may be accessed from academic or public libraries with the assistance of reference librarians. For example, Psychology Information (PsycINFO©) from the American Psychological Association can help locate articles reporting information in psychology or social science. Education Resources Information Center (ERIC©) is an electronic database with many publications relating to teaching and education. These databases are excellent resources for community health nurses.

Electronic databases will help you determine the best strategies for evidence-based community health nursing practice. For example, what types of motivational programs have been most effective to increase exercise participation among community seniors? What strategies have proved effective to improve nutrition among adolescents making food choices from school vending machines? It is always advisable to learn what is published on a topic, such as exercise fitness and older persons or food choices and adolescents, before developing a health program. Always use at least two or three databases to complete a brief electronic review of a topic. The review will provide you with an overview of the current knowledge about the topic. The MEDLINE and CINAHL electronic databases are excellent, organizing a great deal of the current nursing and health care literature along with proceedings from formal conferences and meetings. Additional databases can be considered with the guidance of a reference librarian.

Now is a good time to review your agency or school library website. What electronic databases are available to you? Is CINAHL available? Is MEDLINE available? Locate searching tips and tutorials for each database from your library website or from the databases. How are the tutorials different? Search for information about informatics in both CINAHL and MEDLINE, using the keyword *informatics*. Did you find similar citations? What was different in CINAHL? Why do you think there was a difference?

GOVERNMENT SOURCES FOR HEALTH INFORMATION AVAILABLE ELECTRONICALLY

United States Census Bureau

As presented in Chapter 3, community demographic information is available electronically from the U.S. Census Bureau. A national census is completed every 10 years, by household, to establish information on the population of the United States. Census data are compiled and available electronically at http://www.census.gov. The Census Bureau also completes many annual surveys that are helpful to community health nurses. You can access the census website and choose from a variety of survey findings, in chart or table form, to learn more about your city, county, and state. Annual surveys include economic information in narrative, chart, and table format.

Information available from the census website can facilitate community health planning, program development, and program evaluation. You can access the census data using a city, county, or state name, or using street addresses, census tract numbers, or zip codes. Census information can be compared to previous census data to identify changes in age, gender, and ethnic characteristics of a population. Census data enable the community health nurse to learn about the many characteristics of a community and to identify trends or patterns.

To begin using the census website, take advantage of the electronic tutorial available at http://factfinder.census.gov/home/en/epss/tutorials.html. Once you have completed the tutorial, practice your new skill of accessing census data by locating the census tract where you live. At the census website, in the box provided, type your home address. You will be given choices regarding how you want to view the information for your home address: by county, by census tract, or by city. Choose census tract. View the population chart. In your census tract, are there more males than females? Are there more males than females among persons over age 65? What are the ethnic characteristics? What ethnic group is the largest? Do these data reflect what you have witnessed in your community? Remember, the census tract is a very small portion of the community.

After you have accessed your census tract demographic data for the most recent census survey (2010), return to the home page and choose an earlier decade, such as 1990 or 2000. Enter your census tract again and look for the population charts. What are the gender proportions? How do the gender proportions for the earlier decade compare to the later decade? What about the numbers of children under age 5 and the number of persons over age 65? Trends in population distribution can be noted by reviewing the census surveys. How can this information assist with health program planning?

Do you need a break from the computer screen? If so, I suggest you take a walk in your neighborhood and bring your census tract. Do you notice any differences from the information you reviewed from latest census data and what you witness? Are the ethnic, gender, and racial characteristics of the census tract similar to or different from the characteristics you learned from the census data? How has your census tract changed and how has it remained the same? How can you explain the changes? What implications are there for the changes in your census tract over the decades for community health programs?

The Centers for Disease Control and Prevention

The Centers for Disease Control and Prevention (CDC) is a government agency within the Department of Health and Human Services. The CDC electronically organizes health information that can be accessed at http://www.cdc.gov. Topics on the CDC website include prevalence of communicable diseases, such as influenza; updates for travelers, including tips for airline or cruise ship travel; and immunization information. Immunization requirements for all age groups are listed on the website, and an immunization record chart can be created by placing the cursor on *Vaccines and Immunizations* and following the guide. The CDC website also provides information on *Workplace Health and Safety* and lists resources for activities for health promotion programs at the work site.

Under the CDC, the National Center for Health Statistics (NCHS) offers another source of health information called *"Fast Stats A to Z."* Disease information, vital statistics, and health insurance facts can be accessed on this website found at http://www.cdc.gov/nchs/fastats/Default.htm.

Now is an excellent time to practice using NCHS data. Visit the NCHS website at http://www.cdc.gov/nchs/, choose two topics, and explore information available on the topics. As you place your cursor on different topics, you will see the pointer change to a hand, indicating a link to another source of information. Once you click on a link, you can access another website or web page on the Internet. Click on the Fast Stats link under the Top Ten Links, and then click on Asthma, for example, to learn what information is provided. In addition to statistics describing the annual occurrence of asthma in the population, there are links to organizations and agencies that provide support for persons with asthma. Try exploring another condition listed on the "A to Z" list. What did you learn? How can this website assist community health nurses or community residents? Consider how you might share your retrieval of government health information skills with interested community groups.

Additional sources of government-managed health information available electronically through the CDC include *Morbidity and Mortality Weekly Report* (MMWR), available at http://www.cdc.gov/mmwr/; *Emerging Infectious Disease Journal*, available at http://www.cdc.gov/ncidod/EID/index.htm; and *Preventing Chronic Disease Journal*, available at http://www.cdc.gov/pcd/. Each of these resources provides important health information and can assist you to identify, confirm, and track health problems. Their information is also helpful when planning for programming in communities.

DIRLINE Directory of Health Organizations

The National Library of Medicine offers a database called DIRLINE that provides access to organizations focusing on health. To identify resources available for a particular condition, such as diabetes or heart disease, begin your search at http://dirline.nlm.nih.gov/. DIRLINE is especially easy to use. Place the name of a disease or condition into the search box and click search. Information from this search will be returned in order of relevance. The DIRLINE search engine will identify documents or websites from organizations that contain the word or words you entered. Documents are listed according to how often the search term appears in the document. For practice, search for arthritis in DIRLINE. How many records were returned? If you link to each record, you will find information about the organization, contact specifics, and an abstract that summarizes available information. Now search for a condition that interests you.

Local Government Websites

State and city government websites are excellent sources of information. State websites have health information such as vital statistics, mental health services, and housing assistance. State and county Departments of Health compile information on the health events of the community, such as births, deaths, and marriages. They also maintain records on infectious disease occurrence, such as incidence of diseases, and reports of hospital activity, such as the number of admissions and discharges. City websites provide local information, including geographic locations of city services, such as fire departments, animal control services, and city planning.

Many larger cities have websites, usually sponsored by nonprofit organizations, such as the United Way. These websites contain listings of community health resources, such as clinic locations, services, and eligibility criteria. These electronic sites may have mapping programs to allow creation of a geographic map for a specific area that notes the location of all health and social service agencies. Public libraries frequently create web pages that organize lists of local resources. City and community agency websites may also compile information about the community, including the history of the community. Each of these websites may provide electronic access to a variety of information sources. Electronic websites provide convenient access to a large amount of data to confirm or refute what you witness in your community.

To locate your city or state website, use a general search engine such as Google or Yahoo. Search engines can search and index websites and information on the Internet and provide you with a list of websites pertinent to your topic. To locate the website for your city and state, type the city and state name in the search box of the search engine. If you wish to access only the state website, place only the name of the state in the search box.

To search for your city website, use a search engine such as Google. Place the name of your city and state in the search box on the Google website and click *Go* or press Enter on your keyboard. If you live in Chicago, Illinois, one website that will be returned by the search engine is the City of Chicago website (http://egov. cityofchicago.org/city/webportal/home.do). You are most likely to see the headlines from the daily newspaper as well as a photograph of the Mayor and an accompanying message. Websites and homepages change often, so do not expect to find the same information each time you access a website. Links are available to specific information for residents, businesses, visitors, and tourists. Remember, your cursor will change from a pointer to a hand when you move your cursor over a link. Links also are often different colors than the surrounding text or are underlined. At the City of Chicago website, what information did you find under Health and Human Services? Did you find the locations for the public health clinics? Now access the website for Memphis, Tennessee. Can you find the location of a hospital for children in Memphis? Are there services for senior citizens in Memphis? What other information would be important to you if you were moving to Memphis? Now go to the website for your hometown. Can you find the location of public health clinics? Dental clinics? Services for senior citizens? Are there maps to locate the geographic location of health services?

NONGOVERNMENT SOURCES OF HEALTH INFORMATION AVAILABLE ELECTRONICALLY

Many nongovernment organizations in the United States offer services and support for a variety of health conditions. For example, the March of Dimes and the American Cancer Society are organizations that provide educational materials about specific conditions within their mission. To explore one of these websites, go to the March of Dimes at http://www.marchofdimes.com/. The first page on this website is the home page, which gives you an overview of what is available. You may wish to explore general information about healthy pregnancies or choose to sign up for an electronic newsletter. Discussion groups are available for pregnant women to share information of interest. The website offers access to a section for *Professionals and Researchers*; place your cursor on these words to follow the link. As you link to additional websites and web pages, notice additional newsletters are offered as well as fact sheets of information. Continuing education programs are also available. Explore the list of continuing education programs and consider what might be helpful to a community health nurse working with pregnant teenagers at the local high school. Is there a continuing education course available? What other resources at this site might be helpful?

Visit the American Cancer Society, or another nongovernment organization of your choice, and learn what types of health information are available.

STRATEGIES FOR SUCCESSFUL SEARCHING FOR ELECTRONIC INFORMATION

All search engines offer help pages or tutorials to make searches more effective. For successful searching, first determine the terms that will identify the information you need. You may wish to start with general terms such as violence or use phrase searching, placing quotations around the words in phrase form, such as "violence against women," to increase the precision of your searching.

Boolean Searching

Boolean searching, a mathematical system used in computers, will increase the precision of a search. Boolean terms are word commands including AND, OR, and NOT. When used in the search string, these terms instruct the search engine how to retrieve information indexed by the keywords chosen. For example, a community health nurse searching for information about the existence of crime in a particular community might enter the search string *"crime AND Dallas, Texas."* The search engine would return all information indexed that pertains to crime as indexed in Dallas, Texas. Searching crime alone would return volumes of information on crime everywhere. Searching the location name would return volumes of information on the city or town. The Boolean word AND instructs the search engine to return only resources that have both terms in the documents, resulting in more effective searching.

The OR word enlarges the search yield by identifying all information focused on both terms searched. If a topic is referred to by more than one term, the OR word can be useful to identify information. When searching a topic such as smoking and adolescents, for example, the search string might be *"adolescents OR teenagers" AND smoking* to search for information about smoking that relates to this aggregate. What would be another term you might use in this search string? Using the term "tobacco use" in your search string would also be helpful to find information. Would you search hospitals for this information? Would you search the public school websites?

The NOT word can be used to limit yields when searching by identifying what you do not want. Limit setting is a tool to increase the precision of searches. If you need to learn about resources in your community that are provided by the private sector, the NOT operator might be used to remove government agencies from the returned list of websites. To do this you would add *"NOT .gov"* to the search string. Sites with URLs ending in ".gov" would be eliminated from your search. Tutorials on searching are available on the Internet and from most public library websites and constitute time well spent before searching online. Now is a good time to review how to find a searching tutorial or a search engine.

Search Engines

Although a variety of search engines are available on the Internet, they change frequently. Search engines change names or disappear altogether. Public library websites are good sources for identifying useful search engines, as is the Internet site Search Engine Watch (http://www.searchenginewatch.com). This site monitors the development of search engines, organizes information using technical descriptions of search engine programming, and provides a list and descriptions of current search engines. General search engines also create their own directories and often allow open browsing in their subject-headed directories. Using these directories may help identify the terms to include in your search string.

Review the Search Engine Watch website at http://www.searchenginewatch.com and choose one search engine reviewed. Type the URL of the search engine into the locator bar on your computer screen, and press the enter key. When the website appears, find and read the help page, "about" page, or Frequently Asked Questions (FAQ) page to learn the special abilities and search commands useful for the search engine. Search for education information for your hometown. Use both the AND and the OR words to identify resources for descriptive information and indexed websites. The NOT word might be useful if the search engine is identifying information not needed for your topic.

Directories

A directory is a subject catalog available on the Internet. Like a telephone directory, it is organized, often alphabetically, and provides access to a list (i.e., the index) of websites on the Internet. Directories provide access to websites like an electronic database provides access to articles or documents. One directory available on the Internet is the Librarians Internet Index found at http://www.lii.org. Librarians regularly update and maintain this directory of websites. Main topics index the websites including broad topics such as business, health, law, and science. Indexed under the health heading, you will find more than 400 websites about diseases and conditions, more than 100 websites about drugs, and many more examples of "health" topics. This directory is a reliable source of information because librarians have already evaluated each website.

To practice using a directory, type http://www.lii.org into the locator bar on your computer Internet screen and press enter. Choose the "Health" main topic from the list offered, and then "Patient Education." How many websites are indexed? Read the brief paragraph describing the websites and choose one to explore by placing your cursor on the colored URL for that website at the end of the summary paragraph. How would a community health nurse use this information? Remember, this directory will provide a list of websites to explore on topics chosen by the librarians who maintain this website. This directory is an excellent source for you as you learn about accessing electronic community health information.

REFERENCING AND EVALUATING SOURCES OF ELECTRONIC INFORMATION

Once information has been located through your searches, you may wish to use the bookmarking function on your browser to mark websites for revisiting. In some browsers, the bookmarking function is termed "favorites" and is accomplished by clicking on the favorites command or icon on the menu bar. Other browsers may title bookmarking differently, and some browsers use only an icon, such as a heart. Practice organizing a document or a table to save your information for future use. Gathering electronic health information requires skills of searching, evaluating information, and saving the information to files or charts for future analysis.

It is also important to keep a reference list of electronic sources searched. Your final document must cite correctly all Internet websites accessed. The correct citation for Internet websites, according to the *American Psychological Association Manual*, 5th edition, provides the reader with the address of the website and the date the information was retrieved (APA, 2001). The website for the American Psychological Association format is http://www.apastyle.org/ and offers a link on the left-hand side to "Electronic References"; this is the most current format for citation of Internet or electronic information.

Finally, always evaluate the information you retrieve electronically according to the following criteria:

- *Author.* Who wrote the information? Does the author(s) have credentials to be a content expert? Does the website show institutional affiliation? Has the author written before on this topic or show other evidence of expertise?
- *Credibility and accuracy.* Is the information true and can you confirm it with at least two other sources? Or is this information different from everything else you have found on the topic?
- *Currency.* When was this information last updated? Is it current information, or is more recent information available? Websites often have dates cited at the bottom of the first page to identify when the website was last updated. You will need to look for this date to know if the website is current.
- *Objectivity versus bias.* Information is used to inform the reader; sometimes information is used to influence the reader. As you read information, be aware of potential bias exhibited by the author or website. Some information is produced to influence your opinions; likewise, some information may be omitted to influence your opinion.
- *Navigation.* Is the site easy to navigate? Are you lost constantly and unable to get back to the homepage, or is there so much flashing that you feel overwhelmed by the site? Or does the site make it clear how to find the information you need?

Summary

In this chapter, you have reviewed the development of representative electronic resources that offer demographic data, vital statistics, health data, and sources of health information useful to community health nurses. We reviewed and practiced basic skills of electronic searching, including how to access and locate electronic information, along with strategies for successful searching, and then evaluating information. Clients in the community are more informed each day and will expect the nurses they meet to be equally well informed. Informatics and the skill of electronic information retrieval can promote the partnership of communities and community health nursing practice.

Critical Thinking Questions

1. Compare the population demographics for your home town and two other towns of the same size from different regions of the country. Note the changes from the last decade to the present decade using census data. What are the health implications for changes you see?
2. Which electronic sources of information will be most important for the community health nurse using the latest research evidence to guide practice? Why?

3. Compare and contrast use of an Internet directory such as the Librarians Internet Index versus use of an electronic database such as CINAHL. When would you choose each one? Why?

4. How could the electronic bookmarking function serve the community health nurse in practice? Why is this skill important to teach community residents?

● R E F E R E N C E S

Ackermann, E., & Hartman, K. (2003). *Searching & researching on the Internet & the World Wide Web* (3rd ed.). Wilsonville, OR: Franklin, Beedle & Associates.

American Psychological Association. (2001). *Publication manual of the American Psychological Association* (5th ed.). Washington, DC: Author.

Dee, C. (2005). Making the most of nursing's electronic resources. *American Journal of Nursing,* 105(9), 79–85.

Institute of Medicine. (2003). *Health Professions Education: A bridge to quality.* Retrieved January 14, 2009, from http://www.iom.edu/report.asp?id=5914

Miles, W. D. (1982). *A history of the National Library of Medicine.* Bethesda, MD: U.S. Department of Health & Human Services. Retrieved September 20, 2005, from http://www.libsci.sc.edu/bob/ISP/nlm.htm

National League for Nursing. (2005). Interagency council on information resources for nursing. *Nursing Education Perspectives,* 26(5), 300–309.

National Library of Medicine. (n.d.). The history of NLM. Retrieved September 26, 2005, from http://www.nlm.nih.gov/nlmbin/restrict/about/nlmhistory.html

Nightingale, F. (1860). *Notes on nursing: What it is and what it is not.* New York, NY: D. Appleton and Co.

Skiba, D. J. (2007). Nursing Education 2.0: Are mashups useful for nursing education? *Nursing Education Perspectives,* 28(5), 286–288.

The Public Health Museum in Massachusetts. (n.d.). *Pioneers in public health in Massachusetts.* Retrieved August 10, 2005, from http://www.publichealthmuseum.org/exhibits-pioneers.html

U.S. Census Bureau. (n.d.). *U.S. Census Bureau: History.* Retrieved August 10, 2005, from http://www.census.gov/acsd/www/history.html

Internet Resources can be found on the**Point** at http://thepoint.lww.com/Anderson6e.

Preventing and Managing Community Emergencies: Disasters and Infectious Diseases

Elnora P. Mendias and Deanna E. Grimes

LEARNING OBJECTIVES

This chapter introduces prevention and control of community health emergencies, incorporating principles from disaster preparedness and infectious diseases.

After studying this chapter, you should be able to:

1. Differentiate terminology applied to disaster preparedness.
2. Discuss the range of short-term and long-term negative effects of community disasters.
3. Describe principles of disaster preparedness.
4. Review principles related to the occurrence and transmission of infection and infectious diseases.
5. Apply the chain of transmission to describe approaches to control infectious disease.
6. Describe the legal responsibility for control of communicable diseases.
7. Identify nursing activities for community emergencies at primary, secondary, and tertiary levels of prevention.

Introduction

*W*hat are community emergencies? They are events large enough to have a major impact on community functioning. Because of the nature of these events, organized community efforts must be employed to prevent or control their impact. When such events exceed the community's capacity to manage them, they are called disasters. Community emergencies may occur naturally, such as a hurricane, or may have a human etiology, such as an explosion or an inadvertent or deliberate release of a biologic agent. Community emergencies may occur spontaneously, such as an outbreak of the bird flu or a tornado, or may impact a community over a long period of time as with the HIV/AIDS epidemic. Perhaps no other health issue has the potential to impact the total community—its people and all its systems, including the health care system—as do community health emergencies. Nor does any other health issue have the potential to impact nurses everywhere, irrespective of their practice setting, as do such emergencies. Therefore, nurses need to know essential information to enable them to respond to individual, family, and community needs related to these emergencies.

With its emphasis on partnerships, systems, and people as the core, the community-as-partner model can be appropriately applied to prevention and control of community health emergencies. Well-functioning community systems, with preparedness in mind, improve community lines of defense and resistance, thus decreasing the impact of negative environmental stressors and public reaction to the stressors. The principles implicit in the community-as-partner model, such as building partnerships among the people, health care providers, and relevant systems, are essential for prevention and control of community health emergencies.

Although community health emergencies may encompass many types of events, this chapter is divided into two sections for ease of presentation of content: prevention and control of community disasters, and prevention and control of infectious diseases. Nursing responsibilities and activities are incorporated in each section.

PREVENTING AND MANAGING DISASTERS

Disasters have occurred with tragic frequency throughout history. They have brought about injuries and deaths, environmental destruction, and disruptions in basic community services and systems. Depending on the type of event, a community can lose its ability to provide shelter, power and fuel, food and water, transportation, sanitation, education, communication, employment, recreation, governance, health care, and safety. Disasters can greatly affect a community's health and create immediate and long-term suffering and need. Disasters particularly affect vulnerable groups, including children and the elderly. Some disasters are potentially preventable; others cannot be prevented, but much can be done to ameliorate their effects.

Healthy People 2010 and Disaster Preparedness

Although there is not a Healthy People 2010 focus area for disasters, disaster preparedness is mentioned specifically under the Healthy People 2010 focus area for *Environmental Health: Ensure that State health departments establish training, plans, and protocols and conduct annual multi-institutional exercises to prepare for response to natural and technological disasters* (U.S. Department of Health and Human Services [DHHS], 2000b). Disasters may also affect other Healthy People 2010 health indicators and objectives (Box 10.1).

Components of Community Disaster Management

As in other areas of community health practice, disaster management has its own unique terminology and classification schemes. We define terms and describe types of disasters and their impact on the community in this section.

Definition of Terms

The terms *disaster*, *emergency*, and *hazard* have been differentiated as follows: According to the World Health Organization (WHO, n.d., p. 1), a *disaster* occurs as

BOX 10.1

EXAMPLES OF HEALTHY PEOPLE 2010 OBJECTIVES APPLICABLE TO DISASTER PREPAREDNESS

Access to Quality Care
Increase the proportion of persons who have access to rapidly responding prehospital emergency medical services.
Increase the number of tribes, states, and the District of Columbia having trauma care systems that maximize survival and functional outcomes of trauma patients and help prevent injuries from occurring.

Environmental Health
Improve the quality, utility, awareness, and use of existing information systems for environmental health.

US DHHS, 2000a, 2000b

the result of an event where "normal conditions of existence are disrupted and the level of suffering exceeds the capacity of the hazard-affected community to respond to it." In contrast, an *emergency* occurs as the result of an event where "normal procedures are suspended and extraordinary measures are taken in order to avert the impact of a hazard on the community." If not managed, an emergency may become a disaster. Finally, a *hazard* occurs when an event "has the potential to cause disruption or damage to the community, e.g., earthquake, flood, typhoon, and cyclone. Some hazards may cause emergencies; not all become disasters." Noji (2005) defines a disaster as resulting from "a vast ecological breakdown in the relation between humans and their environment, a serious or sudden event on such a scale that the stricken community needs extraordinary efforts to cope with it, often with outside or international aid." In addition, we may label an event a disaster if it causes millions of dollars of damage, even if there are no direct human injuries or deaths. Other disaster definitions focus on *health needs and capacities.*

Mass trauma or *mass casualty incident* (MCI) are terms often employed to indicate numerous deaths, injuries, disabilities, or emotional distress due to a major disaster (AMA, 2004a, 2005). The terms *Weapons of Mass Destruction (WMD)* or *Weapons of Mass (or Multiple) Effect (WME)* are frequently used to describe devices that produce many casualties and influence health care or critical service access. The mnemonic *CBRNE* (Agency for Healthcare Research and Quality [AHRQ], 2007) refers to WMD causes including: **C**hemical agents, **B**iologic agents, **R**adiological agents, **N**uclear agents, and **E**xplosive agents.

National preparedness plans in the United States rely on surge capacity to meet health care needs during disasters. *Surge capacity* is the ability of health care systems to quickly expand beyond customary services or capacity, in order to meet emergency needs, such as increased beds, personnel, supplies, etc. Nurses in all settings, then, must be prepared to encounter a community emergency.

Types and Causes of Disasters

Disasters are frequently divided into two broad categories: *natural* (caused by environmental or natural forces) and *man-made* (caused by people). Examples of natural disasters include earthquakes; tornadoes, hurricanes, other storms; volcanoes; wildfires or other fires; land or mud slides; tsunamis; droughts; and heat waves (Federal

Emergency Management [FEMA], n.d.). Examples of man-made disasters include chemical spills or explosions, nuclear or radiologic disasters, acts of conflict or war, and terrorist acts (Veneema, 2007). In addition, man-made disasters can be *accidental* or *unintentional*, or *deliberate* or *purposive*.

Health care organizations may experience emergencies related to interruption of normal function (building damage, power outages, interior flooding, etc.); overwhelming patient volume; or patients requiring specific injury care or treatment (triage, decontamination, isolation, or burn, surgical, or critical care, and so on). What poses a health care disaster, then, varies with needs and with available resources and capacities. For example, a plane crash with several severe injuries might be perceived as a health care disaster by a small or isolated facility. A large facility with a full-service emergency department and well-trained emergency personnel, or several smaller facilities working together, however, may have the capacity to handle many trauma victims at once. Or, while flooding or power outages can severely curtail or disrupt normal patient care in community health facilities, a health care disaster may be averted because other nearby resources expand services temporarily to handle increased needs.

Effects of Disasters on Communities

Several characteristics greatly influence whether a disaster can be predicted, prevented, or whether its effects can be controlled. Among these characteristics are the *onset*, *impact*, *duration*, and *location* of the event (Veneema, 2007); the event's *frequency*, *predictability*, *imminence* or *destructive capacity*; and the *potential to prevent or mitigate the effects of the event*. For instance, a gas line rupture and explosion may occur quickly and be unpredictable. Current meteorology, though, permits prediction of a powerful hurricane's storm path, allowing prehurricane response, such as evacuating persons in low-lying areas and planning mitigation activities for during and after the hurricane. An earthquake may be over in a few quick seconds, but a drought may affect an area for months or years, causing long-term harm. Forest fires in heavily populated areas are more likely to result in deaths, injuries, and property damage than are fires in unpopulated or sparsely populated areas.

Disaster epidemiology focuses on a disaster's negative health effects on populations and on the factors contributing to those adverse effects. Health effects vary with the emergency or disaster event. For instance, an explosion can cause injuries from blast trauma, flying glass or other objects, fire, release of toxic chemicals or radiation, electrical shock, suffocation, and so on. In addition to deaths and injuries occurring during disasters or emergencies, numerous studies have linked natural and man-made disasters with shorter- and longer-term negative mental and physical health effects. For instance, a study of adolescents after a fire in a cafe-bar in the Netherlands reports those exposed had significantly higher mental, musculoskeletal, and respiratory symptoms the first year after the fire (Dorn, Yzermans, Spreeuwenberg, Schilder, & van der Zee, 2008). Following the terrorist events in the United States (U.S.) on September 11, 2001 (9/11), multiple studies described negative physical and psychological health effects in diverse populations.

Two Examples of Community Disasters and Their Effects

Two examples of disaster are included because they are well-known worldwide. The December 2004 Indian Ocean tsunami is among the most catastrophic natural disasters in recent memory. Although the earthquake that preceded the tsunami was recognized and the tsunami could have been *predicted*, the sudden *onset* of giant waves caught people unaware and unable to seek higher ground. The tsunami death toll was confirmed at more than 174,000 persons, many of whom were cremated or buried without identification (CDC, 2005). In addition to immediate injury and loss of life and property, many countries in the region experienced devastation of their health systems, with potential long-term impacts on population morbidity and mortality. In Aceh, Indonesia, 53 of 244 health facilities were destroyed or severely damaged, and many health service employees were among the dead or missing. Moreover, the large numbers of persons displaced by the tsunami, flooding, crowding, and a vulnerable population further increased post-tsunami communicable disease risks (WHO, 2005). In addition, the economic structure of the area was severely compromised. Sources of income, such as fishing and tourism, were devastated. Recovery may take years.

In 2005, although *predicted*, the *force* of Hurricane Katrina demolished many U.S. communities in the southern Gulf of Mexico region, especially in the states of Louisiana, Mississippi, and Alabama. Over 1,800 persons are thought to have died, and damages exceeded $81 billion (DHHS, n.d.a). The storm left hundreds of thousands homeless, their communities in ruins. The hurricane's massive effects disrupted local economies, but effects were also felt around the country, including loss of businesses, increased insurance costs, and higher prices for gasoline and natural gas. Following the storm, in New Orleans, Louisiana, a nightmare unfolded. Although the hurricane had been predicted, levee breaches after the storm were *unexpected*, creating rapid flooding of more than 80% of the city. Thousands of residents were left stranded without power, food, potable water, sanitation services, or shelter. Many health hazards emerged as community systems failed. As the days of misery continued, many persons in storm-damaged areas felt bitter and abandoned by their government. What went wrong? Could the events associated with Katrina have been prevented?

Community Planning for Disaster Preparedness

Historically, initial responsibility for planning and responding to U.S. disasters has been the responsibility of individuals and local communities and governments. When these entities become overwhelmed, higher governmental authorities may intervene on request of local authorities. Planning for and responding to disasters must begin at the community level.

Multiple organizations may be involved in disaster planning and disaster management, including health care, law enforcement, emergency services and first aid, financial institutions, emergency shelters, faith-based groups, utility companies, and the postal service. Individuals, serving as volunteers, have also played important roles. Cooperation and coordination among the organizations and levels of government are essential for rapid and effective planning and response.

Among better-known national U.S. disaster-relief organizations are the American Red Cross (ARC), the Federal Emergency Management Agency (FEMA), and the U.S. Department of Homeland Security (DHS). The ARC is a nongovernment agency that provides assistance to victims of overwhelming natural disasters (ARC, n.d.a). The mission of FEMA, a federal agency now part of the DHS, is to "assist first responders and the public to work together to improve national capacity to prevent, mitigate, and recover from all hazards (FEMA, 2009)." The DHS, as a result of the Homeland Security Act of 2002, was created via consolidation of multiple federal agencies into one organization, with the mission to "anticipate, preempt, detect and deter threats to the homeland and to safeguard our people and their freedoms, critical infrastructure, property and the economy of our nation from acts of terrorism, natural disasters and other emergencies" (DHS, n.d.). The DHS has been responsible for national planning and development of many key critical documents, including National Preparedness Goals, a National Response Plan (NRP), and a National Incident Management System (NIMS) (DHS, 2008a). The NRP was replaced by the National Response Framework (NRF) in 2008 (DHS, 2008c). The 2008 NIMS (DHS, 2008b) is available online (http://www.fema.gov/pdf/emergency/nims/NIMS_core.pdf).

Additionally, nongovernmental agencies, such as the ARC as well as local, state, and federal governments have increased efforts to recruit and train health professionals and other volunteers to augment customary services after a disaster. At the national level, some of these include the National Nurse Response Team, the Medical Reserve Corps, Disaster Medical Assistance Teams, and the Community Emergency Response Team. You may wish to check with your local or state health departments or the Board of Nurse Examiners for opportunities to volunteer. Additional training is often provided to volunteers.

Stages/Phases of Disaster Planning

Disaster experts have described several *disaster stages* or *phases* for the planning process. Though different models have been used, one commonly described model has four stages: preparedness, response, recovery, and mitigation. We apply this four-stage model to describe example community and nursing activities later in this chapter.

Agent-Specific and All-Hazards Approaches

Disaster planners may use either agent-specific or All-Hazards approaches in developing their plans. The *agent-specific approach* usually addresses the most likely threats or hazards. An example of the agent-specific approach may be planning for flooding in communities in flood-prone areas, with emphasis on public warning systems, flood prevention efforts, determination of evacuation routes and procedures, public education, and shelter provision. Another example could be planning done by the owners of a chemical plant and the surrounding community to prepare for a specific chemical release, with emphasis on warning systems, protection through sheltering in place, care for the injured or affected, control of the scene and its hazards, and investigation of the incident.

The DHS (2008a) requires a national *all-hazards* approach to disaster preparedness. All-Hazards planning emphasizes emergency or disaster preparedness for all segments of society (government, business, general public, etc.) for any type of emergencies or disasters. This approach identifies five hazard categories for which health professionals should be prepared:

1. *Natural* or *accidental man-made* disasters (e.g., a storm or fire)
2. *Traumatic* or *explosive* disasters: deliberate (e.g., a bomb) or accidental (e.g., a plane crash)
3. *Nuclear* (e.g., nuclear weapon detonation) or *radiation* disasters (e.g., a dirty bomb)
4. *Biologic* disasters: intentional release of pathogens or biologic agents to cause harm, also termed *bioterrorism* (e.g., anthrax), or natural or unintentional exposures (e.g., severe acute respiratory syndrome [SARS] or Avian flu outbreaks)
5. *Chemical* disasters: deliberate or accidental release of a harmful chemical (e.g., cyanide or chloride).

Consider a small island community and its potential disaster causes from an All-Hazards perspective. The island is vulnerable to storms and flooding (potential for natural disasters), with limited access and egress and with a substantial vulnerable population (including the elderly, children, undocumented persons, the immunocompromised, and the poor). The community has a port, railroads, and an airport, and it is located near major chemical facilities and a military base (potential for traumatic or explosive disasters). There is a nuclear power plant not far away, and the island also has large medical facilities (potential for radiologic/nuclear disasters). The port has had experiences with infectious diseases from around the world (potential for biologic disasters). Accidents at nearby chemical plants have resulted in unintentional releases of hazardous gases (potential for chemical disaster). The community's location—in a highly populated region, near a very large city and major business, industrial, financial, health, transportation, shipping, and technology centers—raises fears about intentional disasters. In preparing for all of these potential disaster causes, an All-Hazards response would include broad community collaborative planning and response, including multiple representatives of the community (law enforcement, education, local businesses, power resources, health systems, city government and other city leaders, transportation, communications, planners, service organizations, churches, other disaster organizations, members of the public, etc.). In addition, because of the large population in adjacent counties, and the large numbers of persons living in the region, collaboration with other nearby cities, counties, and the state would facilitate effective planning and preparing for any possible disaster. Multiple issues would need to be addressed, including evacuation, provisions for shelters or sheltering in place, control of infectious diseases, ensuring communication systems, emergency and routine health care, and recovery efforts.

Disaster Plans

Disaster plans should be simple, clear, realistic, flexible, and easy to implement regardless of the nature and extent of the disaster or who must implement the plan. Disaster plans should be tested (disaster drills, equipment checks, etc.), updated regularly, and evaluated periodically and every time used by those implementing the plan. All health care workers should be able to locate and implement the disaster plan at their workplace. In addition to professional responsibilities, nurses should also consider personal preparations and develop a personal disaster plan (Box 10.2).

Responding to a Disaster: The Disaster Paradigm

The Disaster Paradigm (AMA, 2004a, 2005) is a useful model for recognizing and managing a disaster scene. This paradigm establishes the eight priorities following the acronym *DISASTER*.

BOX 10.2

PERSONAL EMERGENCY PREPAREDNESS

The American Red Cross has identified simple emergency preparedness steps:

1. Assemble an emergency supply kit.
2. Prepare your personal emergency plan.
3. Be informed.

Adapted from the American Red Cross, n.d.b

Detect

Is this event a disaster or an MCI? Is it potential terrorism? Is its cause known?

Some disasters or other public health emergencies, such as those on September 11, 2001, at the World Trade Center, may be quickly obvious. Others may be difficult to detect for many reasons, such as: (1) delayed reactions to a biologic or chemical agent; (2) prolonged incubation period for a biologic organism; or (3) nonspecific symptoms which may be easily misdiagnosed. In addition, there may be *multiple causes or agents*, either concomitantly or sequentially.

Incident Command

Should emergency response or emergency management be activated? Is an Incident Command System (ICS) needed? If so, who will be in charge of the scene (e.g., who will be the Incident Commander [IC])?

The ICS is a standardized All-Hazards approach to handling emergencies that provides organizational structure and implementation or adaptation of response processes. The ICS has been used for many years by disaster response groups or organizations, such as fire, police, and emergency management. The ICS is organized according to five primary functions: Command, Operations, Planning, Logistics, and Finance/Administration. The ICS may have a single incident commander or a unified command, with the latter most commonly occurring when the incident is multi-jurisdictional or involves multiple agencies (DHS, 2008c). Hospitals have used an adaptation called the Hospital Emergency Incident Command System (HEICS).

Scene Security and Safety

Is the scene safe and secure?

Generally, a disaster scene is best thought *unsafe until proven otherwise*. Disaster and emergency workers should consider scene safety before entering a disaster scene. If the scene is potentially unsafe for victims or rescuers, entry may be denied or care may be held or halted until the scene is safe. Scene priorities suggested by the AMA (2004b) include: self-protection, followed by protection of health team members, the public, patients, and, lastly, the environment.

The scene must be secured so that only authorized persons leave and enter. If the event was caused deliberately, the scene and the evidence must be preserved.

Safety of responders to the scene is an important consideration. What, if any, *personal protective equipment (PPE)* is needed? The purpose of PPE is to protect people from exposure to a hazardous agent. Key considerations for effective PPE use include the type and amount of agent; how the agent was dispersed and in what setting (indoors or outdoors, large or small area, etc.); the scene activities needed; type of PPE required; and training for proper PPE usage.

Personnel at an emergency or disaster scene (and later at other care sites) must act to protect themselves before they can help others. This self-protection may include wearing PPE appropriate for the type of hazard. Health care workers are familiar with one type of PPE—that specified by Universal Precautions—and may have had additional experience with PPE for specific biologic or radiologic agents (e.g., gowns, gloves, surgical or other masks, protective goggles, booties, lead aprons, etc.). The U.S. Environmental Protection Agency (EPA) provides excellent descriptions of PPE needed by personnel dealing with various hazards (http://www.epa.gov/). For health professionals in health care settings, the

Occupational Safety and Health Administration (OSHA) (http://www.osha.gov/) identifies circumstances requiring health professional PPE usage, and the Centers for Disease Control and Prevention (CDC) recommends guidelines on PPE usage (http://www.cdc.gov/ncidod/dhqp/ppe.html).

Assess Hazards

Are scene hazards known? What hazard(s) are or might be present? Could this event be an act of terrorism?

One must assess both obvious and less-apparent hazards and be aware that disasters can involve multiple or sequential hazards. For example, an explosion can result in a release of toxic gases and fire. Secondary explosive devices may have been planted at a bomb scene and may be set to detonate when the rescuers arrive.

Support

What personnel, equipment, or supplies may be needed?

Depending on the situation, support considerations include personnel, organizations or agencies to be involved, facilities to be used, vehicles, and supplies (AMA, 2004b). Assessment of support needs also includes whether local, state, or federal assistance is needed.

Triage and Treatment

What are the injuries? Is triage (sorting of patients to determine treatment and evacuation priorities, using a standardized method) needed? What treatments are needed?

Many nurses are familiar with the concept of *triage* used in hospital emergency areas. Although triage is best done by those with triage and emergency care training and experience, and many courses exist to provide necessary training, nurses should be familiar with disaster triage models. In an overwhelming mass casualty event or true disaster, the emphasis of triage may shift from meeting the most urgent *individual* need to meeting the needs of the *largest numbers* of victims to maximize the number of lives saved. Because a mass casualty may compromise health systems' or professionals abilities to provide established care standards, the Agency for Health Care Quality (AHRQ) and the Office of the Assistant Secretary for Public Health Emergency Preparedness, U.S. Department of Health and Human Services (DHHS) convened an expert panel to develop standards of care for mass casualty events. The resulting document, "Altered Standards of Care in Mass Casualty Events," (AHRQ, 2005) is available online (http://www.ahrq.gov/research/altstand/).

Although there is no universal disaster triage system, several are well-known and used. One such system is the *Simple Triage and Rapid Treatment (START)* system. The START system uses a systematic approach (flow chart available at http://www.cert-la.com/triage/start.htm) based on three observations (**R**espiration, **P**erfusion, and **M**ental status [RPM]) to triage multiple victims into four categories. Rescuers move systematically through the scene, allotting 30 to 60 seconds or less per victim. The triage assignment is to locate patients in the immediate care priority, correct airway or breathing problems that are life-threatening, apply an immediate tag, then move on to the next victim. An online CERT training course is available (http://www.citizencorps.gov/cert/training_mat.shtm). Table 10.1 indicates examples of triage care and transport priorities.

TABLE 10.1

Examples of Triage Classifications for Care and Transport Priorities

Color and Classification	Characteristics	Care Priority	Transport Priority
Green: Minor/Delayed	May be injured/ill, but is stable and unlikely to deteriorate; able to move and follow commands	Delayed care	Transport after red and yellow
Yellow: Delayed/Urgent	Requires medical care but stable and able to wait, needs observation for deterioration	Urgent care	Transport after Red
Red: Critical/Immediate	Unstable and needs immediate care	Immediate care	Transport first/immediately
Black: Expectant: Dead or dying	Dead or not expected to survive, given available care resources	No care, comfort care	Lowest/Last

Adapted from CERT (n.d.) and AMA, 2004b.

A system recommended in National Disaster Life Support (NDLS) courses is the *M.A.S.S* triage system (Box 10.3), which also sorts by group, then individually, into "ID-ME" categories (AMA, 2005). In this system, M.A.S.S. stands for Move, Assess, Sort, and Send. "ID-ME" stands for Immediate, Delayed, Minimal, and Expectant. Victims' status may change rapidly, either improving or deteriorating. Thus, triage should be an ongoing activity.

Treatment for disaster victims depends on the type of emergency or disaster, scene safety, and resources needed and available. For instance, an explosion may result in blunt trauma injuries, crush injuries, penetrating injuries, blast injuries, burns, psychological distress, and so on. If needs and resources indicate a need for triage, initial treatment at the site of the event will be directed at emergency care and stabilization for the most severe injuries, and first aid or supportive care for those whose care can be delayed. Later treatment may include restorative and rehabilitative care.

Evacuation and Transport of Victims and Casualties

How many persons need evacuation and transportation, in what order, and by what mode of transport?

Evacuation indicates removal of both injured and uninjured persons to a safe environment. In general, triage categories also dictate transportation priority (Table 10.1). In an emergency, school buses, city buses, boats, trailers, planes or helicopters, private cars, and other vehicles may become emergency transport. Care should be taken to

BOX 10.3

MASS TRIAGE SYSTEM

M	Move	Request those able to move and walk to move to a specified safe site. Ask the remaining persons to raise a limb.
A	Assess	Assess individual patients, beginning with those unable to move.
S	Sort	Categorize victims based on urgency of care.
S	Send	Transport injured persons away from the scene.

Adapted from AMA, 2005.

minimize exposure to hazardous agents and contamination of transportation sources and care sites with hazardous agents. Guidelines to reduce further exposure may vary, depending on the agent. For instance, if a hazardous chemical has been released, it is recommended that the triage or "safe area" be upwind and uphill or elevated.

Victims of some hazardous agents may also require decontamination before transport. *Decontamination* involves removal or inactivation of the toxin or agent. Proper decontamination prevents further harm or injury to the victim; minimizes the risk of exposure to rescue workers, other health care workers, other patients, and other persons in the community; and avoids or minimizes environmental contamination. Decontamination should be done by those properly trained and equipped. Multiple resources are available that identify when decontamination is needed and how it should be done. Among these resources are the Agency for Toxic Substances and Disease Registry (ATSDR) (http://www.atsdr.cdc.gov/) and the CDC (http://www.cdc.gov/).

Recovery

What are immediate needs? What are needs several days after the incident? What are long-term needs?

Recovery is defined as "the period during which the community strives to return to a 'normal' function level" (AMA, 2004b, p. 9-1). Immediately after a disaster or emergency, the focus is usually on saving lives. Most lives "are saved in the period immediately following the disaster, with fewer lives saved following the first day of the event" (AMA, 2004b, p. 9-1). Within several days, however, communities need to begin to be able to meet their customary needs. In the long-term, the community may have multiple physical and mental health, economic, environmental, safety, transportation, communication, education, and other needs. However, disaster preparedness has a significant effect on reducing disaster stressors and assisting recovery.

Community and Nursing Activities for Disaster Preparedness

Many nursing skills needed in emergency or disaster situations are familiar to nurses, who have been performing them in the course of their normal duties in their routine work setting. Other skills, such as decontamination following a chemical release, may require specialized knowledge and training. Depending on the disaster and the setting, nurses may function dependently, independently, or interdependently as part of a response team. Although it is beyond the scope of this chapter to teach comprehensive community disaster or emergency preparedness, a number of excellent sources for additional learning have been described. Examples of activities to be performed by the community and nurse are described in Table 10.2.

Competencies

Planning for, preventing, and responding to public health needs caused by disasters and emergencies has long been a role of community health nurses. Since the terrorist events of 9/11, emergency preparedness competencies have been established by several organizations, including the Columbia University School of Nursing, Center for Disease Control and Prevention and the Association of Teachers of Preventive Medicine, the International Coalition for Mass Casualty Education (INCME, now renamed the Nursing Emergency Preparedness Education Coalition [NEPEC]), public health nurses, the Association of State and Territorial Directors of Nursing, and the National Organization of Nurse Practitioner Faculties (Kuntz, Frable, Quereshi, & Strong, 2008).

TABLE 10.2

Stages of Disaster Response: Community and Nursing Roles

	Community Activities	Examples of Nursing Activities
Stage 1: Prevention (Deterrence and early warning)	• Plan and prepare before event is expected, with the aim to prevent • Analyze community vulnerabilities and implement preventive activities • Identify community resources and capacities • Implement effective community warning systems	• Organize and participate in community immunization activities • Participate in agency or community vulnerability assessments and strategies for improvement • Develop/implement prevention strategies for worksites, community sites, home
Stage 2: Preparedness (Continued prevention and preparation for disaster response)	• Implement community disaster education • Evaluate and update policies and procedures • Develop cooperative agreements • Plan drills and training	• Volunteer for emergency response teams • Locate/be able to respond to institutional emergency plans • Develop/update institutional/community emergency plans or protocols • Develop volunteer registry to respond to emergency needs
Stage 3: Response (Management and mitigation)	• Respond to the event (short- and long-term) • Assess community damages, injuries, or needs immediately • Mitigate potential hazards • Provide aid and assistance from within the community and request and secure other needed resources • Involve public health and other agencies for surveillance and hazard control	• Assist with emergency plan activation • Assist with resource mobilization • Assist with public education • Assist with establishment and maintenance of shelters • Provide nursing care (first aid, triage, immunizations, prophylaxis, treatment, etc.) • Assess public health needs of affected communities or populations • Implement disease surveillance, vector control, hygiene measures, safety measures for food and water, etc.

Levels of Prevention

Emergency/disaster planning includes primary, secondary, and tertiary levels of prevention. For instance, evacuation before a major storm, provision of shelter to persons displaced by the storm, and assurance of a safe drinking water supply during and after the storm are examples of primary prevention (efforts to prevent harm or injury to persons in the affected community). Using the same storm analogy, screening for communicable diseases or anxiety reactions among shelter residents would be examples of secondary prevention (early identification and treatment of health problems). Caring for persons dying from storm-related effects, treating persons severely injured by the storm, and providing rehabilitation or psychological counseling services for persons with storm-related health problems would be examples of tertiary prevention.

PREVENTING AND MANAGING INFECTIOUS DISEASES

Despite amazing advances in public health and health care, such as the development of vaccines and improved sanitation, preventing and managing infectious diseases continue to be formidable challenges for health care systems everywhere. One contributor to the challenge is the rapid proliferation of drug-resistant organisms and diseases connected to antibiotic resistance (CDC, 2008a). Up-to-date information on drug resistance can be found at http://www.cdc.gov/drugresistance/diseases.htm. A second contributor is the emergence of new pathogens and new infectious diseases (CDC, 2009a). This is such an important issue that the CDC is now publishing a journal, *Emerging Infectious Diseases*, which is available at http://www.cdc.gov/ncidod/eid/. A third contributor to the challenge of preventing and managing infectious diseases arises from the recent threat that deadly pathogens will be used by terrorists (CDC, n.d.) with information available at http://www.bt.cdc.gov/bioterrorism/. These threats and challenges all have profound implications for nursing practice. Infectious disease control can no longer be limited to the jurisdiction of the public health department or the hospital infection control nurse. Every nurse, regardless of specialty area or practice setting, will be required to be knowledgeable about recognizing, preventing, and controlling infectious diseases. This section provides all nurses with the knowledge necessary to help prevent and control infectious diseases.

Healthy People 2010 and Infectious Diseases

One only needs to examine the Healthy People 2010 objectives to appreciate the magnitude of the infectious disease problem. Three of the 28 focus areas of Healthy People 2010 are devoted to infectious diseases. The focus areas include immunization and infectious diseases (25 objectives), sexually transmitted diseases (17 objectives), and HIV/AIDS (17 objectives). The objectives for each category specify the target populations at risk for the condition and specific prevention and early treatment activities. Examples of the objectives are listed in Box 10.4. Baseline and target data for the objectives can be found on the United States Department of Health and Human Services (2000) Healthy People website (http://healthypeople.gov).

Principles of Infection and Infectious Disease Occurrence

Biologic and epidemiologic principles inherent in infection and infectious disease occurrence are reviewed and major terms are defined in the following sections.

Multicausation

In a simpler time in medical and nursing history, science promulgated cause and effect theories of disease that relied on specifying one cause for each disease. Today, we recognize that all disease causation is complex and multicausal. Infectious diseases are the result of interaction among the *human host*, an *infectious agent*, and the *environment* that impacts the human host. This interaction is often pictured in a triangle of agent, host, and environment. The principle of multicausation emphasizes that an infectious agent alone is not sufficient to cause disease—the agent must be transmitted in the environment to a susceptible host.

Spectrum of Infection

Not all contact with an infectious agent leads to infection, and not all infection leads to an infectious disease. The processes, however, begin in the same way. An infectious agent may contaminate the skin or mucous membranes of a host but not invade the host. The agent may also invade and multiply and produce a *subclinical (asymptomatic) infection* without producing overt symptomatic disease. The host may also respond with symptomatic infectious disease. *Infection*, then, is the entry and multiplication of an infectious agent in a host. *Infectious disease* and *communicable disease* (synonyms, according to Heymann, 2008) refer to the pathophysiologic responses of the host to the infectious

HEALTHY PEOPLE 2010 OBJECTIVES

Immunizations and Infectious Diseases (selected from 25 objectives)

- Reduce or eliminate indigenous cases of vaccine-preventable diseases

Examples: hepatitis B in high-risk groups, bacterial meningitis in children, invasive pneumococcal infections, and hepatitis A

- Reduce meningococcal disease

Also: Lyme disease, new cases of hepatitis C, new cases of tuberculosis and invasive early-onset group B streptococcal disease

- Increase the proportion of persons with chronic hepatitis C infection identified by state and local health departments
- Increase the proportion of all TB patients who complete curative therapy within 12 months
- Increase the proportion of contacts and other high-risk persons with latent TB infection who complete a course of treatment
- Increase the proportion of international travelers who receive recommended preventive services when traveling in areas of risk for hepatitis A, malaria, and typhoid
- Reduce the number of courses of antibiotics for ear infections for young children
- Reduce the number of courses of antibiotics prescribed for the sole diagnosis of the common cold
- Achieve and maintain effective vaccination coverage levels for universally recommended vaccines among young children and adolescents
- Increase the proportion of providers who have measured the vaccination coverage levels among children in their practice population within the past 2 years
- Increase the proportion of children under 6 years of age who participate in fully operational population-based immunization registries
- Increase hepatitis B vaccine coverage among high-risk groups (long-term hemodialysis patients, men who have sex with men, and occupationally exposed workers)
- Increase the proportion of noninstitutionalized and institutionalized adults who are vaccinated annually against influenza
- Reduce vaccine-associated adverse events

Sexually Transmitted Diseases (STDs) (selected from 17 objectives)

- Reduce new cases of gonorrhea
- Eliminate sustained domestic transmission of primary and secondary syphilis
- Reduce the proportion of persons with human papillomavirus (HPV) infection, genital herpes infection, and *Chlamydia trachomatis* infections
- Reduce the proportion of females who have ever required treatment for pelvic inflammatory disease (PID)
- Reduce HIV infections in adolescent and young adult females aged 13 to 24 years that are associated with heterosexual contact
- Reduce neonatal consequences from maternal STDs, including chlamydial pneumonia, gonococcal and chlamydial ophthalmia neonatorum, laryngeal papillomatosis (from HPV infection), neonatal herpes, congenital syphilis, and preterm birth and low birth weight associated with bacterial vaginosis
- Increase the proportion of adolescents who abstain from sexual intercourse or use condoms if currently sexually active
- Increase the number of positive messages related to responsible sexual behavior during weekday and nightly prime-time television programming

B O X   10.4 (continued)

- Increase the proportion of tribal, state, and local STD programs that routinely offer hepatitis B vaccines to all STD clients
- Increase the proportion of youth detention facilities and adult city or county jails that screen for common bacterial STDs within 24 hours of admission and treat STDs before persons are released
- Increase the proportion of sexually active females aged 25 years and under who are screened annually for genital chlamydia infections
- Increase the proportion of pregnant females screened for STDs (including HIV and bacterial vaginosis) during prenatal health care visits, according to recognized standards
- Increase the proportion of all STD clinic patients who are being treated for bacterial STDs (chlamydia, gonorrhea, and syphilis) and who are offered provider referral services for their sex partners

HIV/AIDS (selected from 17 objectives)

- Reduce HIV infection and AIDS among adolescents and adults and all high-risk groups
- Increase the proportion of sexually active persons who use condoms
- Increase the number of HIV-positive persons who know their serostatus
- Increase the proportion of substance abuse treatment facilities that offer HIV/AIDS education, counseling, and support
- Increase the number of state prison systems that provide comprehensive HIV/AIDS, STD, and TB education
- Increase the proportion of inmates in state prison systems who receive voluntary HIV counseling and testing during incarceration
- Increase the proportion of adults with TB who have been tested for HIV
- Increase the proportion of adults in publicly funded HIV counseling and testing sites who are screened for common bacterial STDs (chlamydia, gonorrhea, and syphilis) and are immunized against hepatitis B virus
- Increase the proportion of HIV-infected adolescents and adults who receive testing, treatment, and prophylaxis consistent with current Public Health Service treatment guidelines
- Reduce deaths from HIV infection and AIDS
- Reduce new cases of perinatally acquired HIV infection

Sources: U.S. Department of Health and Human Services. (2000d). *Healthy people 2010: Immunizations and infectious diseases.* Retrieved January 20, 2009, from http://healthypeople.gov/document/html/volume1/14immunization
   U.S. Department of Health and Human Services. (2000e). *Healthy people 2010: Sexually transmitted diseases.* Retrieved January 20, 2009, from http://healthypeople.gov/document/html/volume2/25stds
   U.S. Department of Health and Human Services. (2000c). *Healthy people 2010: HIV.* Retrieved January 20, 2009, from http://healthypeople.gov/document/html/volume1/13hiv

agent, manifesting as an illness. Such a person, when diagnosed, would be considered a *case*. Once infectious agents replicate in the host, they can be transmitted from the host, irrespective of whether disease symptoms are or are not present. Some persons without any disease symptoms become *carriers* and continue to shed pathogens.

Stages of Infection

An infectious agent that has invaded its host and found conditions hospitable will replicate until it can be shed. This period of replication before shedding is called

Stages of Infection

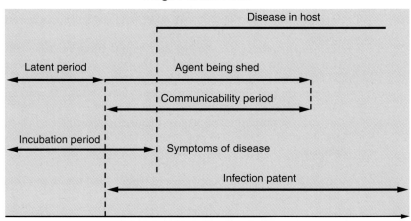

Total period of infection over time

Figure 10.1   Stages of infection. (Adapted from Grimes [1991] p. 19, with permission from Elsevier.)

the latent period, or *latency*. The *communicable period* or communicability follows latency and begins with shedding of the agent. *Incubation period* refers to the time of invasion to the time when disease symptoms first appear. Frequently, the communicable period begins before symptoms are present. The ability to distinguish these stages of infection (Fig. 10.1) is important in controlling transmission.

Spectrum of Disease Occurrence

The principles reviewed to this point apply to individuals and their acquisition of infections and infectious diseases. Control of infectious diseases in a population requires identifying and monitoring the occurrence of new cases (*incidence*) in a population. Some infectious diseases are *endemic* and occur at a consistent, expected level in a geographic area. Such is the case with some sexually transmitted diseases (STDs) and with tuberculosis. *Outbreak* refers to the unexpected occurrence of an infectious disease in a limited geographic area during a limited period of time. Outbreaks of pertussis and salmonellosis are common. *Pandemic* defines the steady occurrence of disease over a large geographic area or worldwide, such as malaria in Africa. *Epidemic* refers to the unexpected increase of an infectious disease in a geographic area over an extended period of time. Epidemics are defined relative to the infectious agent and the history of the disease in the area. One case of smallpox anywhere will constitute an epidemic, whereas 1,000 new cases of gonorrhea will not be considered an epidemic in an area where cases of gonorrhea commonly exceed that number.

Chain of Transmission

Transmission is frequently conceptualized as a chain (Fig. 10.2) with six interconnected links. Each of the links (infectious agent, reservoir, portal of exit, mode of transmission, portal of entry, and host susceptibility) represents a different component that acts to produce transmission. The chain of transmission and its elements are summarized in Table 10.3.

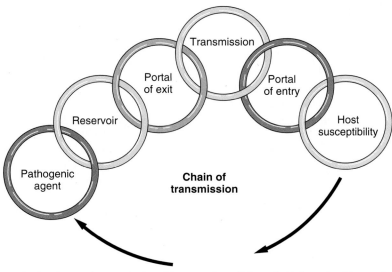

Figure 10.2   Chain of transmission. (Redrawn from Grimes [1991] p. 21, with permission from Elsevier.)

TABLE 10.3

Chain of Transmission

Links of the Chain	Definition	Factors
Infectious agent	An organism (virus, *Rickettsia*, bacteria, fungus, protozoan, helminth, or prion) capable of producing infection or infectious disease	Properties of the agent: morphology, chemical composition, growth requirements, and viability Interaction with the host: mode of action, infectivity, pathogenicity, virulence, toxigenicity, antigenicity, and ability to adapt to the host
Reservoirs	The environment in which a pathogen lives and multiples	Humans, animals, arthropods, plants, soil, or any other organic substance
Portal of exit	Means by which an infectious agent is transported from the host	Respiratory secretions, vaginal secretions, semen, saliva, lesion exudates, blood, and feces
Mode of transmission	Method whereby the infectious agent is transmitted from one host (or reservoir) to another host	Direct: person-to-person Indirect: implies a vehicle of transmission (biologic or mechanical vector, common vehicles, or fomite) Airborne droplets
Portal of entry	Means by which an infectious agent enters a new host	Respiratory passages, mucous membranes, skin, percutaneous injection, ingestion, and through the placenta
Host susceptibility	The presence or lack of sufficient resistance to an infectious agent to avoid prevent contracting an infection or acquiring an infectious disease	Biologic and personal characteristics (e.g., gender, age, genetics), general health status, personal behaviors, anatomic and physiologic lines of defense, and immunity

Infectious Agents

Infectious agents are organisms capable of producing infection in a host. Because the process of transmission is different for every infectious agent, one might envision a different configuration of the chain and its links for every infectious agent. Infectious agents act differently depending on their intrinsic properties and how they interact with their human host. For example, an agent's size, shape, chemical composition, growth requirements, and viability (ability to survive for extended periods of time) have an impact on transmission and the type of parasitic relationship it establishes with its host. Agents are classified as viruses, bacteria, fungi, protozoa, *Rickettsia*, helminths, and prions, based on their characteristics. Knowing the classification is helpful in understanding how specific agents are transmitted and produce disease. Also important is how the agent interacts with its host. What is its mode of action in the body? Does it kill cells as does *Mycobacterium tuberculosis*, or does it interfere with circulation as does the spirochete of syphilis? Or maybe it produces a toxin (*toxigenicity*) as does *Clostridium botulinum* or stimulates an immune response in the host (*antigenicity*) as does the rubella virus. Other considerations for understanding the action of agents include their power to invade and infect large numbers of people (*infectivity*); their ability to produce disease in those infected with the agent (*pathogenicity*); and their ability to produce serious disease in their hosts (*virulence*). Applying the above concepts, the chickenpox virus has high infectivity, high pathogenicity, and very low virulence. On the other hand, *M. tuberculosis* has low infectivity, low pathogenicity, but high virulence if untreated. Smallpox is high on all three concepts. Last, how adaptable is an agent to its human host, and does the agent change (mutate) over time as does HIV?

Reservoirs

The reservoir is the environment in which a pathogen lives and multiplies. Reservoirs can be humans, animals, arthropods, plants, soil, or any other organic substance. Some pathogens have more than one reservoir. Knowing the reservoir is important because in some cases transmission can be controlled by eliminating the reservoir. Understanding the reservoir of bird flu, for example, is important for any plans to prevent future pandemics in humans.

Portals of Exit and Entry

Agents are communicated from the human host through a *portal of exit* and invade through a *portal of entry*. Portals of exit include respiratory secretions, vaginal secretions, semen, saliva, lesion exudates, blood, and feces. Portals of entry frequently correspond with the portal of exit and include the respiratory passages, mucous membranes, open wounds, ingestion, and through the placenta or skin.

Modes of Transmission

Direct transmission implies the immediate transfer of an infectious agent from an infected host or reservoir to a portal of entry in the human host through physical contact such as touching, biting, kissing, or sexual contact. Direct projections of mucous secretions in the way of droplet spray to the conjunctiva; or mucous membranes of the eye, nose, or mouth during coughing, sneezing, and laughing is also considered direct transmission. Direct contact is responsible for the transmission of many communicable diseases, including scabies and STDs.

Indirect transmission is the spread of infection through a vehicle of transmission outside the host. Such vehicles may be contaminated fomites or vectors. *Fomites* can be any inanimate object, material, or substance that acts as a transport agent for a microbe (e.g., water, a telephone, or a contaminated tissue). Reproduction of the infectious agent may take place on or in the vehicle before the transmission of the pathogen. Substances such as food, water, and blood products can provide indirect transmission through ingestion and intravenous transfusions.

Vectors can be animals, insects, or arthropods, and they can transmit infection through biologic and mechanical routes. Biologic transmission occurs when the parasite grows or multiplies inside the animal, vector, or arthropod. Examples of diseases spread by this method of transmission include malaria, hemorrhagic fevers, and viral encephalitis. The mechanical route involves no multiplication or growth of the parasite or microbe within the animal or vector itself. Such is the case when a housefly carries gastrointestinal agents from raw sewage to uncovered food.

Fecal–oral transmission can be both direct and indirect. Examples of indirect transmission include water or food contaminated with fecal pathogens by way of raw sewage or unwashed hands. Unprotected oral–genital–anal sexual activity may result in direct transmission of fecal pathogens.

Airborne transmission mainly occurs through aerosols and droplet nuclei. The time frame in which an airborne particle can remain suspended and the size of the particle greatly influence the infectivity of the organism. Aerosols are extremely small solid or liquid particles that may contain fungal spores, viruses, and bacteria. Droplet nuclei, such as the spray from a sneeze, travel approximately 1 m but usually not farther before the droplets fall to the ground. Within this distance, contaminated droplets may make direct contact with an open wound or with a mucous membrane (e.g., conjunctiva, nose, or mouth), or they may be inhaled into the lung. *M. tuberculosis* is transmitted through inhalation of contaminated droplets.

Host Susceptibility

Not all humans are equally *susceptible* or at risk for contracting an infection or developing infectious diseases. Biologic and personal characteristics play an important role in host resistance (defense against the infectious agent). Just as the young are more susceptible to diphtheria, older adults are at greater risk for bacterial pneumonia. General health status is important as evidenced by the increased risk for gastrointestinal parasites experienced by children living in poverty. Personal behaviors certainly influence susceptibility as does the presence of healthy lines of defense. One is reminded of the importance of the immune system and immunization status when observing the preponderance of infections experienced by the unimmunized and immune-compromised persons.

Breaking the Chain of Transmission

Breaking of one of the links in the chain of transmission is presented in Figure 10.2. Breaking just one link of the chain at its most vulnerable point is, in fact, what is done to control transmission of an infectious agent. Of course, where the chain is broken depends on all of the factors that have just been discussed—characteristics of the agent, its reservoir, portals of exit and entry, how the agent is transmitted, and susceptibility of the host.

Controlling the Agent

Controlling the agent is an area in which technology and medical science have been effective. Inactivating the agent is the principle behind disinfection, sterilization, and radiation of fomites that may harbor pathogens. Anti-infective drugs, such as antibiotics, antivirals, antiretrovirals, and antimalarials, all play an important part in controlling infectious diseases. These drugs not only permit recovery of the infected person, but also play a major role in preventing transmission of the pathogens. Recall that an important step in preventing transmission of tuberculosis and syphilis is to treat the infected person with antibiotics.

Eradicating the Non–Human Reservoir

Common nonhuman reservoirs for pathogens in the environment include water, food, milk, animals, insects, and sewage. Treating these reservoirs or eliminating them, for example, by spraying for mosquitoes, are effective methods of preventing replication of pathogens and, thus, preventing transmission.

Controlling the Human Reservoir

Treating infected persons, whether they are symptomatic or not, is effective in preventing transmission of pathogens that can be transmitted directly to others. Another method of control is to quarantine, which means restricting the activities of those who have been exposed to an infectious agent during the incubation period. Quarantine was used effectively during the outbreak of SARS in 2003, when some hospitals required that their staff, which was exposed to SARS patients, remain at the hospital until proven symptom free at the end of the incubation period.

Controlling the Portals of Exit and Entry

Nurses and other health care providers break the transmission chain at the portal of exit by properly disposing of secretions, excretions, and exudates from infected persons. In addition, controlling portals of exit and entry may involve isolating sick persons from others and requiring that persons with tuberculosis wear a mask in public.

The portal of entry of pathogens can also be controlled in a variety of ways, including using barrier precautions (masks, gloves, condoms); avoiding unnecessary invasive procedures such as indwelling catheters; and protecting oneself from vectors, such as mosquitoes. Universal precaution guidelines are based on the observation that infected people may have no signs or symptoms or may not have any knowledge of their conditions; therefore all people are assumed to be infectious, and health care workers treat them as such.

Improving Host Resistance and Immunity

Many factors, such as age, general health status, nutrition, and health behaviors contribute to host resistance. Immunity, however, is an indispensable defense against infection. There are several different kinds of immunity, each providing resistance in different ways to different pathogens. *Natural immunity* is an innate resistance to a specific antigen or toxin. *Acquired immunity* is derived from actual exposure to the specific infectious agent, toxin, or appropriate vaccine. The two types of acquired immunity are *active* and *passive*. *Active immunity* is when the body produces its own antibodies against an antigen, either as a result of infection with the pathogen or introduction of the pathogen in a vaccine. *Passive immunity* is the temporary resistance

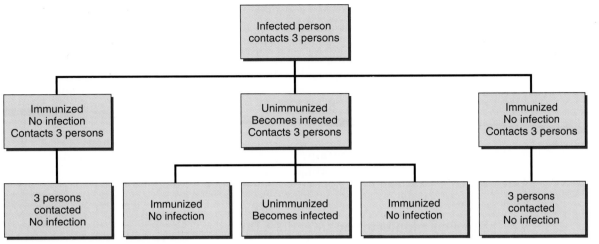

Figure 10.3 Example of herd immunity. Sixty six percent are immunized and distributed evenly in the population: 77% (10/13) are protected.

that has been donated to the host through transfusions of plasma proteins, immunoglobulins, and antitoxins, or transplacentally from mother to neonate. Passive immunity lasts only as long as these substances remain in the bloodstream.

When properly administered according to established guidelines and protocols, vaccines provide acquired immunity in most cases; however, there are exceptions. *Primary vaccine failure* is the failure of a vaccine to stimulate any immune response and can be caused by improper storage that may render the vaccines ineffective, improper administration route, or exposure of light-sensitive vaccines to light. Some immunized persons never seroconvert, due to either failure of their own immune system or some other unknown reason. *Secondary vaccine failure* is the waning of immunity following an initial immune response. This failure occurs in immune-suppressed patients whose immune memory is essentially destroyed.

Herd immunity refers to a state in which those not immune to an infectious agent will be safe if a certain proportion (generally considered to be 80%) of the population has been vaccinated or is otherwise immune. This effect applies only if those immune are distributed among the population. Without the presence of a susceptible population to infect, the organism will be unable to live because the vast majority of the population is immune. An example that demonstrates the principle of herd immunity appears in Figure 10.3.

Public Health Control of Infectious Diseases

Most human diseases can be classified as "personal health problems." Individuals with a personal health problem can be treated by the health care system one person at a time. In contrast, infectious diseases are categorized as public or "community" health problems. Because of their potential to spread and cause communitywide or worldwide emergencies, infectious diseases require organized, public efforts for their prevention and control.

Such organized, public efforts are under the jurisdiction of official public health agencies at the local, state, national, and international levels. Each of these units of government obtains its powers through a complex array of laws. An important concept to remember is that, in areas of health within a state, state laws usually prevail over federal law. The U.S. Constitution does not address health and the Tenth Amendment reserves power to the states over all issues not addressed in the Constitution (Schneider, 2006). Historically, states have accepted this responsibility. For example, all states have laws addressing infectious disease control, such as which diseases must be reported and who has authority to implement quarantines. All states have boards of health and departments of health to implement and enforce state health laws.

The CDC is the public health entity at the national level responsible for infectious disease control. The CDC has the responsibility for monitoring infectious diseases and supporting local and state governments in control of outbreaks or epidemics, if such assistance is needed.

Although there are many aspects of public health control of infectious diseases, four are discussed here: reporting diseases, preventing diseases by vaccination, responding to an outbreak, and risk communication.

Defining and Reporting Infectious Diseases

Standardizing definitions of diseases is important for public health monitoring and surveillance at all levels of government. Diseases are defined and classified according to confirmed cases, probable cases, laboratory-confirmed cases, clinically compatible cases, epidemiologically linked cases, genetic typing, and clinical case definition. Once defined, disease occurrence can be compared across time, populations, and geographic areas and appropriate control efforts can be implemented.

Along with the Council of State and Territorial Epidemiologists, the CDC has designated notifiable infectious diseases, meaning that health care providers who encounter these diseases must report them to the local or regional health department. A list of notifiable diseases published by CDC (2009b) can be found at http://www.cdc.gov/ncphi/diss/nndss/phs/infdis.htm. Because state health departments have the responsibility for monitoring and controlling communicable diseases within their respective states, they determine which diseases will be reported within their jurisdiction. While not all nationally notifiable diseases are reportable in every state or territory, some states have notifiable disease lists that are longer than the CDC's list. As a health professional, you are advised to check the websites of your state health department for specifics about reporting laws in your state. The processes for reporting also vary by state, and this information generally is available on the state health department's website. Generally, providers are encouraged to report cases of infectious diseases to their local or regional health departments, which will then report to the state and to the CDC.

The CDC publishes a weekly listing of notifiable diseases reported by region, state, and nation in *Morbidity and Mortality Weekly Report* (MMWR). MMWR can be found in medical libraries, at local health departments, at infection control departments in hospitals and medical centers, and on the Internet at http://www.cdc.gov.

Preventing by Vaccination

As with other areas of health care, information and recommendations on immunizations and vaccine usage change regularly. Therefore, it is imperative that you seek the most current information on the CDC website and in its publications. Recommendations, policies, and procedures concerning international immunization practices are determined by the World Health Organization (WHO). National governance is provided by the American Academy of Pediatrics (AAP) Committee on Infectious Diseases and the U.S. Public Health Service Advisory Committee on Immunization Practices (ACIP). Occasionally, these agencies differ on their

B O X 10.5

WEBSITES FOR RECOMMENDED VACCINATION SCHEDULES

CDC. (2009). Immunization Schedules. Retrieved January 22, 2009, from
  http://www.cdc.gov/vaccines/recs/schedules/default.htm
CDC. (2009). Child & Adolescent Immunization Schedules Retrieved January 22,
  2009, from http://www.cdc.gov/vaccines/recs/schedules/child-schedule.htm
CDC. (2009). Adult Immunization Schedule: Immunization Recommendation,
  United States-2009 Retrieved January 22, 2009, from http://www.cdc.gov/
  vaccines/recs/schedules/adult-schedule.htm
CDC. (2008). Healthcare Personnel Vaccination Recommendations Retrieved
  January 22, 2009, from http://www.immunize.org/catg.d/p2017.pdf

recommendations. Therefore, it is important to consider the population involved when implementing these recommendations and procedures.

Precautions must be taken when giving any immunization. The most recent recommendations regarding which immunizations to give; to whom they should be given; how they should be given; and how they are to be transported, stored, and administered can be obtained from the CDC. See Box 10.5 for important websites for recommended vaccination schedules for selected population groups.

The CDC produces Vaccine Information Statements (VISs) that explain both the benefits and risks to vaccine recipients, their parents, or their legal representatives. Federal law requires that VISs be handed out before vaccinations are given. These statements can be downloaded from the CDC website at http://www.cdc.gov/vaccines/pubs/vis/default.htm.

Legal documentation of vaccinations is important for future administration and follow-up of hypersensitivity reactions. The health care provider, often the nurse, is responsible for maintaining accurate records, including patient name, date(s) immunized, vaccine type, vaccine manufacturer, vaccine lot number, date of the VIS; and the name, title, and address of the person administering the vaccine (CDC, 2008c).

To monitor actual and potential vaccine-related problems, health care providers must report specific postvaccination "adverse events" to the Vaccine Adverse Event Reporting System (VAERS). Information and reporting forms are available in both the FDA Drug Bulletin and the Physicians' Desk Reference and through a 24-hour recorded telephone message at 1-800-822-7967. Information from the U.S. DHHS (n.d.b) on VAERS is available at http://www.hhs.gov, and CDC (2008b) VAERS information is at http://www.cdc.gov/vaccinesafety/vaers. The National Vaccine Injury Compensation Program reviews all VAERS reports.

The National Vaccine Injury Compensation Program became effective as a result of the National Childhood Vaccine Injury Act of 1986. This system provides assistance for individuals and families who experience a vaccine-related injury, including disability and death.

Responding to an Outbreak

An outbreak of an infectious disease requires organized community efforts to investigate and contain the outbreak as well as to provide care to infected persons. The investigation and containment are generally the responsibility of the local health department, interacting with the health care system that provides treatment to the ill. Systematic and overlapping steps for investigating and containing an outbreak have been identified (Heymann, 2008). These are summarized here:

1. Verify the diagnosis and establish a case definition. This requires recognition and reporting by a health care worker to the health department of the first and subsequent cases of an unusual condition. The report should include characteristics of the case that will aid in the investigation, such as history, physical exam findings, and results of laboratory tests.
2. Confirm the existence of an outbreak. Is the incidence of the infectious disease greater now and in this place than expected? This requires comparing recent new cases with incidence over an appropriate period of time for the area. Mapping the new cases by geographic area may help to confirm the areas where the outbreak is greatest.
3. Identify the characteristics of the affected persons. Record their case histories and identify new cases. Enumerate all cases and their distribution by person, place, and time (i.e., who are they, where are the cases located, when did they get ill. What do these persons have in common demographically, socially, and behaviorally?).
4. Define and investigate the population at risk. Did they eat in the same restaurant, attend the same sporting event, go to the same school, or travel on the same airplane? Once the population at risk is identified, the denominator is known and attack rates can be calculated.
5. Investigate the outbreak and formulate a hypothesis as to its chain of transmission. What was the causative agent, reservoir, mode of transmission, portal of exit, portal of entry, and host susceptibility?
6. Determine the most effective control measures based on the chain of transmission. Implement control measures.

Risk Communication

Local public health agencies have the official responsibility for communicating with the public during infectious disease outbreaks in their jursidiction. Regional and/or state public health agencies may assume such responsibilities if the outbreak extends beyond the boundaries of a local agency. All health professionals who are knowledgeable and/or caring for victims of the outbreak may also be asked to communicate with the public about the event. Effective communication is essential to prevent widespread panic and to elicit support from the public to behave in a fashion that will help to contain the outbreak. Given the importance of conveying the message effectively and in a timely manner, public health professionals are emphasizing the principles of communicating risks to the public, also known as "risk communication."

Characteristics of an infectious disease outbreak create challenges for those responsible for communicating with the public, according to Kindhauser and Thompson (2008). First, infectious disease outbreaks are generally cloaked in uncertainty—uncertainty about the causal agent, about transmission, who is and is not at risk, effective preventive and treatment measures, etc. Facts may unfold incrementally, and yesterday's communication may prove to be wrong. Second, anxiety can be expected. It can have social, economic, and political consequences and lead to unproductive behaviors if ignored. Third, the outbreak may have a social, economic, and political impact beyond the immediate area where it occurred. An example of this in the United States was the detection of one cow with bovine spongiform encephalopathy (BSE), which was estimated to cost the U.S. economy $2 billion in lost beef sales (Kindhauser & Thompson, 2008).

Given these specific challenges, Kindauser and Thompson (2008) have identified five principles for effective risk communication: trust, early announcement, transparency, listening, and planning. These principles are summarized here as a resource for nurses who are frequently asked to provide information to professional and community groups before, during, and after an infectious disease outbreak.

Trust needs little explanation. It is important, however, to recall that trust or distrust are established long before an emergency event occurs. The public who trusts that the nurse or agency spokesperson will be honest about the event is more likely to hear the message and heed the advice. Announcing early is an important prerequisite to maintaining the public's trust as well as alerting the public to preventive measures. Good risk communicators do not wait until all of the facts are collected. They tell what is known as soon as it is known, admitting that they do not yet have complete information. This fulfills the "information vacuum" before it becomes filled with information from less-reliable sources.

Transparent communication is truthful and easy to understand. It reinforces trust. This principle is probably the most difficult to achieve. Health officials and professionals may withhold information due to the worry that they will be blamed or held accountable for the emergency. In addition, if resources, such as vaccines or ICU beds, are limited, the communicator may not want to acknowledge publicly who will or will not receive the resources. With the speed of communication today, the truth will eventually emerge, reinforcing the need for transparency from the onset of the emergency.

Nurses learn early that listening to the patient, the family, and the community is the first step in communicating. Nurses ask questions about what someone knows before trying to provide information to the person, and nurses avoid preaching. One-way communication with the public must be avoided during emergencies of any type. Good risk communicators monitor what people know and are saying during an emergency. They also monitor the press and, lately, the late night talk shows and the Internet blogs. The intent of the monitoring is not to be judgmental but rather to understand the public's perceptions so as to shape the message to that perception.

Communicating effectively with the public during any type of a community emergency is complex and, like all community health work, requires planning. All health care and public health agencies should designate and train knowledgeable persons to communicate with the public during an infectious disease outbreak. Nurses with the knowledge of the community may be the best risk communicators in such a situation.

Community and Nursing Activities for Preventing and Controlling Infectious Diseases

All practicing nurses have a role in primary, secondary, and tertiary prevention of infectious diseases, both for individuals and for the community as a whole. Table 10.4 provides examples of primary, secondary, and tertiary prevention strategies directed at individuals and populations for specific diseases.

TABLE 10.4

Examples of Prevention Activities for Control of Infectious Diseases at the Individual and Population Levels

Infectious Disease	Individual	Population
Primary prevention		
Sexually transmitted disease	Teach safe sex practices	Place condom machines in accessible areas in places where young adults congregate
		Immunize for Human papillomavirus (HPV)
Diseases caused by blood-borne pathogens	Teach barrier precautions to all health care workers	Provide an adequate supply of gloves and sharp containers available in patient care areas
	Teach injecting drug users about dangers of sharing needles	Initiate citywide Needle Exchange programs and Methadone programs
Vaccine-preventable diseases	Ensure that all children who come to the clinic have age-appropriate immunizations	Work with community groups to cosponsor immunization clinics where immunization rates are low
Hepatitis A, gastrointestinal infections	Teach safe food-handling practices at home	Require, as part of the licensing of restaurants, that food handlers take a course in safe food handling
Hepatitis A and B	Immunize against hepatitis B; immunize those at risk against hepatitis A	Mandate that health care workers are immunized for hepatitis A and B
	Provide immune globulin after exposure to hepatitis A or B	
Secondary prevention		
STDs	Screen and treat for all STDs	STD Partner Notification Program
Tuberculosis	Screen close contacts of persons with TB	Initiate a program of yearly testing of health care workers for TB
	Treat persons with a recent skin test - conversion	Provide treatment to all recent converters free of charge at their workplace
HIV/AIDS	Provide testing and treatment for HIV in local clinics	Initiate reporting of HIV cases by name to the local health department to facilitate surveillance of HIV in population
	Ensure that patients adhere to antiretroviral therapy; monitor adherence	
Meningitis	Immunize and provide chemoprophylaxis for persons exposed to meningitis	Provide immunization and chemoprophylaxis to all students in a school following an exposure
Tertiary prevention		
Tuberculosis	Provide therapy for person with active TB	Initiate a Directly Observed Therapy (DOT) program in the community shelters and jails
	Teach patients to take all doses of prescribed antibiotics and monitor adherence	Initiate community education campaigns about the problem of drug resistance associated with incomplete antibiotic use

Summary

In this chapter, we have confronted the challenges posed by two forms of community emergencies: disasters and infectious diseases. Though different, disasters and infectious diseases share characteristics. Both may impact the entire community; both require organized community efforts for prevention and control; and both will impact nurses wherever they practice. The knowledge base for preventing and managing community emergencies is evolving. Nurses are advised to continue to learn about and prepare themselves to live and practice safely and effectively when such emergencies occur.

Critical Thinking Questions

1. You have been asked to participate as a member of your worksite's All Hazards emergency preparedness team. What knowledge and skills do you bring to the team? What skills or knowledge would you need to improve? How would you improve your effectiveness as a team member?

2. As you are driving down a small country road on the way to a community festival, you come on the scene of an accident involving a tanker truck and a train. The truck is on its side, with liquid leaking from its tank. You cannot see the truck driver. Several railroad cars have derailed and are lying on their sides. You can see writing on the cars' sides, which seems to indicate there could be chemicals in the rail cars, though you cannot read the writing from your vantage point. No one else is visible at the scene, although you see people running down the track from the railroad engine toward the derailment site, and you also see another vehicle coming up from behind you. You know you are about 3 miles from the community. What should you do and in what order (what are the scene priorities)?

3. You are employed as a school nurse by Student Health Services at a local college. You are called to a dorm room to see a student who is extremely ill with symptoms that are consistent with meningococcal meningitis. After you send (or escort) the student to the local hospital emergency department for confirmatory diagnosis and treatment, you recognize the implication of the student's infection on the health of the college population.

   a. What multicausal factors for meningococcal meningitis are applicable to the college population? What risk factors are likely to be present in this population?
   b. What is the chain of transmission for meningococcal meningitis?
   c. What is the most effective way of breaking the chain of transmission?
   d. Where can you access information to answer the above questions?
   e. What is your responsibility for reporting this case of meningitis?
   f. How can you learn the requirements and procedures for reporting infectious diseases in your state?
   g. What are the primary, secondary, and tertiary prevention strategies related to meningococcal meningitis that you will implement now and in the future at the college? Which of these strategies are identified in the Healthy People 2010 objectives?

● REFERENCES

Altered standards of care in mass casualty events. (2005). Prepared by Health Systems Research Inc. under Contract No. 290-04-0010. AHRQ Publication No. 05-0043. Rockville, MD: Agency for Healthcare Research and Quality. Retrieved January 9, 2009, from http://www.ahrq.gov/research/altstand/

American Medical Association (AMA). (2004a). *Basic disaster life support* (version 2.5). Chicago, IL: Author.

American Medical Association (AMA). (2004b). *Core disaster life support* (version 1.01). Chicago, IL: Author.

American Medical Association (AMA). (2005). *Management of public health emergencies: A resource for physicians and other community providers*. Washington, DC: Author.

Centers for Disease Control and Prevention. (2005). Health concerns associated with disaster victim identifications after a tsunami—Thailand, December 26, 2004–March 31, 2005. *MMWR*, 54, 349–352. Retrieved February 3, 2009, from http://www.cdc.gov/mmwr/preview/mmwrhtml/mm5414a1.htm.

Centers for Disease Control and Prevention. (2008a). Diseases connected to antibiotic resistance. Retrieved January 20, 2009, from http://www.cdc.gov/drugresistance/diseases.htm.

Centers for Disease Control and Prevention (2008b). Vaccine Adverse Event reporting System (VAERS). Retrieved January 21, 2009 from http://www.cdc.gov/vaccine safety/vaers.

Centers for Disease Control and Prevention. (2008c). Vaccine information statements (VIS). Retrieved January 22, 2009, from http://www.cdc.gov/vaccines/pubs/vis/default.htm.

Centers for Disease Control and Prevention (2009a). Emerging Infectious Disease Journal. Retrieved January 20, 2009 from http://www.cdc.gov/ncidod/eid.

Centers for Disease Control and Prevention. (2009b). Nationally notifiable infectious diseases. Retrieved January 21, 2009, from http://www.cdc.gov/ncphi/diss/phs/infdis.htm.

Dorn, T., Yzermans, J. C., Spreeuwenberg, P. M. M., Schilder, A., & van der Zee, J. (2008). A cohort study of the long-term impact of a fire disaster on the physical and mental health of adolescents. *Journal of Traumatic Stress*, 21, 239–242.

Federal Emergency Management Agency (FEMA). (2009). About FEMA. Retrieved December 30, 2008, from http://www.fema.gov/about/index.shtm

Grimes, D. E. (1991). *Infectious diseases*. St. Louis, MO: Mosby Year Book.

Heymann, D. L. (Ed.). (2008). *Control of communicable diseases manual* (19th ed.). Washington, DC: American Public Health Association.

Kindhauser, M. K., & Thompson, D. (2008). Risk communication during a communicable disease outbreak. In D. L. Heymann (Ed.). *Control of communicable diseases manual* (pp. A20–A27). Washington DC: American Public Health Association.

Kuntz, S. W., Frable, P., Quereshi, K., & Strong, L. L. (2008). Association of Community Health Nursing Educators: Disaster preparedness white paper for community/public health nursing educators. *Public Health Nursing*, 25, 362–369.

Noji, E. K. (2005). *Public health disaster consequences of disasters*. Retrieved January 15, 2009, from http://www.pitt.edu/~super1/lecture/lec20351/index.htm

Schneider, M-J. (2006). *Introduction to public health* (2nd ed.). Boston: Jones and Bartlett.

United States Department of Health and Human Services. (2000a). Healthy People 2010: Access to quality health services. Retrieved August 12, 2005, from http://www.healthypeople.gov/document/HTML/Volume1/01Access.htm#_Toc489432817.

United States Department of Health and Human Services. (2000b). Healthy People 2010: Environmental health. Retrieved January 15, 2009, from http://www.healthypeople.gov/document/HTML/Volume1/08Environmental.htm#_Toc490564712.

United States Department of Health and Human Services. (2000c). Healthy people 2010: HIV. Retrieved January 20, 2009, from http://www.healthypeople.gov/document/html/volume1/13hiv.

United States Department of Health and Human Services. (2000d). Healthy people 2010: Immunizations and infectious diseases. Retrieved January 20, 2009, from http://www.healthypeople.gov/document/html/volume1/14immunization.htm. Healthy People 2010: Public health infrastructure. Retrieved January 20, 2009, from http://www.healthypeople.gov/document/HTML/Volume2/23PHI.htm.

United States Department of Health and Human Services. (2000e). Healthy people 2010: Sexually transmitted diseases. Retrieved January 20, 2009, from http://healthypeople.gov/document/html/volume2/25stds.htm.

U.S. Department of Health & Human Services. (2008a). Hurricane Katrina. Retrieved December 30, 2008, from http://www.hhs.gov/disasters/emergency/naturaldisasters/hurricanes/katrina/index.html.

U.S. Department of Health & Human Services (2008b). VAERS—The Vaccine Adverse Event Reporting System. Retrieved January 21, 2009 from http://vaers.hhs.gov.

U.S. Department of Homeland Security (DHS). (2008). Prevention and Protection. Retrieved January 9, 2009, from http://www.dhs.gov/xprevprot/.

U.S. Department of Homeland Security (DHS). (2008a). Homeland Security Directive 8: National Preparedness. Retrieved January 9, 2009, from http://www.dhs.gov/xabout/laws/gc_1215444247124.shtm

U.S. Department of Homeland Security (DHS). (2008b). National incident management system. Retrieved January 9, 2009, from http://www.fema.gov/pdf/emergency/nims/NIMS_core.pdf.

U.S. Department of Homeland Security (DHS). (2008c). *National response framework*. Retrieved January 9, 2009, from http://www.dhs.gov/xprepresp/committees/editorial_0566.shtm.

Veneema, T. G. (2007). Essentials of disaster planning. In T. G. Veneema (Ed.), *Disaster nursing and emergency preparedness for chemical, biologic, and radiological terrorism and other hazards* (2nd ed.) (pp. 3–19). New York: Springer.

World Health Organization (WHO). (n.d.). Disasters. Retrieved January 15, 2009, from http://www.wpro.who.int/health_topics/disasters/

World Health Organization (WHO). (2005). Tsunami recovery process focuses on long-term development. Retrieved February 3, 2009, from http://www.who.int/mediacentre/news/releases/2005/pr30_searo/en/print.html.

Internet Resources can be found on the**Point** at http://thepoint.lww.com/Anderson6e.

The Process

PART

2

Community Assessment: Using a Model for Practice

ELIZABETH T. ANDERSON AND JUDITH MCFARLANE

LEARNING OBJECTIVES

Preceding chapters have focused on the foundational concepts of community health, epidemiology, environment, culture, ethics, empowerment, health policy, informatics, bioterrorism, and emerging infectious diseases. This chapter and the four that follow focus on the application of the nursing process in the community using a selected model. This chapter takes you through the process of assessing a community using a nursing model.

After studying this chapter, you should be able to:

1. Begin to use a community nursing model in practice.
2. Complete a community health assessment using a selected model.

Introduction

*C*ommunity assessment is a process; it is the act of becoming acquainted with a community. The people in the community are partners and contribute throughout the process. Our nursing purpose in assessing a community is to identify factors (both positive and negative) that impinge on the health of the people to develop strategies for health promotion. As Hancock and Minkler point out, "Health professionals concerned with ... community building have two reasons for implementing effective and comprehensive community health assessments: information is needed for change, and it is needed for empowerment" (Minkler, 2005, p. 139). We will use the community-as-partner model (Fig. 11.1) as a framework for the assessment. (For a specific assessment guide for the workplace, see Appendix A.)

USING A NURSING MODEL TO GUIDE PRACTICE

Boundaries are needed to define areas of concern for nursing, and a conceptual "map" of the nursing process is a necessary guide for action. This is particularly true when the nursing practice focuses on the entire community. The community-as-partner model provides us with both the map and the boundaries and is used

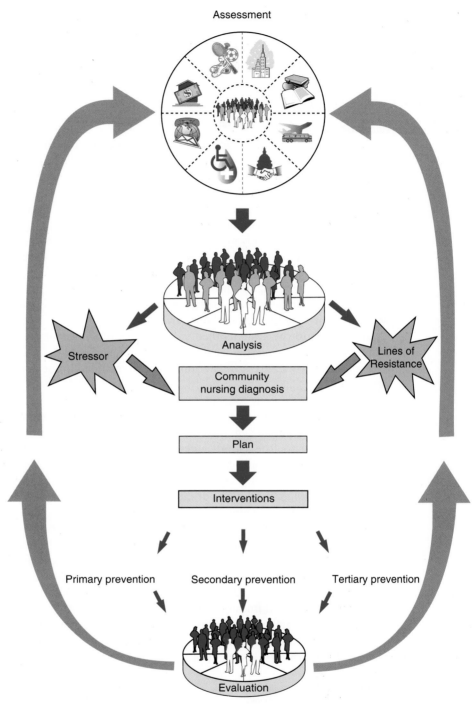

Figure 11.1 Community-as-partner model.

throughout this chapter and subsequent chapters to describe the nursing process applied to the community as a whole. The community-as-partner model is presented in the context of selected community models.

A model with which nurses identified for many years was the medical model (i.e., a disease-oriented, illness- and organ-focused approach to patients, with an emphasis on pathology). However, reliance on the medical model excludes health promotion and the holistic focus that is central to nursing. In addition, important aspects of care, such as psychological, sociocultural, and spiritual areas, are not included in the medical model. Thus, a nursing model should encompass all aspects of health care needs and incorporate long-range goals and planning.

Community-as-Partner Model

Based on Neuman's model of a total-person approach to viewing patient problems (1972), the *community-as-client model* was developed by the authors to illustrate the definition of public health nursing as the synthesis of public health and nursing. The model has been renamed the *community-as-partner model* to emphasize the underlying philosophy of primary health care.

Neuman's total-person approach and, subsequently, the community-as-partner model are considered systems models. You are already familiar with several kinds of systems, for instance, body systems (endocrine, neuromuscular); social systems; and filing systems. Systems have a common purpose, interrelated parts, and boundaries. The whole system is considered greater than the sum of its parts, and there is emphasis on the interaction of those parts to make up the whole. An individual, group, or community can be considered an open system in that there is constant interaction with the environment through boundaries.

In addition to the systems theory, Neuman's model incorporates Selye's stress adaptation theory, *gestalt* theory from psychology, and field theories. For application to community work, stress adaptation has been included in the community-as-partner model.

Definitions of the four concepts that are central to nursing—person, environment, health, and nursing—provide a framework for the community-as-partner model. *Person* is a population or an aggregate. Everyone in a defined community (total population) or aggregate (the elderly, teens, nurses) represents the person. In effect, *environment* may be thought of as community (i.e., a network of people and their surroundings). The links between the people in the community may be where they live, the work they do, their ethnicity or race, the way they live, and any other factors that they have in common (Baum, 1998). *Health* in this model is seen as a "resource for everyday life, not the objective of living. [It is] a positive concept emphasizing social and personal resources, as well as physical capacities" (World Health Organization, 1986). *Nursing*, based on definitions of the other three concepts, is prevention. That is, all of nursing is considered preventive: primary prevention is aimed at reducing possible encounters with stressors or strengthening the lines of defense (e.g., sunscreen to prevent skin cancer; immunizations); secondary prevention occurs after a stressor crosses the line of defense and causes a reaction, and it is aimed at early detection to prevent further damage (e.g., breast self-examination); and tertiary prevention aims to maintain and restore a more-or-less healthy state (e.g., rehabilitation, meditation).

TAKE NOTE

The types of prevention may seem confusing, and sometimes they are! For instance, meditation, listed under tertiary prevention because it can be practiced after a major bodily insult (breast cancer followed by chemotherapy and radiation), can also be considered a form of primary prevention. Meditation diminishes the effects of stress overall and may actually strengthen the lines of defense.

Consider the community-as-partner model (Fig. 11.1). There are two central factors in this model: a focus on the *community* as partner (represented by the community assessment wheel at the top, which incorporates the community's people as the core) and the use of the *nursing process*. The model is described in some detail to assist you in understanding its parts; this will guide your practice in the community. Refer now to Figure 11.2, the community assessment wheel for the following discussion.

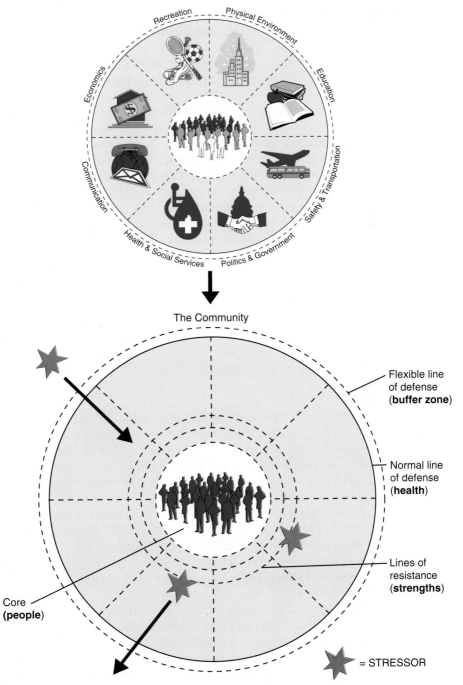

Figure 11.2   The community assessment wheel, featuring lines of resistance and defense within the community structure.

The core of the assessment wheel represents the *people* who make up the community. Included in the core are the demographics of the population as well as their values, beliefs, and history. As residents of the community, the people are affected by and, in turn, influence the eight subsystems of the community. These subsystems are physical environment, education, safety and transportation, politics and government, health and social services, communication, economics, and recreation.

The solid line surrounding the community represents its *normal line of defense*, or the level of health the community has reached over time. The normal line of defense may include characteristics such as a high rate of immunity, low infant mortality, or middle-income level. The normal line of defense also includes usual patterns of coping, along with problem-solving capabilities; it represents the health of the community.

The *flexible line of defense*, depicted as a broken line around the community and its normal line of defense, is a buffer zone representing a dynamic level of health resulting from a temporary response to stressors. This temporary response may be neighborhood mobilization against an environmental stressor such as flooding or a social stressor such as an unwanted adult bookstore. The eight subsystems are divided by broken lines to remind us that they are not discrete and separate but influence (and are influenced by) one another. (Remember: A principle of ecology is that everything is connected to everything else. This also applies to the community as a whole.) The eight divisions both define the major subsystems of a community and provide the community health nurse with a framework for assessment.

TAKE NOTE

Take a moment to examine the selection of subsystems that have been identified. Can you think of any that have been omitted? Think of the community where you live. What examples of each subsystem can you identify?

Within the community are *lines of resistance*, internal mechanisms that act to defend against stressors. An evening recreational program for young people implemented to decrease vandalism and a freestanding, no-fee health clinic to diagnose and treat sexually transmitted diseases (STD) are examples of lines of resistance. Lines of resistance exist throughout each of the subsystems and represent the community's strengths.

Stressors are tension-producing stimuli that have the potential of causing disequilibrium in the system. They may originate outside the community (e.g., air pollution from a nearby industry) or inside the community (e.g., the closing of a clinic). Stressors penetrate the flexible and normal lines of defense, resulting in disruption of the community. Inadequate, inaccessible, or unaffordable services are stressors on the health of the community.

Stressors and lines of resistance (strengths) together become part of the community nursing diagnosis by giving rise to the *degree of reaction*. The degree of reaction is the amount of disequilibrium or disruption that results from stressors impinging on the community's lines of defense. For instance, if there is a case of measles (stressor) in an elementary school and the lines of resistance are strong (99% of students are up-to-date on immunizations), the degree of reaction (potential outbreak of measles) will be minimal. The degree of reaction may be reflected in mortality and morbidity rates, unemployment, or crime statistics, to name a few.

> ### TAKE NOTE
>
> There are many models applicable to practice in the community. Two in particular are used by community health nurses: Pender's health promotion model and Green and Kreuter's PRECEDE–PROCEED model. You will find these sources listed in the Further Readings section of this chapter.

> ### TAKE NOTE
>
> The outcome of a stressor impinging on a community is not always negative. Often, it is positive. For example, in the face of a crisis, people may band together and develop a community group to deal with the crisis. This group may continue to function after the crisis is over—strengthening the community and continuing to contribute to its "health." (A community recovery committee formed after Hurricane Ike in Galveston, Texas, continues to provide input and support to the city as positive changes are implemented.)

> ### TAKE NOTE
>
> Community assessments are not done in a vacuum. You are probably already familiar with some aspects of the community by virtue of your involvement in caring for people who reside there, perhaps in a clinic or a nearby hospital. In addition, this is not a solo job; many people will contribute to the assessment, so try not to get discouraged by the seeming enormity of the task. Tackle it in increments.
>
> (Regarding information contained in tables, our intention is to provide you with numbers, percentages, rates, and so on, along with their source. These figures, however, are for illustration only and do not reflect current data related to the areas where they are found. For your assessment, be sure to use the latest figures and include the date within the citation.)

BEGINNING THE COMMUNITY ASSESSMENT

Begin by identifying your community. Recall that a system is a whole that functions because of the interdependence of its parts. A community, too, is a whole entity that functions because of the interdependence of its parts, or subsystems. The community assessment wheel (see Fig. 11.3) will be your overall framework, while the assessment is facilitated by using the model in survey form. The windshield survey shown in Table 11.1 was adapted from an earlier version that has been expanded to include each component of the community assessment wheel. Note that the guide has three parts: (1) the community core; (2) the community subsystems; and (3) perceptions. In addition, there are columns for the listing of observations and data. From now on we will refer to the survey as the windshield survey.

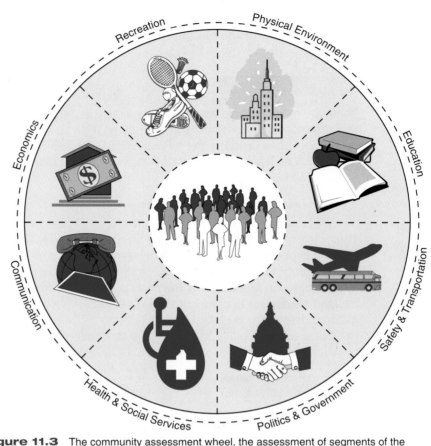

Figure 11.3   The community assessment wheel, the assessment of segments of the community-as-partner model.

TAKE NOTE

Your community health nursing course time limitations may not permit each student to complete an entire community assessment. In fact, it is a rare instance when an individual completes a community assessment alone, as community assessment requires teamwork. Therefore, teams of students may be assigned to assess one or two community subsystems. At the end of the course, each team will present its assessment, and the total community assessment may be completed. A similar situation may arise in agencies when health care providers from a variety of disciplines are assigned one aspect (one subsystem) of a community to assess.

The community of Rosemont, comprising Census Tracts (CT) 4104 and 4107, will be used to illustrate the use of the model in conducting a community assessment (as well as subsequent analysis, diagnosis, planning, intervention, and evaluation). Although we have chosen an urban community defined by census tracts, the guide can be used to assess any community regardless of size, location, resources, or population characteristics. It can also be used to assess a "community within a community," such as a school, an industry, or a business. Examples of these communities are included in Part 3 of this book. In addition, this guide can be used to assess an aggregate (i.e., a

TABLE 11.1

Windshield Survey*

	Observations	Data
I. Community Core 1. History—What can you glean by looking (e.g., old, established neighborhoods; new subdivision)? Ask people willing to talk: How long have you lived here? Has the area changed? As you talk, ask if there is an "old-timer" who knows the history of the area		
2. Demographics—What sorts of people do you see? Young? Old? Homeless? Alone? Families? What races do you see? Is the population homogeneous?		
3. Ethnicity—Do you note indicators of different ethnic groups (e.g., restaurants, festivals)? What signs do you see of different cultural groups?		
4. Values and Beliefs—Are there churches, mosques, temples? Does it appear homogeneous? Are the lawns cared for? With flowers? Gardens? Signs of art? Culture? Heritage? Historical markers?		
II. Subsystems 1. Physical Environment—How does the community look? What do you note about air quality, flora, housing, zoning, space, green areas, animals, people, man-made structures, natural beauty, water, climate? Can you find or develop a map of the area? What is the size (e.g., square miles, blocks)?		
2. Health and Social Services—Evidence of acute or chronic conditions? Shelters? "Traditional" healers (e.g., *curanderos*, herbalists)? Are there clinics, hospitals, practitioners' offices, public health services, home health agencies, emergency centers, nursing homes, social service facilities, mental health services? Are there resources outside the community but accessible to them?		
3. Economy—Is it a "thriving" community or does it feel "seedy?" Are there industries, stores, places for employment? Where do people shop? Are there signs that food stamps are used/accepted? What is the unemployment rate?		
4. Transportation and Safety—How do people get around? What type of private and public transportation is available? Do you see buses, bicycles, taxis? Are there sidewalks, bike trails? Is getting around in the community possible for people with disabilities? What types of protective services are there (e.g., fire, police, sanitation)? Is air quality monitored? What types of crimes are committed? Do people feel safe?		
5. Politics and Government—Are there signs of political activity (e.g., posters, meetings)? What party affiliation predominates? What is the governmental jurisdiction of the community (e.g., elected mayor, city council with single-member districts)? Are people involved in decision making in their local governmental unit?		
6. Communication—Are there "common areas" where people gather? What newspapers do you see in the stands? Do people have TVs and radios? What do they watch/listen to? What are the formal and informal means of communication?		
7. Education—Are there schools in the area? How do they look? Are there libraries? Is there a local board of education? How does it function? What is the reputation of the school(s)? What are major educational issues? What are the dropout rates? Are extracurricular activities available? Are they used? Is there a school health service? A school nurse?		
8. Recreation—Where do children play? What are the major forms of recreation? Who participates? What facilities for recreation do you see?		
III. Perceptions 1. The Residents—How do people feel about the community? What do they identify as its strengths? Problems? Ask several people from different groups (e.g., old, young, field worker, factory worker, professional, minister, housewife) and keep track of who gives what answer.		
2. Your Perceptions—General statements about the "health" of this community. What are its strengths? What problems or potential problems can you identify?		

Note: Supplement your impressions with information from the census, police records, school statistics, chamber of commerce data, health department reports, and so on to confirm or refute your conclusions. Tables, graphs, and maps are helpful and will aid in your analysis.

*This survey form was renamed "Learning about the Community on Foot" to underscore the necessity of walking around the community. Also, when one of the authors (Elizabeth T. Anderson) used it in rural Mexico, the area being assessed was not accessible by automobile. For ease of citation and referral, we will continue to use "windshield survey" as its title.

defined group within the community [e.g., teenagers, battered women, the elderly, or children under age 5]) by providing the context in which this group is found. The *process* of assessment, regardless of where it is applied, always remains the same.

> ### TAKE NOTE
>
> Some students choose to format their assessment with observations and data reported in narrative form with data presented in tables. Others simply include their information directly in the table. As you will learn, there is no one way to collect and report data in the community. Do, however, agree with your team on a model-based format such as those illustrated here and adhere to it.

Assessment is a skill that is refined through practice. Everyone feels awkward and unsure as he or she begins (remember the first time you took a blood pressure?); this is normal. The first step is always the most difficult.

COMMUNITY CORE

We think of the core as something that is essential, basic, and enduring. The core of a community is its people—their history, characteristics, values, and beliefs. The first stage of assessing a community, then, is to learn about its people. In fact, partnering with people in the community is an integral part of working in the community. Table 11.2 lists the major components of the community core along with suggested locations and sources of information about each component. Because every community is different, information sources available about one community may not be available for another.

The History of Rosemont

The Rosemont property was originally deeded to a Miss Ima Smith, who received a land grant of 3,370 acres in 1827. For almost 100 years, the area remained as prairie, dotted with cattle ranches and small farms. In 1920, John Walker and William Bell formed a land corporation and began developing the Smith property. The first area that was improved and deed restricted was named Rosemont after a legendary town in Scotland. After development, Rosemont prospered and attracted newcomers to the area. Numerous prominent families made their homes in Rosemont, including a state governor, a Nobel laureate, and a president of the United States. However, during the economic depression of the 1930s and the years before and during World War II, a drastic decrease in building activities occurred. Many stately homes deteriorated and either became multifamily dwellings or were left to decay. Eventually, economic forces succeeded in breaking deed restrictions, and residential areas were forced to accept the introduction of industry and small businesses. As a result, property values plummeted, leaving quaint boutiques and antique shops to exist alongside an increasing number of nightclubs and nude modeling studios.

From 1950 to 1970, Rosemont witnessed the influx of a large population of young adults, commonly referred to as "hippies," who used the large, spacious homes for group living. This practice of communal living attracted drug addicts and runaways. Rosemont gradually assumed the reputation of tolerating "nontraditional" lifestyles—a factor that precipitated an influx of a large population of gay men.

TABLE 11.2

Community Core Data

Components	Sources of Information
History	Library, historic society Interview "old-timers," town leaders

Demographics
  Age and sex characteristics
  Racial distribution
  Ethnic distribution
	Census of population and housing
	Planning board (local, city, county, state)
	Chamber of commerce
	City hall, city secretary, archives
	Observation

Household types by
  Family
  Nonfamily
  Group
	Census

Marital status by
  Single
  Separated
  Widowed
  Divorced
	Census

Vital statistics
  Births
  Deaths by
    Age
    Leading causes
	State department of health (distributed through
	  city and county health departments)

Values and beliefs	Personal contact Observation (see Table 11.1) (To protect against stereotyping, avoid the library for this portion of the assessment.)
Religion	Observation Telephone book

Because of low property values and affordable rent during the mid- to late 1970s, large groups of Vietnamese and Mexicans also settled in Rosemont. Simultaneously, established families and single professionals, weary of the lengthy commute from suburbia to the inner city, began returning to Rosemont—a trend that continues today. Today, old homes are being refurbished, businesses are being revitalized, and pride, once lost, is being reclaimed.

Demographics and Ethnicity

Tables 11.3 and 11.4 show age, sex, race, and ethnicity data for CT 4104 and CT 4107 as well as for the nearest city and county. Gathering data on city, county, state, and nation affords comparisons that may be important for the analysis. (The census lists only numbers of people; you must calculate percentages.) Tables 11.5 and 11.6 list data on family types and marital status. (We calculated the percentages.)

TAKE NOTE

During the next step of the nursing process, analysis, you will need data about the other comparable entities, so collect all needed data now.

TABLE 11.3

Population Age and Sex Characteristics for CT 4104, CT 4107, City of Hampton, and Jefferson County

Age (years)	CT 4104 Males	CT 4104 Females	CT 4104 Total %	CT 4107 Males	CT 4107 Females	CT 4107 Total %	Hampton Number	Hampton Total %	Jefferson County Number	Jefferson County Total %
Under 5 years	370	362	10.6	29	11	0.6	123,150	7.8	189,246	8.4
5–19	1,200	991	31.9	241	195	6.5	377,345	23.9	569,991	25.3
30–34	395	437	12.2	1,965	911	42.6	514,705	32.6	716,431	31.8
35–54	837	970	26.2	1,758	721	36.7	339,453	21.5	484,380	21.5
55–64	222	370	8.6	221	181	5.9	116,835	7.4	157,705	7
65 and over	270	450	10.5	175	349	7.7	107,361	6.8	135,176	6
TOTAL	3,294	3,580	100	4,389	2,368	100	1,578,849	100	2,252,929	100

Data from Census of Population and Housing, selected characteristics.

TABLE 11.4

Population Race and Ethnicity for CT 4104, CT 4107, City of Hampton, and Jefferson County

	CT 4104 Number	CT 4104 Total %	CT 4107 Number	CT 4107 Total %	Hampton Number	Hampton Total %	Jefferson County Number	Jefferson County Total %
White	852	12.4	5,871	88.5	970,489	61.5	1,562,091	69.4
Black	3,732	54.3	305	4.6	434,014	27.5	467,177	20.7
Asian/Pacific Islander	1,321	19.1	54	0.7	32,335	2.1	45,432	2
Hispanic	625	9.1	321	4.7	131,763	8.3	163,774	7.3
American Indian	242	3.5	38	0.6	3,203	0.2	4,923	0.2
Other	111	1.6	58	0.9	7,045	0.4	9,532	0.4
TOTAL	6,874	100	6,757	100	1,578,849	100	2,252,929	100

Data from Census of Population and Housing, selected characteristics.

TABLE 11.5

Population Family Types for CT 4104 and CT 4107

	CT 4104 Number	CT 4104 Total %	CT 4107 Number	CT 4107 Total %
Family	5,706	83	2,443	36.2
Nonfamily	1,168	17	4,103	60.7
Female-headed household	721	994		
Male-headed household		447	2,189	
Group quarters			211	3.1
TOTAL	6,874	100	6,757	100

Data from Census of Population and Housing, selected characteristics.

TABLE 11.6

Persons Age 15 and Over by Sex and Marital Status for CT 4104 and CT 4107

	CT 4104			CT 4107		
Marital Status	**Male**	**Female**	**Total %**	**Male**	**Female**	**Total %**
Single	348	408	15.2	2,418	1,016	53.5
Married	1,510	1,498	60.1	796	768	24.4
Separated	120	245	7.2	113	72	2.8
Widowed	52	119	3.4	68	198	4.3
Divorced	294	407	14.1	572	397	15
TOTAL	2,324	2,677	100	3,967	2,451	100

Data from Census of Population and Housing, selected characteristics.

Vital Statistics

Table 11.7 lists birth and death statistics for CT 4104 and CT 4107 as well as for the city, county, and state. Using a similar format, Table 11.8 lists the leading causes of death. Please note: It is always preferable to report rates because you can then make comparisons. However, if you do not know the population at risk (the denominator), it is not possible to calculate rates. Some of these mortality data in Table 11.8 do not allow the calculation of rates for that reason. See Chapter 3 for help in calculating rates.

Values, Beliefs, and Religion

Included in the community core are the values, beliefs, and religious practices of the people. All ethnic and racial groups have values and beliefs that interact with each community system to influence the people's health. Review Chapter 7 for methods to help you understand these cultural elements of the community. Notice that Table 11.2 cautions against the exclusive use of the library for information about values, beliefs, and religious practices; the reason is that books and articles frequently offer broad generalizations to describe the practices of ethnic and racial

TABLE 11.7

Selected Birth and Death Vital Statistics for CT 4104, CT 4107, City of Hampton, and Jefferson County

	CT 4104	CT 4107	Hampton	Jefferson County	State
Births	210	117	30,726	56,865	363,325
Deaths (rates)*					
Infant	7(33)	2 (17)	372 (12)	698 (12.3)	2,064 (5.7)
Neonatal	5 (23)	2 (17)	245 (7.9)	471 (8.3)	1,226 (3.4)

*Rates are per 1,000 live births.
Data from State Vital Statistics, Department of Health.

TABLE 11.8

Deaths by Selected Causes for CT 4104, CT 4107, City of Hampton, and State of Texarkana

Cause of Death	CT 4104		CT 4107		Hampton		State		
	Number	%	Number	%	Number	%	Number	%	Rate*
Heart disease	16	22.2	10	23.8	3,186	33.4	42,968	28.7	211.2
Malignant neoplasms	17	23.6	11	26.1	2,078	21.8	33,298	22.2	163.7
Cerebrovascular diseases	6	8.3	2	4.7	690	7.3	10,721	7.2	52.7
Accidents	4	5.6	4	9.5	585	6.2	7,602	5.1	37.4
Chronic lower respiratory diseases	0	0	0	0	79	0.8	7,284	4.9	35.8
Diabetes mellitus	0	0	2	4.8	139	1.4	5,195	3.5	25.5
Diseases of early infancy	7	9.7	1	2.4	248	2.6	NI	NI	NI
Homicides	6	8.3	1	2.4	592	6.2	NI	NI	NI
Cirrhosis of liver	0	0	1	2.4	163	1.7	2,092†	1.4	10.3
Pneumonia	2	2.8	1	2.4	210	2.2	3,708	2.5	18.2
Suicides	3	4.2	1	2.4	195	2	2,093	1.4	10.3
Congenital anomalies	0	0	2	4.8	99	1	NI	NI	NI
Nephritis and nephrosis	0	0	0	0	13	0.1	NI	NI	NI
Tuberculosis	1	1.4	0	0	17	0.2	NI	NI	NI
All other causes	10	13.9	6	14.3	1,239	13	31,631	21.1	155.5

*Rates per 100,000 estimated population. (Note: It is always preferable to report rates because you can then make comparisons. However, if you do not know the population at risk (the denominator), it is not possible to calculate rates. The above mortality data for the census tracts and for the City of Hampton do not allow the calculation of rates.)
†Includes chronic liver disease for state.
NI, not included in "Leading Causes of Death" in state.
Data from Hampton Vital Statistics, City of Hampton health department, and from the State Department of Health.

groups (e.g., the lifestyles of urban African Americans) or discuss one practice of one ethnic group (such as breastfeeding practices of Mexican-born Hispanics). Each community is unique, with values, beliefs, and religious practices that are rooted in tradition and continue to evolve and exist because they meet the community's needs.

To validate the published, secondary demographic data, use your survey to establish the presence and geographic location of different racial and ethnic groups. It is during this phase—assessment of the physical system—that we enter the community to learn and experience the values, beliefs, and religious practices of the community.

SUBSYSTEMS

Our partner, the Rosemont community, is located within the City of Hampton and is in Hampton's central business district. It is bounded by Way Drive on the west, Buff's Bayou on the north, Live Oak Boulevard on the south, and Hampton Street on the east. Figure 11.4 is a map of the Rosemont community. Using the windshield survey (see Table 11.1) as a guide, we step into the community.

Figure 11.4   Rosemont community streets and boundaries.

Physical Environment

Just as the physical examination is a critical component of assessing an individual patient, so it is in the assessment of a community. And just as the five senses of the clinician are called into play in the physical examination of a patient, so, too, are they needed at the community level. Table 11.9 provides the components of the physical examination, both of an individual and a community, and compares tools and sources of data for each.

TABLE 11.9

Physical Examination Components and Sources of Data

	Sources of Data	
Components	**Individual**	**Community**
Inspection	All senses Otoscope Ophthalmoscope	All senses Windshield survey Walk through community
Auscultation	Stethoscope	Listen to community sounds/residents
Vital signs	Thermometer Sphygmomanometer	Observe climate, terrain, natural boundaries, and resources "Life" signs such as notices of community meetings; density
Systems review	Head-to-toe	Observe social systems, including housing, businesses, churches, and hangouts
Laboratory studies	Blood tests X-rays Scans, other tests	Almanac; census data Chamber of commerce planning studies and surveys

Inspection

Rosemont Boulevard bisects the community and serves as a major north–south thoroughfare for residents traveling to or through the community. It is tree-lined and divided by a grassy median into sections. Many businesses, especially restaurants, are located along Rosemont Boulevard. Many of the restaurants are of the specialty health-promoting types that serve quiche, sprout sandwiches, and herbal teas. Other businesses along the boulevard include gas stations; office buildings; art-supply stores; a veterinarian; small art galleries; a nursery; one Mexican *barbacoa* stand in a grocery store; florists; a bank; a pharmacy; and various shops specializing in leather goods, books, and handcrafted items. (See the Economics section of this chapter for a summary of business units.)

The major east–west thoroughfare through Rosemont, Pecan Drive, is also lined with businesses and, with fewer trees, presents a more urban face. At the east end can be seen nude modeling studios; small restaurants specializing in various ethnic foods (Greek, Pakistani, Mexican, Vietnamese, and Indian, to name a few); and numerous small art shops. The Rosemont Health Center is located in this area. Further west on this street is a large theater that attracts many first-run productions. There are a couple of adult movie houses and the ubiquitous specialty restaurants (in this area, they are of the type that caters to the business or professional crowds—quiet tea rooms that play classical music). Along this street, too, are many large old houses, many of which have been converted into antique shops, flower shops, and other small stores. There is no large industry in Rosemont. The area behind the two business-filled thoroughfares that divide the community seems like a different world. The streets are narrower, and some are cobbled; old oak and pecan trees are abundant, and, in many areas, the branches of the trees meet over the streets to form protective canopies.

The streets other than the thoroughfares are narrow, and most of them have sidewalks, as is typical of old neighborhoods in Hampton. In general, the streets and sidewalks are in good repair and free from debris; however, because there is little off-street parking, many residents park on the streets, causing traffic congestion at times when most residents are home (primarily nights and weekends).

Vital Signs

The climate of Rosemont (and the Hampton Standard Metropolitan Statistical Area [SMSA]) is mild and moderated by sea winds. Summers are hot (the temperature is 90°F or higher approximately 87 days a year) and humid (averaging 62%), but evenings are cool, and there is rarely a hard freeze in the winter. Flora, both temperate and tropical, abounds—live oaks, hibiscus, and pines may grow in one block, for example.

The terrain is generally flat, with little variation in grade. It is 20 feet above sea level. The only naturally occurring water in the area is Buff's Bayou, a concrete-lined "river" that serves to carry off excess rain and drainage to reduce chances of flooding in Hampton. The bayou ends in the Hampton Ship Channel, which leads to the sea.

Rosemont is the third most densely populated area in Hampton, with 14.4 people per acre. An area in CT 4104 that contains the subsidized-housing complex is the most densely populated in all of Hampton, with 221 people per acre.

The variety of local stores reflects the diversity of interests in Rosemont. Posters advertising a meeting of the Gay Political Caucus share bulletin-board space with senior citizens' meetings; church announcements; educational programs at the community college's "Sundry School;" Vietnamese relocation services; the community's STD clinic; and a musical show by "El Barrio" from the Mexican–American area. Rosemont is a community of rich diversity, a microcosm of Hampton.

Figure 11.5   Rosemont community greens and parks.

The churches of Rosemont also reflect its diversity—virtually all denominations are represented. From the large Methodist and Presbyterian churches on its borders to the small storefront churches serving refugees, Rosemont contains resources for all major religious groups.

Systems

Most of Rosemont is developed; there is little space not in use. Four small neighborhood parks, a narrow strip along the bayou, and the land around the community college comprise the green space available to the community (Fig. 11.5), although most houses have well-kept lawns with trees and shrubs. Table 11.10 presents land use data for Rosemont.

TABLE 11.10

Rosemont Land Use

	CT 4104		CT 4107	
Land Use	**Number of Acres**	**Total %**	**Number of Acres**	**Total %**
Single-family dwellings	161.2	28.03	95.4	31.78
Multifamily dwellings	46.4	8.06	46.5	15.49
Commercial	210.2	36.55	61.2	20.39
Industrial	44.9	7.8	0.2	0.06
Public	6.8	1.18	11.1	3.69
Open	52.9	9.2	53.2	17.72
Water	6.3	1.09	4.7	1.56
Undeveloped	46.3	8.05	14.6	4.86
Right-of-way	0	0	13.2	4.39
Total acres	575	100	300.1	100

Data Book, Rosemont Community Development, City of Hampton, Planning Department.

TABLE 11.11

Average Value of Housing and Rent for Years 1990 and 2000 for CT 4104, CT 4107, City of Hampton, and Jefferson County

	CT 4104		CT 4107		Hampton		Jefferson County	
	1990	2000	1990	2000	1990	2000	1990	2000
Average value of housing	$43,400	$47,630	$62,400	$71,600	$61,900	$79,300	$70,500	$87,000
Average rent	$284	$476	$346	$650	$337	$575	$489	$590

Data from Census of Population and Housing, selected characteristics.

The majority of houses in Rosemont are old, reflecting the early development of the area. Within certain sections, the houses resemble each other (e.g., all one-story, wood-frame houses with porches); however, there may also be great heterogeneity from one block to the next. In the northeast quadrant is a large subsidized-housing area of run-down apartments with broken windows and poorly kept streets, whereas in the southwest quadrant houses have been remodeled and well maintained. Also in the northeast is an area covering several blocks of what are called "shotgun houses" (the story is told that one can shoot a shotgun from the front door, and the shot will go out the back door); placed side by side, they are tiny and poorly maintained. See Table 11.11 for housing information.

During the day, most of the people seen on the streets move quickly and purposefully as though on business or an errand. Those who could be described as "strolling" are elderly people or young men, usually alone. Few children are seen during the day except in the schoolyards, which are not on the main thoroughfares. Dogs bark as one walks through the neighborhoods, and cats sun themselves in windows; however, few pets run loose in the area.

At night, Rosemont assumes a different flavor along Pecan Drive; all of the restaurants are open, and many have outdoor patios. Smells of fajitas, curry, exotic spices, and charbroiling fill the air. "The Strip," as Pecan Drive is called, comes alive with sounds of rap, disco, country, and rock music, along with the stroking of a sitar or quiet strumming of a guitar.

Most of the clients in these restaurants and nude modeling "studios," according to residents, come from outside of Rosemont. Many are attracted by the food, and some by the freewheeling sex reputed to be available in the area. Many of the residents express disdain for the Strip, calling it a "tourist attraction," and they believe it is contributing to the deterioration of Rosemont. They state that "outsiders" and "cowboys" exploit and prey on unsuspecting tourists and that the unsavory reputation of the area is not the fault of the people who live there. An absence of zoning laws has facilitated the establishment of some of the less-than-desirable businesses in the area.

The physical examination of Rosemont reveals it to be a community of contrasts: churches and nude modeling studios; subsidized city housing units and restored homes from a more affluent time; old people and young; White and Black (and all shades between); quiet tree-lined streets and busy thoroughfares; sedate tea rooms and garish adult movie theaters; families and singles; and the rich and poor.

Health and Social Services

One method of classifying health and social services is to differentiate between facilities located outside the community (extracommunity) and those within the

TABLE 11.12

Health and Social Services

Component	Sources of Information
Health Services	
Extracommunity or intracommunity facilities.	Chamber of commerce
Once identified, group into categories (e.g., hospitals and clinics, home health care, extended care facilities, public health services, emergency care).	Planning board (county, city)
	Phone directory
	Talk to residents
For each facility, collect data on	Interview administrator or
1. Services (fees, hours, and new services planned and those discontinued)	someone on the staff
	Facility annual report
2. Resources (personnel, space, budget, and record system)	
3. Characteristics of users (geographic distribution, demographic profile, and transportation source)	
4. Statistics (number of persons served daily, weekly, and monthly)	
5. Adequacy, accessibility, and acceptability of facility according to users and providers	
Social Services	
Extracommunity or intracommunity facilities.	Chamber of commerce
Once identified, group into categories (e.g., counseling and support, clothing, food, shelter, and special needs).	United Way directory
	Phone directory
For each facility, collect data on areas 1–5 listed above.	

community (intracommunity). Once the health and social service facilities are identified, group them into categories, perhaps by type of service offered (e.g., hospitals, clinics, extended care); by size; or by public versus private usage. Table 11.12 suggests a classification system as well as possible major components of each facility requiring assessment.

Extracommunity Health Facilities

Hospitals
Jefferson County has 50 hospitals with a total of 12,321 beds, 4,321 of which are in the Hampton Medical Center, a complex that includes all medical subspecialties as well as sophisticated diagnostic and treatment services. The Medical Center is located 7 miles from Rosemont. All patients admitted to the Medical Center must be referred by a physician; self-referral is not permitted. (Self-referral allows the individual to choose and acquire medical care independently.) Although the existence of the Medical Center is common knowledge among Rosemont residents, few people know anyone who has sought or received care there. Numerous private hospitals are located in Jefferson County, most of which are in Hampton. All private hospitals require third-party reimbursement for services rendered. (Third-party reimbursement means payment for services by an entity other than the patient. For example, Medicare, Medicaid, insurance, and Workmen's Compensation are third-party reimbursers.) In addition to private hospitals, most communities use tax revenues to support at least one hospital for the general public. In Jefferson County, the public hospital is Jefferson Memorial.

Jefferson Memorial is a full-service facility located 5 miles south of Rosemont. Care units and clinics at Memorial include medical, surgical, pediatrics, maternity, gynecology, trauma and burns, psychiatry, and emergency rooms (ERs). People can self-refer to Jefferson Memorial. According to the director of the ER, 290 people are seen daily in the ER (approximately 100,000 people annually). Of these, some 40% are admitted. Follow-up care is provided by the Memorial's outpatient clinics. The Memorial is supported by city and county taxes as well as by fees collected for services. Health care provider fees, as well as treatments and diagnostic services, are in addition to the base fee. All fees are on a sliding scale according to income and family size. Rosemont residents use Memorial but complain of lengthy waits of up to 8 hours and of having to undergo repeated assessments as they are moved from one health care provider to another.

Hospital personnel recognize the lengthy waiting period and fragmentation of care, but they cite budget constraints and a shortage of qualified providers as major obstacles to improving care. No services have been discontinued at Memorial, and no new services or staff positions are budgeted for the next 2 years.

Private Care Providers, Group Practices, and Specialty Clinics

A full selection of general medical and specialty care is available in Jefferson County through private practitioners, group practices, and specialty clinics. Payment is usually third-party reimbursement. Two health maintenance organizations (HMOs) are located in Jefferson County. Rosemont residents with adequate finances use a variety of private practitioners and specialty clinics. The residents usually self-refer after a favorable recommendation from a neighbor, friend, or work colleague.

Public Health Services: The Health Department

To monitor, maintain, and promote the public's health, each state has a state health department and accompanying regional, county, and sometimes city health departments. National, state, and local tax revenues are used to support public health services. There is a Hampton Health Department as well as a Jefferson County Health Department. Because Rosemont is within the city limits of Hampton, the services of the Hampton Health Department are assessed.

The Hampton Health Department offers all medical outpatient services through its seven satellite clinics. The Sunvalley Clinic, located 6 miles from Rosemont and the closest to the area, provides the following services:

- Immunizations
- Well and ill infant, child, adolescent, and adult care
- Antepartum/postpartum care
- Family planning
- Nutrition counseling
- Screening and testing for genetic and acquired conditions such as sickle-cell anemia, diabetes, and phenylketonuria (PKU)
- Dental assessment, cleaning, and restoration
- Mental health counseling and referral
- Health education
- Maternal and infant home visitation after early hospital discharge (defined as earlier than 48 hours after delivery)
- Child abuse, battered spouse, and abandoned person counseling and referral
- STD screening and follow-up (including HIV testing)

Additional services include a pharmacy, laboratory, and radiation department. Payment for most services is on a sliding scale; remaining services are free to all city residents. Free services include immunizations as well as screening and treatment for STDs. The majority of Rosemont residents who use the health department attend antepartum or postpartum clinics. The staff nurse in the maternity clinic estimates that, of the 75 women seen in the prenatal clinic each week, 20 to 25 are Rosemont residents.

The major service-delivery problem cited by nurses in the maternity clinics is the long waiting period (frequently 8 to 10 weeks) between a woman's initial request for an appointment and the scheduled appointment date. Because many women wait until they are 6 or 7 months pregnant to request antepartum care, the first available appointment time may be after the woman's expected delivery date. Consequently, a large number of women from Rosemont deliver at Jefferson Memorial having received no antepartum care. The administrator of the Sunvalley Clinic felt additional education, support, and monitoring services for pregnant patients and new mothers to be a top service priority.

No services have been discontinued in the recent past. With regard to the question of services that are needed, the elderly were identified as a target group. Plans were under way to establish a nursing clinic for the elderly as well as a wellness program to be offered at day care for the elderly and at senior centers. There are presently more than 10 such facilities for seniors within the city of Hampton.

Numerous Rosemont residents use the health department services, especially the Sunvalley Clinic. Problems cited include lack of a direct bus connection to the clinic (three bus transfers are required) and "impersonal" service. Because patients are not assigned to a primary care provider, it is customary for them to see a different health care provider at each visit. Maternity patients have an additional concern. Each woman must make her own delivery arrangements, and frequently women who qualify for antepartum care at Sunvalley Clinic do not meet eligibility requirements for delivery at Jefferson Memorial. Consequently, women must search for a facility that will admit them for labor and delivery. All too often, they are forced to deliver at home, a situation documented by Sunvalley nurses and confirmed by several Rosemont residents.

Home Health Agencies

The Visiting Nurses Association (VNA) of Hampton is the largest home health agency in Jefferson County. Services of the VNA include home health care by registered nurses, physical and occupational therapists, speech therapists, social workers, and home health aides. The VNA accepts paying clients and third-party reimbursements. Paying clients are charged on a sliding scale according to income and family size. Patients who are unable to pay a fee can request financial assistance from several community social service agencies such as the United Way.

Numerous other home health agencies are located in Hampton and Jefferson County. Although more limited in scope of service, all offer home health services and require fees or third-party reimbursement for payment.

Long-Term, Extended-Care, and Continuing-Care Facilities

There are two long-term facilities within 8 miles of Rosemont: the Pinewoods Rest Center and the Windsail Nursing Home. Each facility is classified as an intermediate-care facility and is licensed by the state health department. A profile of the services, resources, and characteristics of the residents for each facility is presented in Table 11.13. In addition, several hospitals offer extended-care services.

Emergency Services

The Poison Control Center provides information to individuals and health care providers on harmful substances and methods of assessment and treatment. The center provides educational materials and programs for schools and interested groups.

TABLE 11.13

Services, Resources, and Resident Characteristics at Pinewoods Rest Center
and Windsail Nursing Home during the Preceding Year

	Pinewoods Rest Center	**Windsail Nursing Home**
Services	Convalescent nursing care; physical, occupational, and speech therapy	Convalescent nursing care
Full-time personnel	Six RNs, four licensed visiting nurses (LVNs), three nurse aides, one administrator	Three RNs, two LVNs, one nurse aide, one administrator
Licensed bed capacity	96	38
Patient days	33,524	12,965
Occupancy rate	0.96	0.93
Certified bed capacity*	96	38
Median age of residents	79	76
Average duration of stay	4 years	6 years

*Recommended occupancy rate for nursing home beds is 90%.
Data from Jefferson County Planning Council, Pinewoods Rest Center, and Windsail Nursing Home record books.

The Medical Emergency Ambulance Service (MEAS) is financed by Hampton city taxes, public donations, Jefferson County contributions, and organized fundraisers. The MEAS first-aid services are free and available 24 hours a day to all residents of Rosemont. (The MEAS operates in conjunction with the local fire stations. See the Safety and Transportation section of this chapter for a description of fire protection services.)

The MEAS closest to Rosemont has two ambulances; one is used daily, and the other serves as a backup. The MEAS averages 90 to 110 calls a month, with a response time of less than 8 minutes. (Table 11.14 presents specific reasons for ambulance service to people in Rosemont during the last 3-month period.) Calls are received through the central fire department and dispatched by radio to the nearest MEAS team. Each MEAS team consists of 25 people: 3 paramedics having completed 100 hours of class work and 200 hours of hospital experience, and 22 emergency medical technicians (EMTs) with basic paramedic training and additional experience in intravenous therapy and intubation. Both paramedics and EMTs are certified. In addition to emergency service, the MEAS team offers CPR and first-aid classes to community groups.

TABLE 11.14

Reasons for Medical Emergency Ambulance Service (MEAS) to Persons
in Rosemont during the Preceding 3-Month Period

Reason	**Total %**
Cardiac-related problems and cerebrovascular accidents	25
Falls and household accidents	19
Respiratory problems	12
Dizziness and weakness	12
Lacerations	11
Fractures and dislocations	9
Abdominal pain	7
Mental–psychiatric disorders	5

Data from MEAS paramedic records.

Special Services

Frequently, special facilities exist to serve specific groups such as the physically or mentally disabled. After surveying the immediate extracommunity area, no such facilities were located within a 10-mile radius of Rosemont.

Intracommunity Health Facilities

According to the Health Systems Agency (HSA) of Jefferson County, CT 4104 is a medically underserved area; CT 4107 is not.

The type and number of practitioners offering health services in Rosemont are listed in Table 11.15. A need for gynecologic and obstetric services was frequently expressed by female residents. Numerous people cited the need for family practitioners as well as bilingual health care providers. (One of the nurse practitioners speaks Spanish, but none speaks Vietnamese.) Rosemont residents with financial resources tend to select from extracommunity medical services, whereas indigent residents rely on medical services within the community. All private practitioners require payment when services are rendered or third-party reimbursement; the nurse practitioners use a sliding scale to calculate fees. In addition to private practitioners, two clinics—the Third Street Clinic and the Rosemont Health Center—are located in Rosemont.

Third Street Clinic

The Third Street Clinic was founded in 1968 by concerned citizens and church leaders in Rosemont. The clinic, located in the center of CT 4104, was initially financed by public donations and church-sponsored fundraisers. All professional time and supplies were donated. Today, the Third Street Clinic serves 30% to 40% of Rosemont residents and has an annual operating budget of $750,000, a reduction of $220,000 from 2 years ago. The majority of funds are from federal and state grants as well as from client fees and Medicare and Medicaid reimbursements. Although patients are charged according to a sliding scale, no one is denied care. Services provided at Third Street Clinic are summarized in Table 11.16. The clinic provides no acute or trauma care services. The staff includes one part-time physician, two part-time nurses, one social worker, one administrator, and a clerk. Both nurses speak Spanish, but none of the staff speaks Vietnamese. Optometry students and supervising faculty provide services 1 day a week, and one nurse-midwife provides antepartum care two mornings a week. The clinic is open Monday through Friday, 8 AM to 5 PM. On average, 125 people are seen weekly. Medical professionals and

TABLE 11.15

Practitioners in Rosemont

Type	Number
Dentist	6
General medical	1
Optometrist	2
Orthodontist	1
Osteopath	2
Podiatrist	1
Chiropractor	3
Nurse practitioner	2

Data from windshield survey, Chamber of Commerce, and phone directory.

TABLE 11.16

Services and Number of People Served at Third Street Clinic

Service	Description	Patient Visits (Weekly Average)
Family planning	Physical examinations, education, and prescriptions filled	24
Well-child examinations	Physical assessment, referral for illness, immunizations, and screening	19
Antepartum and postpartum	Physical assessment and monitoring	42
Optometry	Eye examinations and prescriptions filled	9
Podiatry	Assessment and treatment	6
Chronic disease counseling and treatment	Treatment and care instructions for hypertension, diabetes, and cardiovascular conditions	31

citizens form the board of directors. According to the clinic's director, immediate medical needs for the residents of CT 4104 include the following:

- Ill infant, child, adolescent, and adult assessment, treatment, and follow-up
- Dental assessment and restoration
- Counseling, referral, and, when possible, treatment for drug abuse and alcoholism
- Group health teaching, especially for pregnant women, parents of young children, and adolescents
- Wellness and self-care classes for all age groups
- Support groups for single parents and senior citizens

There are no consistent health education or counseling services. Transportation services from area neighborhoods to the clinic, as well as dental and home nursing care, were discontinued 2 years ago after grant reductions. The major problem confronting the clinic is the recruitment of health care providers, especially nurses and physicians. Clinic services cannot be expanded (or maintained at the present level) unless additional health care providers are recruited and retained.

Most Rosemont residents are aware of the Third Street Clinic, and many use the clinic's services routinely. The major impediment to clinic use is the 1- to 2-mile walk to the clinic for many residents (there is no direct bus connection for most people). Rosemont residents feel welcome at the clinic, and low staff turnover has fostered positive relationships between the staff and the community. Residents did, however, express a need for additional services at the clinic.

Rosemont Health Center
The Rosemont Health Center, centrally located in CT 4107, is a nonprofit clinic devoted to the diagnosis and treatment of STDs (including HIV infection). The clinic is open Monday to Saturday, 6 PM to 10 PM., and Sunday, 2 PM to 10 PM. The center reports 20% of the syphilis cases and 60% of the gonorrhea cases in Jefferson County. Approximately 600 patient visits occur monthly (200 new cases, 200 repeat cases, and 200 follow-ups). All 75 professional staff members are volunteers and donate 4 to 10 hours of service a month. The director of the clinic is employed part-time. The state donates penicillin, tetanus cultures, and Venereal Disease Research Laboratory (VDRL) tests. Initially, there were no fees for services. Now, a sliding scale fee is assessed to defray costs of equipment, rent, and utilities. No person is denied care. Ninety percent of the patients were gay men when the clinic opened. However, in recent years the demographic makeup of the clientele has shifted to more closely

resemble the entire population of the area. Each patient is issued an identification number and card that is used with each visit. People in psychological crisis are referred to the city health department for counseling. Most patients drive or walk to the clinic.

The director of the health center discussed the immediate need for expanded counseling and support groups, especially for people who are HIV positive. A second need is for an orientation program and information update sessions for staff members, most of whom are former patients. The majority of patients are from the Rosemont area, although an increasing number of patients are commuting to the clinic from Hampton and surrounding Jefferson County. Patients surveyed in the waiting room rated the care as excellent; appointments are rarely canceled by patients.

Observations at the clinic revealed a warm, caring atmosphere where people were treated with respect and were provided privacy when needed. However, there was no visible emergency cart. There were no standard policy and procedure manuals and no posted protocol for an adverse treatment response (such as penicillin reaction) for the many volunteers who worked there.

Extracommunity Social Service Facilities

Because social service agencies are frequently located in office buildings, their location in the community may be difficult to determine during a windshield survey. It is preferable to use a directory such as the type compiled by the Chamber of Commerce or local planning board to begin identifying social service organizations relatively close to the community being assessed. If the community does not have a Chamber of Commerce, use the telephone directory.

Counseling and Support Services

The Hampton Comprehensive Counseling Center was founded in 1971 by concerned citizens of Hampton and Jefferson County for the purpose of providing counseling to adolescent drug users. Today, the center offers a comprehensive mental health program for all residents of Hampton. The center is located 2 miles south of Rosemont. Although people can self-refer to the center, most patients are referred from schools, clinics, and private practitioners. Fees are based on a sliding scale; third-party reimbursements are not accepted. Last year's operating budget was $1,800,000. The majority of revenue comes from clients, although numerous churches and social service agencies sponsor individuals and families. The staff consists of six professionals and two clerks. Services are outlined in Table 11.17. An

TABLE 11.17

Services Offered at the Hampton Comprehensive Counseling Center

Service	Description
Diagnosis	Screening procedure for the mentally handicapped; recommends services required for clients' needs
Information and referral	Liaison teams coordinate services with state schools for the mentally retarded and state hospitals for the mentally ill
Counseling and therapy	Group and play therapy provided
Alcohol and drug abuse services	Counseling services
Psychiatric evaluation and medical services	Psychiatric department provides evaluations and medications for clients
Emergency service	Handles crisis calls 24 hours/day, 7 days/week
Education and consultation	Center staff works with other community groups, including schools, police, and social service agencies, to solve local problems

Data from Hampton Comprehensive Counseling Center.

average of 300 patients are seen each month. The director describes the patient population as white and middle- to upper income, with more men than women. Most patients use private transportation to arrive at the clinic. No additional services are planned because the center staff believes they are adequately meeting the needs of the population. Rosemont residents queried were unaware of the existence of the counseling center, and no one knew of anyone having used the center, although all residents interviewed knew of several adolescent drug users.

The YMCA Youth Development Center borders Rosemont and offers a variety of educational and recreational programs. Adjacent to the "Y" is the YMCA Indo-Chinese Refugee Program, an agency that seeks to facilitate the resettlement of Asian immigrants. Major services include cultural orientation, job counseling and placement, and courses in English as a second language. The agency services have experienced a 200% increase in usage during the past 3 years. Presently, more than 100 people use the facility daily. Although all four staff members are bilingual, the staff is too small to meet the needs of the Vietnamese community—a large proportion of which lives in Rosemont. The staff believes the immediate need is for counseling and therapy programs for alcohol and drug abuse as well as teaching basic survival skills (e.g., finding a job, housing, and medical care). The staff estimates that 40% to 50% of the Asians using their services are from Rosemont. Asian residents in Rosemont agree that the "Y" is responsive to their needs, but, when asked, they do acknowledge long waiting periods (sometimes weeks) for classes and counseling.

Clothing, Food, Shelter, and Basic Welfare Services
Most churches and synagogues in the area have a food pantry, and many can arrange emergency shelter and provide clothing and essential transportation services. People are usually helped on a walk-in basis, but sometimes the church is referred to a family or individual in need. In Hampton, a special organization, The Metropolitan Ministries, serves as an interfaith link between the religious communities of Hampton and community residents in need of social services. The Metropolitan Ministries coordinates services, thereby avoiding duplication, and refers people to the program that can best meet their immediate needs.

TAKE NOTE

In most communities, churches must be contacted individually for a listing of services. In addition to the churches, synagogues, and mosques, numerous clothing resale shops are located in shopping areas close to Rosemont. Residents are very knowledgeable about available retail stores and actively promote preferred merchants.

The Jefferson County Welfare Department and the Hampton Welfare Department screen and process applicants for food stamps, housing subsidies, and financial aid. Each welfare department has a division of child protection that investigates reports of child abuse and neglect. The division provides casework services, foster home placement, and emergency shelter for women and children, as well as parenting classes and child-therapy groups. Welfare departments are funded by federal, state, and local tax revenues.

Special Services
The United Way lists 42 private and public-supported social service agencies located in Hampton or Jefferson County. The United Way directory includes identifying

information for each agency, as well as services and fees. Agencies on the roster include the Society to Prevent Blindness, American Lung Association, March of Dimes, Hampton Area Woman's Center, Paralyzed Veterans Association, and the International Rescue Committee.

T A K E   N O T E

In your community assessment material, this would be an ideal location to append a list of social service agencies, along with identifying information (such as address, phone number, major services, and contact person). Brochures describing services, eligibility, and so on are useful to include as well.

Intracommunity Social Service Facilities

Two churches in Rosemont, South Main Methodist and St. Martin Episcopal, have extensive social outreach programs, including preschool and day care services; benevolence funds for food, clothing, and shelter; and numerous support groups (e.g., Parents Without Partners, Singles, and Solitaires). St. Martin has a seniors' center open 8 AM to 6 PM daily. The seniors enjoy a variety of recreational and educational programs and a hot noon meal. In addition, volunteers assist with shopping and errands, minor home repairs, light housekeeping, and meals for seniors who are permanently or temporarily incapacitated. Noticeably absent from St. Martin were any support groups or programs directed at the large gay male population. When asked about this, staff members responded, "That problem does not exist in this community." South Main does offer a coffee klatch on Friday night and plans to offer additional services to the gay male population, although there is strong resistance from the older parishioners.

On the north side of CT 4107 is Lambda Alcoholics Anonymous (AA), a program specifically for gay men and women, a group originally not allowed to join Alcoholics Anonymous. Lambda AA in CT 4107 is an active group, with the present participation exceeding 200 people. All socioeconomic groups are represented in the meetings, and members take turns leading the support groups.

Economics

The economic subsystem includes the "wealth" of Rosemont (i.e., the goods and services available to the community) as well as the costs and benefits of improving patterns of resource allocation. It should be evident that extracommunity factors, such as the state of the United States and world economies, affect in great measure the local economy. Nevertheless, intracommunity economic factors impinge on all other subsystems, so they must be included in the assessment. Table 11.18 lists the suggested areas for studying a community's economy, along with sources of the data. The census data can be used to summarize most of these economic indicators. Two key indicators of a community's economic health are the percentage of households below the poverty level and the unemployment rate.

Financial Characteristics of Households

The two census tracts that comprise the Rosemont community vary greatly in income characteristics. The census data show the median income for households

TABLE 11.18

Economic Indicators and Sources of Information

Indicators	Source
Financial Characteristics	
Households	
Median household income	
% households below poverty level	
% households receiving public assistance	Census records
% households headed by females	
Monthly costs for owner-occupied households	
and renter-occupied households	
Individuals	
Per capita income	
% of persons who live in poverty	Census records
Labor Force Characteristics	
Employment Status	
General population (age 18+)	
% employed	Chamber of commerce
% unemployed	Department of Labor
% not participating in employment (retired)	Census records
Special groups	
% women working with children under age 6	
Occupational Categories and Number (%) of Persons Employed	
Managerial	
Technical	
Service	
Farming	Census records
Production	
Operator/laborer	
Union Activity and Membership	Local union(s) office

in CT 4104 to be $34,798, whereas in CT 4107 it is $28,247. Table 11.19 lists the household income for the community and Hampton, comparing 1990 and 2000 figures. Midyear data may be used to continue looking at trends, but until the completion of the 2010 census, there will not be 10-year data for comparison.

TABLE 11.19

Income Indices for the Years 1990 and 2000 for CT 4104, CT 4107, and City of Hampton

	CT 4104		CT 4107		HAMPTON	
Income Indices	1990	2000	1990	2000	1990	2000
Median household income	$25,878	$28,247	$21,238	$34,798	$29,378	$42,598
% of families with incomes below poverty level	13.3	20.6	18.3	12.1	14.2	12.1
% of female-headed households	NA	29.6	NA	19.8	12.7	27.1

NA, data not available.
Data from Census of Population and Housing, selected characteristics.

Businesses

Several high-rise office buildings are located on the northern boundary of the area along the Audubon Parkway, including the National General Life Insurance complex of three towers, the new National Tower, the National Service Corporation, and the Second Mortgage Corporation's building. Way-on-the-Bayou, a new office complex, is also being constructed at the corner of Way Drive and Buff's Bayou. These buildings all feature spacious landscaped grounds, modern architecture, and covered parking. Some of the residents of the area are employed in these offices; however, most employees, according to local residents, live outside of Rosemont.

The major area businesses include the Rose Milk Company factory at the northern edge of the area on Way Drive, the Sheet Metal Workers Union Local No. 54 at the corner of Way Drive and Jackson, and American Life Insurance Company on Green.

All of the main thoroughfares in the area are lined with locally owned businesses such as grocery stores, craft stores, antique shops, cleaners, and small restaurants (see the Physical Description section). In addition, these kinds of businesses are also dispersed throughout the area within the residential districts. The Hampton Lighting and Power Service Center is located near the northern edge of the area. Hampton's vehicle maintenance department and its street repair department are also located on West Pleasant in the northern part of the Rosemont area. There is also a considerable number of publishing houses (probably the largest concentration in Hampton) on the northern edge of the area, as well as the broadcast studios of the local CBS station (KHAM-TV).

According to local residents, the economic impact of these businesses on the Rosemont area is minimal because most residents are employed outside of Rosemont, and, although they do patronize neighborhood convenience stores, they tend to shop for major purchases in other areas of the city. The residents also indicated that the vast majority of the businesses do not directly participate in the life of the community. Selected industries of the area are listed in Table 11.20.

When there are major businesses within a community that employ a substantial number of community residents, a thorough assessment is required. See Chapter 19 for further information about workplace assessment.

Labor Force

Employment Status

As mentioned earlier, the unemployment rate is a key indicator of the economic health of the community. The labor force of a community is composed of people

TABLE 11.20

Selected Industries in Rosemont

	CT 4104		CT 4107	
	Number	Total %	Number	Total %
Manufacturing	92	10	430	15
Wholesale and retail trade	450	48	1,084	37
Professional and related services	387	42	1,423	48
TOTAL	929	100	2,937	100

Data from Census, selected characteristics.

TABLE 11.21

Rosemont Labor Force for CT 4104, CT 4107, City of Hampton and Jefferson County

	CT 4104	CT 4107	Hampton	Jefferson County
People age16 and over	4,580	6,470	1,189,136	2,519,937
Labor force	1,825	5,472	850,389	1,653,892
Percentage of people age16 and over	39.8	85.4	71.5	65.6

Data from Census of Population and Housing, selected characteristics.

TABLE 11.22

Class of Workers for CT 4104, CT 4107, and Jefferson County by Percentage of Work Force

	CT 4104	CT 4107	Jefferson County
Private wage and salary	67%	76%	82.6%
Government	18%	12%	11.2%
Local government	13%	12%	6.0%
Self-employed	2%	6%	0.2%
TOTAL	100%	100%	100%

Data from Census of Population and Housing, selected characteristics.

aged 16 years and above. Table 11.21 summarizes key data relating to the workforce of the Rosemont community as well as the City of Hampton and Jefferson County. The majority of workers are categorized under "private wage and salary," as shown in Table 11.22.

Occupation
General occupational categories are included in the census. Table 11.23 lists the occupations of the citizens of Rosemont.

TABLE 11.23

Occupations for Rosemont (CT 4104 and CT 4107)

	CT 4104		CT 4107	
	Number	%	Number	%
Managerial, professional, and related	117	7.1	2,238	42.1
Technical, sales, administrative support	198	12.1	1,813	34.1
Service	724	44.2	560	10.5
Farming	28	1.7	11	0.02
Precision production	186	11.3	463	8.7
Operators, fabricators, laborers	387	23.6	230	4.3
TOTAL	1,640	100	5,315	100

Data from Census of Population and Housing, selected economic characteristics.

Differences between the two census tracts that constitute Rosemont are clearly seen in the occupational makeup of the community. Whereas almost half of the workers in CT 4104 are categorized under "service," a similar percentage of workers in CT 4107 are classified under "managerial and professional specialty."

Safety and Transportation

Table 11.24 lists the major components of safety and transportation that affect the community.

Protection Services

Fire, police, and sanitation services are provided by the City of Hampton. Rosemont residents pay for these services through their city taxes. Therefore, these services are extracommunity, located outside the community of Rosemont.

TABLE 11.24

Safety and Transportation

Indicators	Sources of Information
Safety	
Protection services	Planning office (city, county, and state)
Fire	Fire department (local)
Police	Police department (city and county)
Sanitation	
Waste sources and treatment	} Waste and water treatment plants
Solid waste	
Air quality	Air control board (state, regional, and local offices)
Transportation	
Private	
Transportation sources	} Census data: Population and housing characteristics
Number of persons with a transportation disability	
Public	
Bus service (routes, schedules, and fares)	} Local and city transportation authorities
Roads (number and condition; primary, secondary, and farm-to-market roads)	State highway department
Interstate highways	
Freeway system	
Air service (private and publicly owned)	Local airports (Note: Local airports are frequently owned and operated by city government.)
Rail service	In the United States, Amtrak is the primary source of intercity rail transportation

Fire Protection

The fire department and MEAS are combined in Hampton. (For a description of the MEAS, see the Health and Social Services section.) The fire station serving Rosemont maintains two fire trucks, one air boat (for evacuations during flooding), and 20 personnel. Firemen must complete 335 hours of basic certification courses. The fire captain reports a response time of less than 10 minutes. During the 90 days before the assessment, the station responded to 45 fires. This compares to 39 responses during the same period of the previous year. Forty responses were to homes—the major culprit being grease fires that started in the kitchen. Other leading causes of fires include lighted cigarettes and children playing with matches. In addition to responding to fires, personnel perform safety checks of homes; teach fire-prevention to school and community groups; and distribute window stickers that specify the location of children, elderly citizens, and pets for emergency alert during a fire.

Police Protection

The police department serving Rosemont has a staff of 27 full-time employees, including 21 police officers and 6 civilians (4 dispatchers and 2 record clerks). Equipment includes five marked and four unmarked patrol cars, two motorcycles, and a complete computerized data storage and retrieval system. This station has one holding cell where people are detained until they can be transported to the Hampton Jail. According to the dispatcher, response time to Rosemont is 4 to 6 minutes. Crime statistics for CT 4104 and CT 4107 are presented in Table 11.25.

The most frequent crimes are burglaries and thefts, which the police captain believes are committed mainly by nonresidents of Rosemont. Speeding and driving while intoxicated (DWI) are also frequent crimes in Rosemont; although, after the addition of two motorcycle police officers 2 years ago, the number of traffic accidents has decreased by 38%. The police department offers the following services to Rosemont residents:

- Housewatch—When residents are out of town, the police will check their house three times a day for up to 30 days.
- Identification—The police department loans an engraver to citizens who wish to engrave personal belongings. The department also provides household possessions registration and pamphlets on how to protect one's home from burglary.

TABLE 11.25

Crime Statistics for CT 4104 and CT 4107

	2003		2004		2005	
	CT 4104	CT 4107	CT 4104	CT 4107	CT 4104	CT 4107
Murder	10	3	5	3	7	2
Rape	34	17	17	5	12	4
Robbery	328	186	345	157	320	146
Aggravated assault	94	29	76	25	57	20
Burglary	345	339	329	337	320	325
Theft	384	363	370	359	328	322
Vehicle theft	109	327	112	378	101	315
TOTAL	1,304	1,264	1,254	1,264	1,145	1,134

Data from City of Hampton police department.

- Fingerprinting—Fingerprinting is done and a record of the prints is provided to the person for personal identification as well as for immigration requirements. The police department is presently pursuing a special project, a citywide campaign to fingerprint all children and adolescents. A copy of the fingerprint record is given to parents, and the original remains with the police. After several weeks of radio and TV announcements, police personnel are now present at local shopping centers every weekend to explain and complete the fingerprinting process. This special project is in response to citizen concern and requests for police assistance in locating an increasing number of missing children.
- Animal Protection Officer—The City of Hampton has a leash and fence law for dogs. The animal protection officer picks up stray animals and detains them in the city kennel until the owner or an adopter can be found.
- Public Education—Crime prevention programs are offered to community and school groups.

Residents of Rosemont repeatedly voiced concern about their personal safety. Elderly citizens expressed fear of being mugged and related stories of friends who have been harassed and robbed during the day as they walked to and from local stores. (One grocery store owner reported that he has stopped cashing Social Security checks because so many patrons had been mugged after leaving his store.) The feeling of being a prisoner in one's own home was repeatedly expressed, as were questions regarding what people could do to protect themselves.

Gay men described experiences of perceived harassment by police as well as incidents of marked delay (up to 30 minutes) in police response time to requests for help. Residents reported that brawls, quarrels, and physical violence are becoming commonplace in Rosemont. The citizens are concerned for themselves and others; they want a safe place to live.

Sanitation

Water Sources and Treatment. The terrain of Rosemont is flat with minimal changes in elevation. Stagnant pools of water are common—a situation that promotes mosquito populations during the warm months. Drainage is toward the northeast and into Buff's Bayou, the only open stream in Rosemont. All storm water and sewage are gathered into Hampton's sewage system. There is no separate system for storm water disposal. As a result, raw sewage backs up during heavy rains, and residents complain about the smell and problems associated with toilets that cannot be flushed.

Sewage from Rosemont is treated at the 5th Street Plant. A sewage moratorium exists for Rosemont owing to overcapacity at the 5th Street Plant. Consequently, only single-family dwellings can be built on plotted lots. Builders requesting permits for multifamily dwellings are given the option of delaying building indefinitely or being assessed a fee based on projected occupancy of their building and the associated gallons of sewage that will be produced. The assessed fee is used to increase the capacity of the treatment plant. However, even if the assessed fee option is chosen, it may be 3 to 4 years before the permit is issued.

Potable (drinkable) water for Rosemont comes from Lake Hampton, located 20 miles north of the city. Residents are concerned about possible contamination of the drinking water with lead and other heavy metals. There is no routine testing of the drinking water except to meet state health department requirements for chlorine content. Fluoride is not added to Rosemont's drinking water, and it is not present naturally.

Solid Waste. Garbage is collected weekly from City of Hampton–provided individual household plastic cans at curbside; residents state that the service and frequency are adequate. The major complaint is that illegal dumping of large items, such as refrigerators, stoves, and so forth, has increased, and, despite numerous calls to proper authorities, the trash is not cleaned up with any regularity. Parents are concerned that children attracted by abandoned machinery and appliances may be hurt as they explore. In addition, inoperable automobiles are abandoned in parking spaces on the streets, and months can pass before the cars are removed by the city.

Air Quality

The Federal Air Quality Act of 1967 provided for the establishment of air-quality control regions. Regional offices maintain an inventory of air-pollution sources and monitor air status. In a similar fashion, individual states formed advisory boards that developed air-quality standards and long-range air-quality programs. Local air-monitoring stations sample and record information levels on such pollutants as ozone, carbon monoxide, sulfur dioxide, and nitrogen dioxide. In addition, some 30 to 40 suspended particles in the air (solids) are measured and recorded, as are certain gaseous substances (e.g., ammonia).

To assess the air quality of Rosemont, the Air Control Board was contacted; its recent reports document a rise in air pollution, which is attributed to an increase in industrial growth and a high population density. Some 25 miles east of Rosemont is a large industrial complex, and, although the daily emissions from the industries are within acceptable limits, certain wind and temperature patterns act to compound emissions. This causes a visible yellow haze to form that shrouds Rosemont and surrounding communities many days of the year. Area residents complain of eye irritation and increased frequency of respiratory conditions. The chemical reactions that lead to the haze and the contribution of automotive and industrial emissions, as well as potential health effects associated with the haze, are unknown and are presently being researched.

TAKE NOTE

Air pollution is a frequently used term; it is defined as the presence of one or more contaminants in such concentration and of such duration that they may adversely affect human health, animal life, vegetation, or property.

Despite the pollution increase and industrial growth, there has been no significant increase in the amount of pollutants introduced into the atmosphere surrounding Rosemont. This is attributed to compliance of industries with the Air Control Board regulations and the permit system for new industries. Citizens can contest industry construction permits and, through this process, provide a forum for public opinion and objections that regulation boards take into consideration during the permit decision-making process. Citizens are also entitled to complain to the board regarding a specific industry's emissions; the board will then investigate and file a report.

During the past year, Rosemont has experienced three air stagnation advisories. Because the pollution concentration is greater than usual, people with respiratory conditions such as bronchitis and emphysema are advised to remain indoors and limit outside activities until the air stagnation clears.

> *T A K E   N O T E*
>
> Air stagnation occurs when a layer of cool air is trapped by a layer of warmer air above it; the bottom air cannot rise and pollutants cannot be dispersed.

The board believes citizens are ill informed regarding the meaning of and the appropriate actions that should be taken during air stagnation advisories as well as each citizen's responsibility in minimizing pollution. For example, citizens seem unaware that transportation sources (such as automobiles and buses), not industry, are the major contributors of air pollution problems and that a citizen who burns leaves or trash is releasing tiny particles of matter into the air that can irritate the eyes, nose, and lungs. To promote public awareness and understanding, the local office makes presentations to organizations, schools, and citizen groups. Numerous public television and radio programs were planned for the year after the assessment.

Transportation

The primary means of transportation in Rosemont include walking, bicycle riding, automobiles, Hampton city buses, Hampton city vans (special transportation for the elderly and handicapped), and school buses.

Private

The major source of private transportation is the automobile. Table 11.26 presents the types of transportation used to commute to work, and Table 11.27 indicates the number of people aged 16 years or older who have a transportation disability. According to the census data, mean travel time to work for Rosemont residents is 17.7 minutes as compared to 26.6 minutes for Hampton residents.

Public

The major source of public transportation within Rosemont and surrounding communities is the Hampton bus system. The city provides east–west bus service at half-hour intervals during the day on Pecan Drive and Live Oak Boulevard. The same service is provided on north–south routes for Way Drive, Rosemont Boulevard, and Hampton Street. For people who qualify (such as the elderly or handicapped), the

TABLE 11.26

Transportation Sources to Work Used by Residents of CT 4104, CT 4107, and City of Hampton

	CT 4104		CT 4107		Hampton	
	Number	**%**	**Number**	**%**	**Number**	**%**
Drive alone	1,351	42.8	3,279	63.8	NA	75.7
Car pool	749	23.7	808	15.7		14.6
Public transportation	721	22.8	567	11		4.1
Walk	231	7.3	300	5.8		1.8
Other means	79	2.5	130	2.5		1.4
Work at home	27	0.9	58	1.2		2.4
TOTAL	3,158	100	5,142	100		100

NA, data not available.
Data from Census of Population and Housing, selected characteristics.

TABLE 11.27

Noninstitutionalized People 16 Years of Age or Older by Transportation
Disability Status for CT 4104 and CT 4107

	With Disability		Without Disability		Total	
	Number	%	Number	%	Number	%
Age 16–64						
CT 4104	221	5.9	3,495	94.1	3,716	100
CT 4107	15	0.3	5,908	99.7	5,923	100
Age 65 and over						
CT 4104	197	21.3	728	78.7	925	100
CT 4107	55	10.5	469	89.5	524	100

Data from Census of Population and Housing.

bus company provides door-to-door service from the person's home to essential
services such as food shopping or medical care visits. The cost of this service varies
from $1.00 to $2.00 per trip, according to geographic area. Although all users agree
the service is reliable, it is only available Monday through Friday, 8:30 AM to 5:00 PM,
and reservations are required several days in advance—a requirement that is impossible to meet in some situations such as during acute illnesses.

Roads
Jefferson County (of which Rosemont is a part) has adequate primary, secondary,
and farm-to-market roads. In addition, several miles of a freeway system circle
Hampton. Two major interstate highways transect Hampton, and the state highway
department has budgeted $2 billion for highway construction and maintenance for
Jefferson County over the next 20 years. Recently, the residents of Jefferson County
voted for an additional tax devoted entirely to improving intracounty transportation.
Rosemont residents complain of congested freeways and damaged roads that go
without repair for months. The need was expressed for a road system that efficiently
handles local traffic.

Air Service
Jefferson County has four small, privately owned airports. The City of Hampton
owns and operates two airports that provide national and international service.

Rail Service
Amtrak connects Hampton to other major cities in the state as well as to other states.
METRO light rail began operation in Hampton on January 1, 2004. It was the first
phase of a projected 73 miles of service by 2025. The rail runs near, but not through,
Rosemont, serving downtown Hampton, a major sports stadium, two universities,
the museum district, a city park, and the medical center. Fare is $1.00 one way, and
for $2.00 the rider can purchase a 24-hour pass for unlimited rides.

Politics and Government
Rosemont falls within the city limits of Hampton, which has a mayor-council form
of government. There are 14 council members (5 at-large), one of whom represents
Rosemont and nearby communities. Each serves a 2-year term. The city council
meets at City Hall on the first Tuesday of each month. The meetings are open to
the public, and Rosemont residents often attend.

The city council and mayor comprise the policy-making body as well as the administrative head of Hampton. Their duties include the following: maintaining competent staff to operate all city services (the health department and police, for instance), passing ordinances, and appropriating funds to carry out policies.

The councilman for District Three, which includes Rosemont, is James Browning. Councilman Browning was elected by a wide margin of votes and has been popular with the Rosemont community because he spearheaded the fight against sexually oriented businesses (the "SOB Fight," as it is popularly called). This issue has not been settled, and the citizens are supporting Councilman Browning's reelection, so he may continue the fight.

The active participation in the Hampton council of Councilman Browning is only one indicator of Rosemont's politics. There are several politically oriented organizations and civic clubs in the area, all of which seek to improve the quality of life in Rosemont and help to support intercommunity activities.

A brief synopsis of several organizations that are politically active in Rosemont is presented in Table 11.28. (Contact person, address, and phone number should be included in such lists but have been omitted from this description.)

Several other groups in the community are less visible and active unless an issue of particular interest becomes "hot." For instance, many voluntary agencies, such

TABLE 11.28

Organizations Politically Active in Rosemont

Organization	Description
Neartown Business Alliance (Founded 1949)	Owners of businesses in the area meet monthly and work to promote the area and its businesses. The alliance contributes to campaigns of supporters of Rosemont
Gay Political Caucus (Founded 1964)	This is a very active and visible group. It works to influence elections through voter registration, campaign work, and education. It has been credited with the election or defeat of certain candidates. Membership is open to all interested in community improvement. It meets on third Tuesday, 7:00 PM
Rosemont Firehouse (Founded 1973)	This is a coordination and referral group; it operates a 24-hour crisis hotline. It is sponsored by donations from most of the area's churches as well as the civic groups, and most of the workers are community volunteers
Rosemont Watch (Founded 1978)	The Watch works to prevent crime in the area through education and visible activities such as "Block Awareness Week." It coordinates activities with the Hampton City Police. All citizens are encouraged to become involved. It meets monthly
Seniors for a Safe Community (Founded 1980)	Composed primarily of retired people (but open to all interested residents), this group was formed to address the problem of the mugging or robbing of senior citizens, especially on the days when Social Security checks arrived. The original small group has expanded, as have their goals, so now they are actively involved in promoting a better quality of life for all in the community (with a special emphasis on the elderly). This group is active in the "SOB Fight" and also works closely with Rosemont Watch

as the American Lung Association—Hampton Chapter, are located in the community and can be called on to assist specific campaigns (e.g., smoking-prevention programs in the schools or antipollution campaigns aimed toward extracommunity sources). The Community Services Directory lists all such organizations both by interest (heart, lung, crime, and so on) and general area (Rosemont groups can usually be found under "Southwest, near downtown").

Political activism is evident throughout Rosemont. During election years, there are campaign posters everywhere; talk at gathering places (barbershops, grocery stores, bars) inevitably turns to politics; and numerous rallies are held in support of candidates or issues. In Rosemont, there appear to be two major political factions. Voting records show CT 4107 residents to be more liberal than residents in CT 4104. This may reflect the fact that CT 4107 has more affluent, younger, and more professional residents than CT 4104.

Communication

Communication may be formal or informal. Formal communication usually originates outside the community (extracommunity) as opposed to informal communication, which almost always originates and is disseminated within the community. Salient components of formal and informal communication, as well as sources of data, are presented in Table 11.29.

Formal Communication

Hampton has one major newspaper, *The Hampton Herald*. Additional daily newspapers include a business journal, *Current Issues*; an African-American-oriented paper; *Progress*; one Spanish-language paper, *La Prensa*; and a Vietnamese tabloid. Hampton has 12 AM radio stations and 10 FM stations, 6 commercial TV stations, and 1 educational network. Cable television is available to Rosemont residents on a monthly subscription basis. Residents receive home mail delivery.

TABLE 11.29

Communications

Components	Sources of Information
Formal	
Newspaper (number, circulation, frequency, and scope of news)	Chamber of Commerce
	Newspaper office
Radio and television (number of stations, commercial versus educational, and audience)	Telephone company
	Yellow Pages
Postal service	Telephone book
Telephone status (number of residents with service)	Census data on phone use
Informal	
Sources: bulletin boards; posters; hand-delivered flyers; and church, civic, and school newsletters	Windshield Survey
Dissemination (How do people receive information?)	Talking to residents
Word of mouth	Survey
Mail	
Radio, television	
Internet may be considered both formal and informal	Personal computer, workplace, public library, "Cyber" cafes

Informal Communication

Bulletin boards and posters dot community and municipal buildings in Rosemont. Posters are placed on trees and tacked to buildings throughout the community, and a rainbow of flyers can be seen tucked into fences and doors. Radio and television announcements herald forthcoming events and offer open forums on community issues. The Rosemont Civic Association publishes a bimonthly, four-page newsletter to notify residents of upcoming meetings and social activities. Polls and surveys are a regular feature of the newsletter, which is distributed free to all residents.

Key informants within Rosemont include the Civic Association secretary, local ministers, and fire and police personnel as well as community civic board members. People can be seen chatting throughout Rosemont, and, when asked how information is received, they mention all of the above formal and informal sources.

Education

The general educational status of a community can be summarized using census data. Census information lists the number of residents attending schools, years of schooling completed, and percentage of residents who speak English. To supplement this broad assessment, information is needed about major educational sources (e.g., schools, colleges, and libraries) located inside the community. Table 11.30 is a guide for assessing a community's educational sources.

TAKE NOTE

It is sometimes difficult to decide which educational sources to include in the assessment. Community usage is probably the single most important indicator. Primary and secondary schools attended by the majority of children in a community, regardless of intra- or extracommunity location, are major educational sources and require a thorough assessment, whereas schools composed primarily of students from outside the community do not require such extensive appraisal.

TABLE 11.30

Education

Components	Sources of Information
Educational Status	
Years of school completed	Census data—Social characteristics section
School enrollment by type of school	Census data—Social characteristics section
Language spoken	Census data—Social characteristics section
Educational Sources	
Intracommunity or extracommunity (collect data for each facility)	Local board of education
Services (educational, recreational, communication, and health)	School administrator (such as the principal or director) and school nurse
Resources (personnel, space, budget, and record system)	School administrator
Characteristics of users (geographic distribution and demographic profile)	Teachers and staff
Adequacy, accessibility, and acceptability of education to students and staff	Students and staff

TABLE 11.31

Years of School Completed for CT 4104, CT 4107, and City of Hampton

	CT 4104	CT 4107	Hampton
Persons 25 years and over	3,459	4,948	888,269
Elementary			
0 to 4 years	611	26	41,695
5 to 7 years	665	164	66,775
8 years	409	101	37,373
High school			
1 to 3 years	800	278	136,179
4 years	661	914	240,320
College			
1 to 3 years	181	1,173	160,999
4 or more years	132	2,292	204,928
% High school graduates	28.2	88.5	68.3

Data from Census of Population and Housing, social characteristics.

Educational Status

Table 11.31 presents the years of schooling completed by adults in CT 4104 and CT 4107. In a similar format, Table 11.32 lists school enrollment by type of school, and Table 11.33 presents the number and percentage of community residents who speak English poorly.

Intracommunity Educational Sources

Temple Elementary School
Temple Elementary School is located on the corner of Pecan and Magnolia Drives, close to the center of CT 4104. Asphalt lots bound three sides of Temple; two are used for vehicle parking, and one is for play. A small patch of grass persists on the remaining side, a fenced-in area that contains several large trees, a swing set, and

TABLE 11.32

School Enrollment and Type of School for CT 4104, CT 4107, and City of Hampton

	CT 4104	CT 4107	Hampton
Type of school			
Public nursery school	94	44	20,735
Private nursery school	77	44	15,427
Public kindergarten	194	14	21,863
Private kindergarten	25	14	4,833
Public elementary (1 to 8 years)	1,258	186	198,367
Private elementary (1 to 8 years)	10	136	18,440
Public high school (1 to 4 years)	482	92	94,099
Private high school (1 to 4 years)	12	25	7,154
College	92	922	78,472
Total enrolled in schools (age 3 years and over)	2,120	1,258	413,536

Data from Census of Population and Housing.

TABLE 11.33

Ability to Speak English for CT 4104, CT 4107, and City of Hampton

	Percentage Who Speak English Poorly or Not At All	
	Age 5–17	Age 18 Years and Over
CT 4104	75.9	73.8
CT 4107	11	19.3
Hampton	21.4	26.2

Data from Census of Population and Housing.

three teeter-totters. Several broken windows were seen, and no graffiti was noted. Temple is in its 74th year of continuous operation teaching grades kindergarten to eighth. Present enrollment is 924; 42% of the students are black, 33% are Asian, 18% are Hispanic, and 5% are white. Most of the children live in Rosemont and either walk to school or ride the school bus (provided for children living farther than 2 miles from Temple).

As part of the Hampton School District (HSD), Temple receives funding from the district revenues obtained from local property taxes, state coffers, and the federal budget. State monies to HSD are based on average daily attendance of students at each school. Most policies affecting Temple are formed and enforced by the HSD Board. The board is composed of eight nonsalaried people, each elected from one of eight regions in the school district. Each term of office is 4 years. Board member Jane Roberts represents Rosemont; at the time of assessment, she was in the second year of her 4-year term. Responsibilities of the HSD board include prescribing qualifications of employees, establishing salary schedules, setting goals and objectives for the district, establishing the policies to implement the goals and objectives, and evaluating the performance of the district in relationship to adopted goals and objectives. The general superintendent is the administrative head of the board and is salaried and recruited by the Board.

Principal. Temple's principal cited truancy and the related problem of academic failure as the school's major problems. According to office records, some 6% to 8% of the student body is absent each day, and most of those absent are not ill. Compounding the problem is the fact that many parents do not have telephones. As a result, it is not uncommon for a student to be absent for 2 or 3 days before parental contact is made. (In most cases, it is found that the parent assumed the child was in school.) The principal believed that truancy is most common among seventh and eighth graders, especially among Hispanic boys.

Regarding bilingual education for non-English-speaking students, the principal believes that all classes should be in English and that the presence of bilingual education at Temple only slows the progress of the children who are learning English. There are two bilingual teachers at Temple; they reported that they have a list of over 100 students who have requested and have been assessed as needing the bilingual program.

Teachers. Teachers repeatedly stated the need for improved communication with parents. They believe that parents need to have current information about their child's learning needs and school performance as well as knowledge of specific techniques for fostering academic achievement. (School policy allows for two 20-minute parent–teacher conferences yearly—a time allotment that was rated as extremely inadequate by the teachers.) The teachers reported that 22% of the student body at Temple failed last year. Major impediments to learning were listed as poor English-speaking skills and understanding of English, stressful home environments, and inadequate adult supervision at home. Teachers felt overwhelmed and frustrated; the average employment stay at Temple is 2 years.

School Nurse. The school nurse at Temple is present 2 days a week; she is at West Hampton High the remaining 3 days. A review of the daily clinic register for the preceding 6 weeks noted a clinic attendance of 141; the majority (72%) of those visiting suffered from stomachache or headache. Although none of the stomach ailments required early dismissal, 60% of the headaches were associated with fever and necessitated early dismissal from school. Remaining complaints were sore throats and minor cuts or falls. All children were screened biannually for vision and hearing problems. The nurse recognized the need for yearly screening but said she lacked the necessary time. She stated that if school policy would permit the recruitment and training of a parent volunteer(s), then yearly screening would be feasible. In addition to vision and hearing testing, all children are screened for head lice twice a year; children found to be infected are dismissed from school and are not readmitted until they have been successfully treated.

Some 62% of the students participate in the free lunch program. The nurse expressed concern that several children who appear undernourished (displaying, e.g., low weight for height and small arm circumference for age) do not qualify for the lunch program, whereas others who appear to be well nourished do qualify. Eligibility is based on family size and income.

Major health problems as described by the nurse include lack of hygiene (children frequently come to school dirty and inadequately clothed for cold weather); dental caries; high (30% to 40%) annual incidence of head lice, especially in primary grades (kindergarten, first grade, and second grade); incomplete immunization status (92% of the children have up-to-date immunizations); and lack of parent follow-through for needed medical care and treatment during illnesses.

To assess dental status, the nurse performed oral assessment of children who came to the clinic during one 4-week period. She found that 62% of the children had discolored areas or cavities in the pits of their teeth or between teeth. Most of the children stated they had never been to a dentist, and many reported frequent tooth pain and difficulty chewing.

The nurse does not do any health teaching in the classroom because school policy mandates that the nurse be present in the clinic at all times. The ruling causes considerable frustration because the nurse's participation in the teaching and promotion of health habits is restricted to one-to-one clinic encounters (a time when the child is ill and not receptive to learning). When asked about staff and teacher usage of the clinic, the nurse discussed at length the need for health information expressed by both teachers and staff. Questions regarding exercise, stress, and diet modifications are common. The nurse would like to assess and identify specific health needs of staff and teachers.

Community Service. As a community service, Temple sponsors scout troops and basketball and softball teams and provides a meeting place for several newly formed church and community action groups. In addition, Monday through Thursday nights, Temple houses extension courses from Hampton Community College. A full range of subjects is offered, including academic, vocational, and enrichment courses. Present enrollment exceeds 1,200, an increase of 22% from the previous year.

All Rosemont residents were familiar with Temple Elementary; most had children who attended Temple, or they themselves had attended Temple as children. Residents felt that Temple was a community landmark and a symbol of unity that links one generation to the next. The primary complaint, repeated by several families, was a perceived insensitivity of Temple's staff and teachers to ethnic and racial differences and needs. For example, all school notices are written in English, and all programs offered by the Parent Teachers Organization (PTO) are presented in English. Both Asian and Hispanic parents have brought specific concerns and needs to the staff and teachers at Temple but have repeatedly been told that all parental requests must come from appropriate PTO committees—an organization that seems alien to many Asian and Hispanic parents.

Day Care
One day care center is located in CT 4104—the Busybee Nursery. There are no day care facilities in CT 4107. Housed in a renovated building, Busybee accepts children aged 2 to 5 years. Some 60 children are cared for by five staff members, and 43 children (primarily toddlers) are on the waiting list. The center is licensed by the state. Rosemont residents repeatedly lamented the lack of day care facilities. Many parents felt forced to leave their young children with other mothers or teenagers who have dropped out of school. Several mothers reported leaving their children daily with a babysitter who cares for 8 to 10 children.

Library
The Rosemont library is conveniently located adjacent to the main shopping district and offers a variety of adult, teen, and youth book programs, films, and special educational activities. Notices of all programs are published in the Rosemont Civic Association newsletter and posted on local bulletin boards.

Extracommunity Educational Sources

High school students from Rosemont attend Central Hampton High, a complex that houses 4,800 students and is located 8 miles from Rosemont. Concerned about truancy and grade failure, Central Hampton began a "Failproof" program 2 years ago. Some 82% of students and their parents have participated. As a result, school scores on state and national proficiency tests have improved, and truancy has decreased. The principal described numerous community outreach services offered by the school, including recreational programs in the evening and on the weekends, as well as a full complement of adult education courses.

The nurse at Central Hampton is present 5 days a week. The majority of visits to the clinic (an average of 30 daily) involve allergy-related complaints, gastrointestinal upsets, and minor sprains or strains that occur during physical exercise class. Because of HSD policies, the school nurse is prohibited from offering health education in the classroom.

The nurse's major concern is the increased number of teenage pregnancies and the HSD board's decision of 2 years ago not to permit sex education information in the classroom. Classes in sexuality, sexually transmitted disease, contraception, and decision making in the area of sexual activity had been offered at all high schools in Hampton before the new ruling. The nurse does not know the sequence of events that resulted in the sex education decision. A second major concern is the increased use of alcohol among students. A drug awareness curriculum was prepared by the state board of education and will be implemented during the next semester as part of the biology course.

Numerous private preschool and grade schools are available in Hampton, and some are used by the residents of Rosemont, especially by people in CT 4107. Some

20 colleges and universities are located in Hampton and Jefferson County; most offer a variety of general education and specialty training programs. One unique aspect of the area's educational resources is Hampton Community College, a junior college that provides classes in 21 public schools in Hampton and Jefferson County. Numerous residents state that they prefer Hampton Community College to other area resources because of its convenient locations, low tuition, and employment-oriented approach to education.

Recreation

The recreation facilities within and adjacent to Rosemont are listed in Table 11.34 and pictured in Figure 11.5 (page 185). With the exception of the schoolyards, there is very little recreational area for children and almost none for adults and teenagers. Although there are funds in the budget of the Hampton Parks and Recreation Department for the acquisition of property, there are no plans for any development in the Rosemont area. However, the city has recently begun an improvement program along the banks of Buff's Bayou to create a "River Walk" similar to those in other cities with rivers. It will be several years before the project is completed.

The Rosemont Sports Association provides quality organized recreation opportunities for the local community. Programs consist of teams for bowling, softball, flag football, tennis, and so forth. The Rosemont Sports Association, however, is open only to members who pay a fee of $20 per year.

Churches of Rosemont (two were visited—see the Social Services section) offer a wide variety of activities for all ages. Exercise classes, craft classes, Mother's Day Out, preschool classes, senior citizens' groups, and many other programs are available to members. Although other community residents are welcome to take advantage of these activities, the people interviewed at the churches reported that their participants are almost all church members.

Several residents spoke of an area along the northern bank of Buff's Bayou (just east of Way Drive) that is used as a gathering place by residents who live nearby. Families take their children there on summer evenings, so parents can visit while the children play. The only facilities at this area are benches that have been placed along the grassy area.

TABLE 11.34

Recreational Facilities in Rosemont and Adjacent Areas

	Acreage	Location	Facilities
San Juan	2.6	1650 Pleasant	Shelter building, playground equipment, softball field, and baseball field
Richards	1	1414 Redbud	Shelter building, playground equipment, picnic area, and basketball court (swimming pool recently filled in)
Applehurst	1.9	600 Water Oak	Recreation center, rest room, playground equipment, picnic area, tennis, basketball, and volleyball courts
Jeckle Park	0.08	1500 Maple	None
Buff's Bayou	?	"Greens" along the bayou	Park benches and jogging/bicycle trail

Data from City of Hampton, Parks and Recreation Department, interview with JB [Director], May 1994.

A bicycle/jogging trail follows the bayou for several miles and is popular with the health-conscious residents who use it frequently, especially in the early morning and late evening hours. Some people have expressed fear of being mugged while using this trail, but there have been no official reports of crime in this area over the past year. The trail and all the land along the bayou are maintained by the city of Hampton.

The area residents of the east side tend to congregate for recreation on sidewalks and in neighborhood bars. The one playground in the area, other than the one at Temple Elementary, is located adjacent to the Audubon Parkway Village (the low-rent housing complex), and it is used exclusively by the residents of that complex. The playground equipment is in very poor repair, and there is virtually no grass left in the area. The Parks and Recreation Department has no plans to upgrade or replace the equipment or to replant the grass.

There is one movie theater and one theater for stage production in Rosemont, but movie theaters are accessible and near almost all areas surrounding the community. Other forms of evening entertainment are reflected in the numerous bars and restaurants that feature live music (as was mentioned in the physical examination of the community).

Extracommunity recreational facilities abound. A large city park that includes museums, a zoo, a band shell, and picnic areas is less than a mile to the south of Rosemont. Another city park in downtown Hampton, called Serenity Park, is less than a mile to the northeast.

Virtually every major league sport has a team in Hampton. The sports arenas are some distance from the area, but there is adequate bus service to them.

An abundance of music and theater is available to those who can afford it. Hampton has a symphony orchestra, a ballet, both grand and light opera, and a legitimate stage company, to name a few options. In addition, water activities, such as boating and fishing, are as close as 30 miles away. According to several residents of Audubon Parkway Village, a special day out includes crabbing along the bay—which is often a successful endeavor to fill the dinner pot as well as provide fun for the whole family.

Summary

The community assessment is never complete; however, we must pause at some point. Because we have addressed all parts of the model, this is where we will stop. A description of each community subsystem has been recorded. Note that at every step of the assessment, people in the community were included. Not only did we interview the professionals (e.g., school nurses, principal, police chief, and so on), but clients of the subsystems were also included (parents, shoppers, patients, and people on the street). The assessment, like all steps in the process, is carried out in partnership with the community. The next step is analysis, a process that synthesizes the assessment information and derives from it diagnoses specific to the community.

Crucial to community assessment is a model, or map, to direct and guide that process. The model (community assessment wheel) provided a framework, and the windshield survey tool guided the assessment of Rosemont. In the Further Readings list, several other approaches to community assessment are presented. As you are aware, there are other models you may wish to consider as you continue your practice of community health assessment.

Critical Thinking Questions

1. You are a member of many communities. Describe at least three communities of which you are a part. What makes each a community?

2. Describe one community you have identified above using the community assessment wheel. Find some basic demographic information about the community on the Internet. Does it differ with your own view of that community?

3. What opportunities exist for you to become involved in your community? Are these related to your role as a community health nurse?

● References

Baum, F. (1998). Measuring effectiveness in community-based health promotion. In J. K. Davies & G. Macdonald (Eds.). *Quality, evidence and effectiveness in health promotion.* New York: Routledge.

Hancock, T., & Minkler, M. (2005). Community health assessment or healthy community assessment. In M. Minkler (Ed.) *Community organizing and community building for health* (pp. 138–159). New Brunswick, NJ: Rutgers University Press.

Neuman, B. N. (1972). A model for teaching total person approach to patient problems. *Nursing Research*, 21(3), 264–269.

World Health Organization. (1986). *Ottawa charter for health promotion.* WHO Regional Office for Europe. Copenhagen, Denmark: Author.

■ Further Readings

Beverly, C. J., McAtee, R., Costello, Chernoff, R., & Casteel, J. (2005). Needs assessment of rural communities: A focus on older adults. *Journal of Community Health*, 30(3), 197–208.

Clark, N., & Buell, A. (2004). Community assessment: An innovative approach. *Nurse Educator*, 29(5), 203–207.

Corso, L., Wiesner, P. J., & Lenihan, P. (2005). Developing the MAPP community health improvement tool. *Journal of Public Health Management and Practice*, 11(5), 387–392.

Escoffery, C., Trowbridge, J., & Miner, K. R. (2004). Conducting small-scale community assessments. *American Journal of Health Education*, 35(4), 237–241.

Green, L. W., & Kreuter, M.W. (1999). *Health promotion planning: An educational and ecological approach* (3rd ed.). Mountain View, CA: Mayfield.

Kretzman, J. P., & McKnight, J. L. (1993). *Building communities from the inside out: A path toward finding and mobilizing a community's assets.* Chicago: ACTA Publications.

Pender, N. J., Murdaugh, C. L., & Parsons, M. A. (2006). *Health promotion in nursing practice* (5th ed.). Upper Saddle River, NJ: Prentice Hall.

Serafini, P. (1976). Nursing assessment in industry: A model. *American Journal of Public Health*, 66(8), 755–760.

Williams, R., & Yanoshik, K. (2001). Can you do a community assessment without talking to the community? *Journal of Community Health*, 26(3), 233–247.

Zahner, S. J., Kaiser, B., & Kapelke-Dale, J. (2005). Local partnerships for community assessment and planning. *Journal of Public Health Management and Practice*, 11(5), 460–464.

Internet Resources can be found on the**Point** at http://thepoint.lww.com/Anderson6e.

Community Analysis and Nursing Diagnosis

ELIZABETH T. ANDERSON AND JUDITH MCFARLANE

LEARNING OBJECTIVES

This chapter focuses on the second phase of the nursing process, analysis, and the associated task of forming community nursing diagnoses.

After studying this chapter, you should be able to:

1. Critically analyze community assessment data.
2. Formulate community nursing diagnoses.

Introduction

*A*nalysis is the study and examination of data. These data may be quantitative (numerical) as well as qualitative. All aspects need to be considered. Analysis is necessary to determine community health needs and community strengths, as well as to identify patterns of health responses and trends in health care use. During analysis, any need for further data collection is revealed as gaps and incongruities in the community assessment data. The end point of analysis is the community nursing diagnosis.

COMMUNITY ANALYSIS

Analysis, like so many procedures we carry out, may be viewed as a process with multiple steps. The phases we use to help in the analysis are categorization, summarization, comparison, and inference elaboration. Each is described below.

Categorize

To analyze community assessment data, it is helpful to first categorize the data. Data can be categorized in a variety of ways. Traditional categories of community assessment data include the following:

- Demographic characteristics (family size, age, sex, and ethnic and racial groupings)
- Geographic characteristics (area boundaries; number and size of neighborhoods, public spaces, and roads)

- Socioeconomic characteristics (occupation and income categories, educational attainment, and rental or home ownership patterns)
- Health resources and services (hospitals, clinics, mental health centers, and so forth)

However, models are being used increasingly in the organization and analysis of community health data because they provide a framework for data collection and a map to guide analysis. Because the community assessment wheel (see Fig. 11.2) was used to direct the community assessment process in the Rosemont example, that same model can be used as a framework for analysis. Consider the core as the major focus for analysis with the subsystems representing the context. Stressors and strengths (lines of resistance) may be contributed by either the core, the subsystems, or both.

Summarize

Once a categorization method has been selected, the next task is to summarize the data within each category. Both summary statements and summary measures, such as rates, charts, and graphs, are required.

> ### T A K E   N O T E
>
> Many health care agencies and educational institutions have access to computerized information systems—systems through which formatted data can be retrieved in a variety of forms—including summary health statistics. For example, data entered into a computer system as census figures can be configured into population pyramids, and census and vital statistics information can be programmed to calculate birth, death, and fertility rates. Calculations that previously required hours to complete are now computed in seconds. In your practice, make it a point to inquire as to the availability of computer systems and, if possible, use computer processes to complete quantitative data analysis. In addition, your local health department may be able to furnish the rates for you (for instance, the infant mortality rate [IMR]). Note, however, that the denominator used may not be the community as you have defined it.

Compare

Additional tasks of data analysis include the identification of data gaps, incongruencies, and omissions. Frequently, comparative data are needed to determine if a pattern or trend exists or if data do not seem correct and if revalidation of original information is required. Data gaps are inevitable, as are mistakes in recording data; the important task is to analyze data critically and be aware of the potential for gaps and omissions. It is helpful to have professional colleagues as well as community residents review the analysis. Every person has a unique perspective; it is only through the sharing of views that a whole and comprehensive picture of community assessment data can evolve.

> ### T A K E   N O T E
>
> The word *data* is plural for datum (a real or assumed thing used as a basis for calculations). So, when referring to data, use the appropriate (plural) verb form. For example, the data *were* collected by all members of our group; or, these data *reflect* a downward trend in the IMR.

Using the data from your community, compare them with other similar data. For instance, you calculate (or discover) an IMR of 12 per 1,000 live births. How does this compare with the city? The state? The nation? Is it for the entire infant population of your community? Is the IMR different based on race? (Note: This is a good time to review Chapter 2 to assist you with epidemiologic reasoning as you try to make sense of your data.)

Another important comparison—across time—is helpful to detect trends. If data are available for several years, you can compare those different times to discover whether the problem is improving. An example would be IMRs.

Other resources for comparison are the documents dealing with objectives—for the nation and for individual states. Healthy People 2010 presents national figures, such as incidence and prevalence when available, for our major health problems and proposes goals and objectives for each (U.S. Department of Health and Human Services, 1997). Healthy People 2010—along with state and, if available, local health planning documents—can be invaluable to you both as you analyze your data and as you develop a plan based on those data.

Draw Inferences

Having categorized, summarized, and compared the data you have collected, the next phase is to draw logical conclusions from the evidence (i.e., to draw inferences that will lead to the statement of a community nursing diagnosis). It is in this phase that you synthesize what you know about the community (i.e., what do these data *mean*?). These conclusions or inferences will identify the community's stressors and strengths in succinct phrases. These phrases, then, form the basis for a community nursing diagnosis.

The next section of this chapter walks you through analysis of the data we collected in the community assessment of Rosemont. Following these analysis examples, information on how to form community nursing diagnoses is presented (see the Community Nursing Diagnosis section later in this chapter).

ROSEMONT SAMPLE COMMUNITY ANALYSIS

The analysis of the Rosemont assessment data, as in the assessment process, begins with the community core, because it is the core (the people and their health) that is of interest to the community health nurse. Recall that the core is affected by (and affects) all of the subsystems depicted in the model surrounding it. Some subsystems will influence certain problems more than others, but it is important to assess the subsystems because of their contribution to the causes and alleviation of problems in the core.

Community Core

An analysis of Rosemont's core is presented in Table 12.1. Community core data include many demographic measures, a type of data especially amenable to graphs and charts. The adage "one picture is worth a thousand words" is particularly meaningful for demographic characteristics.

Perhaps the most graphic illustration of the age and sex composition of a population is the population pyramid. Population pyramids for census tracts (CTs) 4104 and 4107 appear in Figure 12.1. A population pyramid for Rosemont is shown

TABLE 12.1

Analysis of Rosemont's Core

Categories of Data	Summary Statements/Measures	Inferences
History		
	Cultural and ethnic diversity	Community revitalization
	Renovation of businesses and homes	Community pride
	Pride and concern evident	
Demographics		
Age		
CT 4104	42.5% of population <19 years	Large % of children and adolescents
	53% of population >19 years or <65 years	High dependency ratio*
	10% of population >65 years	Large % of elderly compared to Hampton and Jefferson County
Data gap: Need prior census data to determine if demographics are consistent or changing		
CT 4107	7.5% of population <19 years	Small % of children and adolescents
	15.2% of population <19 years or >65 years	Low dependency ratio
	7.7% of population >65 years	
Data gap: Need census data on 5-year increments to construct population pyramids		
Sex		
CT 4104	48% of population is male	Equal % of males and females
	45% of population aged 20–64 is male	
CT 4107	65% of population is male	High % of males
	69% of population aged 20–64 is male	
Data gap: Need prior census data to determine if demographics are consistent or changing		
Race/ethnicity		
CT 4104	Diversity: black 54%; Asian 19%; white 12%; Hispanic 9%	Racial and ethnic diversity
CT 4107	Homogeneity: white 89%	Racial and ethnic homogeneity
Data gap: Need census data from 1990 to determine if demographics are consistent or changing		
Household types		
CT 4104	83% of households are families	Family households dominate
CT 4107	36% of households are families	Nonfamily households dominate
Marital status		
CT 4104	15% single, 60% married, 14% divorced	Small % of single adults
		Majority of adults married
CT 4107	53% single, 24% married, 15% divorced	Large % of single adults
		Small % married
Data gap: Need prior census data to determine if demographics are consistent.		
Vital Statistics (Refer to Chapter 3 for rate calculation)		
Births	Rate per 1,000	(When compared to Hampton and Jefferson County data)
CT 4104	30.5	A higher birth rate
CT 4107	17.3	A lower birth rate
Hampton	19.4	
Jefferson County	25.2	
Data gap: Need general fertility rate and age-specific birth rate		
Deaths	Rate per 1,000	(When compared to Hampton and Jefferson County Data)
CT 4104		
	Infant 33.3	A higher death rate for all ages
Neonatal	23.8	
	Fetal 76.2	
CT 4107		
Infant	17.1	A higher infant and neonatal rate
Neonatal	17.1	
Fetal	8.5	
Crude	6.2	

Categories of Data	Summary Statements/Measures	Inferences
Data gap: Need vital statistics from previous 3 to 5 years to determine if rates are consistent or changing		
Hampton		
Infant	12.1	
Neonatal	7.9	
Fetal	12.6	
Crude	6.0	
Jefferson County		
Infant	12.3	
Neonatal	8.3	
Fetal	15.3	
Crude	7.3	
Causes of Death	See Table 11.8	(When compared to Hampton and Jefferson County data)
CT 4104		A much higher % of deaths due to diseases of infancy, homicides, suicides
CT 4107	See Table 11.8	A higher % of deaths due to cerebrovascular disease A lower % of deaths due to heart disease

*Dependency ratio describes the potentially self-supporting portion of the population and the dependent portions at the extremes of age. The dependency ratio is usually computed as follows:

$$\frac{\text{population under age 20 + population age 65 and over}}{\text{population age 20 to 64 years of age}} \times 100$$

The dependency ratio for CT 4104 is 91, meaning for every 100 persons aged 20 to 65 (supposedly self-supporting because of age), there are 91 persons under age 20 or over age 65 needing support (because of age). In contrast, the dependency ratio for CT 4107 is 19.

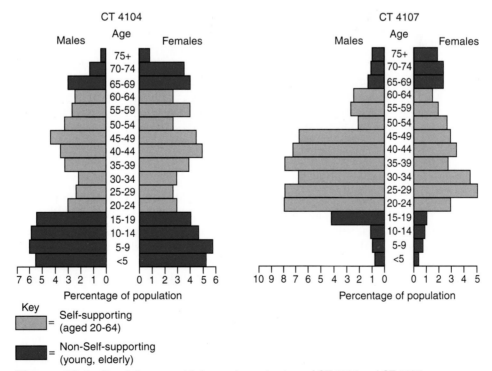

Figure 12.1 Population pyramid: Age and sex structure of CT 4104 and CT 4107.

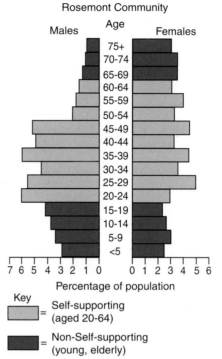

Figure 12.2 Population pyramid of Rosemont: Age and sex structure.

in Figure 12.2. Several other graphic display methods (pie chart, frequency graph, bar chart, and map) may be used. An example of each is included in Figure 12.3.

T A K E   N O T E

The population pyramid is formed of bars; each bar represents an age group. Usually 5- or 10-year age groups are used, although adaptations can be made for smaller or larger age ranges. Bars are stacked horizontally, one on another, with bars for males on the left of a central axis and those for females on the right. The percentage of males and females in a particular age group is indicated by the length of the bars, as measured from the central axis. All age groups in a pyramid should use the same interval.

To construct a population pyramid, use Table 12.2 to calculate the percentage contribution of each age and sex class and Table 12.3 for actual pyramid construction. Note that parts of the population pyramids in Figure 12.1, those depicting people younger than 20 years and older than 65, are shaded; this was done to denote the dependent portions of the population.

Studying the population pyramids for CT 4104 and CT 4107 reveals striking age and sex differences, and this illustrates an important lesson. If the demographics of Rosemont had been presented as one population pyramid (see Fig. 12.2), important age and sex differences might have been minimized or have gone unrecognized, and their associated age- and sex-related health needs would be left unmet. This hazard in data analysis is referred to as aggregating or pooling

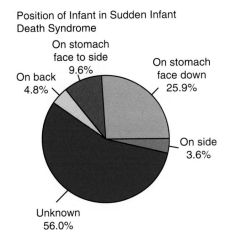

Position of Infant in Sudden Infant Death Syndrome

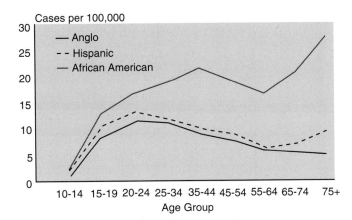

Suicides by Race and Age Group, 1994-1996

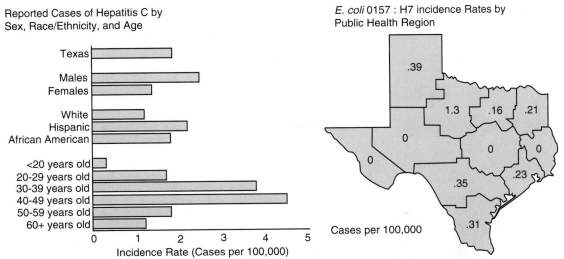

Reported Cases of Hepatitis C by Sex, Race/Ethnicity, and Age

E. coli 0157 : H7 incidence Rates by Public Health Region

Figure 12.3 Graphic models to display assessment data (Texas Department of Health [1998]. Epidemiology in Texas 1997 Annual Report. Austin, TX: Author.).

the data. It is important to divide data along all possibly meaningful lines, so important information is not overlooked. Be alert to this problem as you proceed with your analysis.

Studying the inferences presented in Table 12.1, in conjunction with the population pyramids in Figures 12.1 and 12.2, the following statements can be made about Rosemont's core. In CT 4104, there exists the following:

- A large percentage (42.5%) of children and adolescents
- A high dependency ratio
- An equal percentage of adult men and women aged 20 to 64 years
- A larger percentage (10%) of elderly than Hampton or Jefferson County
- A small percentage (15.2%) of single adults
- A moderate percentage (60.7%) of married adults
- A predominance (83%) of family households
- A mixed racial/ethnic composition with 54% black, 19% Asian, 12% white, and 9% Hispanic

TABLE 12.2

Calculations for a Population Pyramid

Community Name, Census Tract, or Geographic Boundaries: _____
Total Population: _____

Ages (Years)	Males		Females	
	Number	% of Total Population	Number	% of Total Population
		Total		
		Younger than 5		
		5–9		
		10–14		
		15–19		
		20–24		
		25–29		
		30–34		
		35–39		
		40–44		
		45–49		
		50–54		
		55–59		
		60–64		
		65–69		
		70–74		
		75 and over		

TABLE 12.3

Calculations for a Population Pyramid

Population Pyramid For: _____

Males						Females
					75 and Over	
					70–74	
					65–69	
					60–64	
					55–59	
					50–54	
					45–49	
					40–44	
					35–39	
					30–34	
					25–29	
					20–24	
					15–19	
					10–14	
					5–9	
					Younger than 5	

8	6	4	2	0	2	4	6	8

Percentage of population.

- A high infant and neonatal death rate:
  - IMR (33 per 1,000 live births)
  - Neonatal mortality rate (24 per 1,000 live births)
- A higher birth rate (31 per 1,000 population) than Hampton (19 per 1,000 population) or Jefferson County (25 per 1,000 population)
- A higher crude death rate (10 per 1,000 population) than Hampton (6 per 1,000 population) or Jefferson County (7 per 1,000 population)
- A much higher percentage of deaths caused by diseases of early infancy, homicide, suicide, and tuberculosis than Hampton or Jefferson County
- A slightly higher percentage of deaths caused by cerebrovascular disorders than Hampton or Jefferson County

In contrast, it can be seen that CT 4107 has the following factors:

- A small percentage (7.5%) of children and adolescents
- A low dependency ratio
- A larger percentage (7.7%) of elderly than Hampton or Jefferson County
- A high percentage (69%) of adult males aged 20 to 64 years
- Racial and ethnic homogeneity, with 89% of the population white
- A predominance (64%) of nonfamily households
- A large percentage (53%) of single adults
- A small percentage (24%) of married adults
- A lower birth rate (17 per 1,000 population) than Hampton, Jefferson County, or the state
- A higher infant mortality (17 per 1,000 live births) and a higher neonatal mortality (17 per 1,000 live births) than Hampton, Jefferson County, or the state
- A lower crude death rate (6.2 per 1,000 population) than Hampton or Jefferson County
- A higher percentage of deaths from accidents, diabetes mellitus, and congenital anomalies than Hampton, Jefferson County, or the state
- A lower percentage of deaths due to heart disease than Hampton or Jefferson County

Having analyzed the core characteristics of Rosemont, it is evident that major differences exist between CT 4104 and CT 4107, although both are part of Rosemont. In the following sections, this finding will be explained in more detail as each subsystem in our community assessment wheel model is analyzed.

Physical Environment

To study the physical components of Rosemont, data were collected that began with community inspection in the windshield survey and concluded with a systems review and laboratory studies (in other words, census and chamber of commerce data). Table 12.4 presents an analysis of the physical examination data.

Studying the inferences in Table 12.4, the following statements about Rosemont's physical components can be made:

- Rosemont is a community of contrasts and diversity.
- Densely populated residential areas, composed mainly of older homes, abut businesses of various types.
- Industry is minimal and is concentrated entirely in CT 4104.
- Housing values increased greatly in CT 4107; in both CT 4104 and CT 4107, only rents rose greatly.

TABLE 12.4

Analysis of Rosemont's Physical Examination Data

Categories of Data	Summary Statements/ Measures	Inferences
Inspection		
Windshield survey (Learning about the community on foot)	A community of contrast: bustling business areas and quiet neighborhoods	Ethnic and business diversity Congested streets lined with homes or businesses
	Ethnic diversity evident in foods	Minimal industry Little "open" space
Vital Signs		
	Flat terrain and mild climate	Mild climate, abundant flora
	Densely populated (14 persons per acre)	Densely populated (14 persons per acre)
	Posters abound, sharing information and heralding forthcoming events	Note: In CT 4104, there are 221 persons per acre at one housing development
Systems Review		
Land usage		
CT 4104	37% of land in commercial usage, 28% single family, 8% multifamily, and 9% open	CT 4104 has almost twice the commercial usage of land (37%) compared to CT 4107 (20%)
CT 4107	20% of land in commercial usage, 32% single family, 15% multifamily, and 18% open	CT 4107 has twice the percentage of open space (18%) compared to CT 4104 (9%)
Housing Values		
CT 4104	From 1990 to 2000, average home values increased 9.7% and average rents increased 67.6%	Sharp contrast between average home values; in CT 4104, average home value is $47,630, compared to $71,600 in CT 4107
CT 4107	From 1990 to 2000, average home values increased 14.7% and average rents increased 87.8%	Average rent is higher in CT 4107, a reflection of "gentrification" in the area

Note: No data gaps identified; data for this area are complete.

Health and Social Services

An analysis of the health and social services in Rosemont is presented in Table 12.5. Because the data were categorized initially as extra- and intracommunity health and social services, the same format has been used in the analysis. Notice that statements from health care providers have been reported separately from those of health care recipients. This distinction has been made because health care providers frequently have a different concept of the adequacy, accessibility, and acceptability of health services than health care recipients. Be sure to collect and analyze data from both perspectives.

After reviewing Table 12.5, the following statements can be made about Rosemont's health services:

- The Sunvalley Clinic, operated by the city health department, has inadequate antepartum services for Rosemont women; this results in
  - Many women delivering at Jefferson Memorial with no antepartum care
  - Women forced to deliver at home because they do not meet eligibility requirements at Jefferson Memorial

TABLE 12.5

Analysis of Health and Social Services in Rosemont

Categories of Data	Summary Statements/Measures	Inferences
Health Facilities		
Extracommunity		

Hospitals	Most are referral or private. One public hospital, Jefferson Memorial, has problems of
	   Long waits ($\geq$8 h)
	   Fragmented care
	   Inaccessibility
		Only one public hospital; users complain of lengthy waits and fragmented care

Private care	Numerous options, including HMOs	Variety of private care options

Health department (Sunvalley Clinic)	Health providers feel Sunvalley Clinic has
	   Inadequate antepartal services; women wait 8–10 weeks for an initial appointment that is often after their expected date of confinement
	Inadequate nursing services to meet elderly's needs
	Rosemont residents feel the clinic is
	   Inaccessible (no direct bus connection)
	   Impersonal (no primary care providers)
		Inadequate antepartal services
		Many women deliver at Jefferson Memorial with no antepartal care
		Many women are forced to self-deliver at home because they do not meet eligibility requirements at Jefferson Memorial
		Inaccessibility and unacceptability of Sunvalley services

Data gap:
Number of Rosemont residents using
Well and ill infant, child, adolescent, adult services
Mental health counseling and referral services
User's perception of adequacy, accessibility, and acceptability of the above services

Home health	One large Visiting Nurse Association (VNA) Numerous home health agencies; most require fee-for-service or third-party reimbursement.	Numerous options for home health care

Data gap:
Frequency and type of VNA services used by Rosemont residents

Continuing care	Two long-term licensed facilities close (8 miles) from Rosemont	Two long-term licensed facilities

Data gap: Adequacy of facilities as perceived by health administrators, staff, and patients

Emergency services: Medical emergency ambulance service (MEAS)	Cardiac and cerebrovascular accident (CVA) are major reasons for MEAS visits to Rosemont	Cardiac and CVA are major reasons for MEAS visits, followed by accidents and home falls

Data gap:
Number of persons using MEAS and their age, sex, race, and ethnic characteristics
Intracommunity Health Services

Health care practitioners	Rosemont has no Obstetric, gynecologic, or family practitioners Bilingual health practitioners	Lack of OB/GYN and family practitioners No bilingual health practitioners

table continues on page 226

TABLE 12.5 (continued)

Categories of Data	Summary Statements/Measures	Inferences
Clinics		
Third Street Clinic	Health care providers feel immediate health needs include	Inadequate health services for Ill persons (all ages)
	Ill infant, child, adolescent, and adult assessment, treatment, and follow-up	Dental assessment and restoration
	Dental assessment and restoration	Counseling and treatment for substance abuse
	Counseling, referral, and treatment for substance abuse	Health education
	Group health teaching	Self-help/support groups
	Support groups for single parents and senior citizens	
	Additional needs of the clinic include recruitment and retainment of health care providers	
	Many Rosemont residents use the clinic routinely; people feel welcomed and comply with medical care	Rosemont residents state that care at Third Street Clinic is acceptable and accessible
	Residents agree that additional services are needed	

Data gap:
Number of persons requesting services that health care providers believe are needed
Characteristics of people requesting medical care services

Rosemont Health Center	Director of clinic feels immediate needs are	Highly acceptable, accessible, and affordable care for sexually transmitted diseases
	Formation of counseling and support groups	Inadequate counseling and support groups
	Orientation program and inservice for staff (all are volunteers)	Lack of orientation and inservice for the staff
		Lack of procedure manuals and posted protocols for emergency care
		Lack of safety procedures including visible emergency cart and proper syringe disposal

Data gap:
What do staff perceive as needs?
What do residents perceive as needs?

Social Facilities
Extracommunity

Hampton Community Counseling Center (HCCC)	HCCC offers counseling to adolescent drug users	HCCC is close to Rosemont and offers needed counseling for substance abuse, yet HCCC is not used by Rosemont residents
	Most patients are middle- or upper-class males; all are white	
	Staff believe they are meeting community needs	
	Rosemont residents are not aware that the center exists	
YMCA Indo-Chinese Refugee Program	Cultural-orientation programs for Asian immigrants; staff perceive immediate needs are for programs on the following:	Insufficient number of cultural programs resulting in long waiting periods and frustration
	Substance abuse	
	Basic life survival skills (e.g., employment, self-health care)	

Categories of Data	Summary Statements/Measures	Inferences
	Many Rosemont residents use the YMCA services; all agree the programs are excellent but state the waiting period for classes is long and frustrating	
Intracommunity		
Churches		
South Main	Extensive social service programs; social program for gay men despite resistance from older members	Social outreach programs offered by both churches. Only South Main offers program for gay men although older members of South Main resent the program
Westpark	Extensive social service program. No social programs for gay men	
Lambda Alcoholic Anonymous (AA)	Active AA program for gay men: membership exceeds 120	Active chapter of Lambda AA

- There are no practicing private obstetric, gynecologic, or family practitioners nor are there any nurse-midwives in Rosemont.
- The Third Street Clinic has inadequate health services, specifically a lack of
  - Assessment and treatment of people who are ill
  - Dental assessment and restoration
  - Counseling and treatment programs for substance abuse
  - Health-education programs responsive to residents' needs
  - Support and self-help groups as needed and requested by residents
- The Rosemont Health Center offers acceptable, accessible, and affordable services for sexually transmitted diseases (STDs); however, there is a lack of
  - Orientation and education for the staff
  - Procedure manuals and posted protocols for emergency care
  - A visible emergency cart

The following deductions can be made about Rosemont's social services:

- Hampton Community Counseling Center (HCCC) is located close to Rosemont but is not used by Rosemont residents, although residents repeatedly expressed a wish for substance-abuse counseling programs.
- The YMCA Indo-Chinese Refugee Program is heavily used by Asians in Rosemont; however, present programs of cultural orientation are inadequate to meet the demand. Both the YMCA staff and Rosemont residents see a need for additional programs.
- South Main and Westpark churches offer numerous social service programs; however, only South Main offers a social program especially for the gay male population—a program that is resisted by older parishioners.
- An active chapter of Lambda AA is located in Rosemont.

Economics

An analysis of the economic and financial characteristics of Rosemont is presented in Table 12.6. The analysis begins with individual wealth indices (such as income), proceeds to indicators of business and industrial wealth, and concludes with employment status of community residents. As with other subsystems, the categories for data assessment have become categories for data analysis.

TABLE 12.6

Economic Indicators of Rosemont

Categories of Data	Summary Statements/ Measures	Inferences
Financial Characteristics of Households		
Median household income (2000)		
CT 4104 $28,247		Median household income in CT 4107
CT 4107 $34,798		is considerably higher than in
Hampton $42,598		CT 4104
% of families with incomes below poverty level (2000)		
CT 4104 20.6%		In CT 4104, one fifth of all families have
CT 4107 12.1%		incomes below the poverty level
Hampton 12.1%		
% of families on public assistance/welfare		
CT 4104 36.4%		In CT 4104, 36.4% of all families are on
CT 4107 4.3%		public assistance/welfare compared
Hampton 3.4%		to 4.3% in CT 4107 and 3.4% in Hampton
Business/industry characteristics (2000)		
CT 4104	Nearly equal percentage of wholesale/retail (48%) and professional (42%)	In CT 4104, equal percentage of wholesale and professional businesses
CT 4107	Predominance of professional (48%) over wholesale/retail (37%)	In CT 4107, professionals predominate
Labor force characteristics (2000):		
Age (% of persons >16 years of age)		
CT 4104 39.8%		Only 40% of persons in CT 4104 are of
CT 4107 85.4%		employable age (>16) compared to
Hampton 71.5%		85% in CT 4107 and 71% in Hampton
Occupational groups		
Managerial/professional		
CT 4104 7.1%		Striking differences between CTs by
CT 4107 42.1%		managerial occupational categories
Technical/sales		In CT 4104, 67% of workers are in
CT 4104 12.1%		service or operator occupations
CT 4107 34.1%		compared to CT 4107 with 14.8%
Service		In CT 4107, 76% of workers are in
CT 4104 44.2%		managerial or technical occupations
CT 4107 10.5%		compared to 19% in CT 4104
Operators/laborers		Almost a quarter of workers in CT
CT 4104 26.3%		are operators/laborers
CT 4107 4.3%		

Note: No data gaps identified; data in this area are complete.

After studying Table 12.6, the following statements can be made about the economic status of Rosemont. Striking differences exist in the financial characteristics between households in CT 4104 and CT 4107.

In CT 4104, it was found that:

- The median household income of $28,247 is only 34% of the median income in CT 4107 and Hampton.
- One fifth of families (20.6%) have incomes below the poverty level.

- Thirty percent of all households are headed by females.
- One-third of all families receive public assistance/welfare.

In CT 4107, the following factors exist:

- The median household income of $34,798 is much greater than that of CT 4104, but less than that of Hampton.
- Twelve percent of families have incomes below the poverty level.
- Twenty percent of all households are headed by females.
- Only 4.3% of families receive public assistance/welfare.

Striking differences also exist between the labor force characteristics of CT 4104 and CT 4107.
In CT 4104, it was found that:

- Only 39.8% of the population is of employable age (16 years or older).
- Most people (67.8%) work in service or operator/labor occupations.

CT 4107 presented a contrasting picture:

- Of the population, 85.4% is of employable age (16 years or older).
- Most people (76.2%) work in managerial or professional positions.

Safety and Transportation

An analysis of the safety and transportation services in Rosemont is set forth in Table 12.7. Reviewing the data, the following statements can be made about Rosemont's safety (protection) services and associated concerns:

- Grease fires are the major cause of house fires.
- Thefts and burglaries are the major reported crimes, followed by robbery and vehicle theft; elderly people and gay men feel especially victimized. Both groups related numerous stories of harassment and violence.
- There is no fluoride in Rosemont's drinking water, neither is there routine testing for arsenic or heavy metals, substances that residents fear are contaminating the water.
- Abandoned vehicles and dumping of machinery and appliances places residents, especially children, at increased risk of accidental injury.
- Air pollution has increased; the Air Control Board believes that citizens are inadequately informed about air pollution advisories as well as personal actions that can be taken to decrease pollution.

Regarding Rosemont's transportation services, the following deductions are made:

- A large percentage of residents in CT 4107 drive to work alone (64%) compared to those in CT 4104 (43%); however, 47% of the residents in CT 4104 use car pools or public transportation to get to work, compared to 27% in CT 4107.
- When compared to CT 4107, a substantially larger percentage of the population in CT 4104 has a transportation disability, especially among those over age 65.

Politics and Government

A rich diversity of political organizations exists in Rosemont. However, at this point in the nursing process—analysis—it is sufficient to describe the organizations and identify key persons. Consider your information about the political system and form

TABLE 12.7

Analysis of Safety and Transportation Services in Rosemont

Categories of Data	Summary Statements/Measures	Inferences
Safety		
Protection Services		
Fire	45 fires during past 90 days; of these, 40 occurred in homes (usually a grease fire)	Major cause of fires within last 90 days was grease

Data gap:
Obtain additional data (12 months) and determine if grease fires are major cause
Document age, sex, and racial characteristics, as well as time of day and associated circumstances

Police	Crime statistics for past 4 years show thefts as the leading crime, followed by burglary. Frequency of occurrence is high for both census tracts. Robbery is twice as prevalent in CT 4104 compared to CT 4107, and vehicle theft is three times more common in CT 4107. Residents expressed fear and related stories of muggings and violence directed especially toward the elderly and gay male populations	Thefts and burglaries are the major crimes; the elderly and gay men feel especially victimized

Data gap:
Assess residents' knowledge about self-protection measures against crime
Assess residents' interest and past participation in crime prevention programs
Assess available crime prevention programs

Sanitation		
Sewage	Sewage moratorium exists owing to overcapacity of present facility	Inadequate sewage treatment facilities resulting in building restrictions
Potable water	No fluoride in drinking water	Lack of fluoride in drinking water
	No routine testing of drinking water for arsenic or heavy metals (elements that residents believe may be contaminating the water)	No routine tests of drinking water for arsenic or heavy metals

Data gap:
Assess history of fluoride issue. Has fluoride been proposed, voted on? What is the present position of the health department, city council, civic associations, and the general public?
Regarding arsenic and heavy metals: Is Lake Hampton tested for arsenic or heavy metals? What is the position and plan of the health department, city council, and civic associations?

Solid waste	Increased illegal dumping of machinery and appliances; unoperable autos are parked on the streets for months before removal by the City of Hampton	Potential for accidents (with consequences such as trauma and suffocation) as people explore abandoned objects and automobiles

Data gap:
Document laws and fees for illegal dumping. Are signs posted to notify persons of law and associated fines? What actions have been taken by residents, civic associations, businesses?

Air	Rise in air pollution attributed to increase in industrial growth and population density. Residents complain of eye irritation and increased number of respiratory conditions	Increased air pollution
	Air Board feels citizens are inadequately informed regarding actions needed during an air stagnation advisory and individual responsibility to decrease pollution	Citizens may be inadequately informed regarding personal actions needed during an air stagnation advisory to - decrease air pollution

Data gap:
Assess if public awareness programs have occurred. If so, when, and what was the response? What do residents understand about air pollution, air advisories, and their role in decreasing air pollution? Do residents desire more information about air pollution?

Categories of Data	Summary Statements/Measures	Inferences
Transportation *Private (to work)* CT 4104	43% of people drive alone, 24% carpool, and 23% use public transportation	Almost half (43%) drive alone to work, with equal percentages (24%) carpooling or using public transportation
CT 4107	64% of people drive alone, 16% carpool, and 11% use public transportation	Most people (64%) drive alone to work, some carpool (16%), and only a few use public transportation (11%)
Transportation Disability CT 4104	6% of persons aged 16 to 64 and 21% of over age 65 have a disability	When compared to CT 4107, a large percentage of residents in CT 4104 have a transportation disability, especially those over age 65
CT 4107	0.3% of persons aged 16 to 64 and 11% of those over age 65 have a disability	

of government to be reference material that will be useful at the next stage of the nursing process—program planning with the community.

Communication

Ample formal and informal communication sources exist in Rosemont. No analysis is required of the data. Consider the communication data to be reference material that will be useful at the next stage of the nursing process—program planning with the community.

> ### T A K E   N O T E
>
> If sufficient information is collected regarding a community's communication system (refer to Table 11.29 in Chapter 11 for components to assess), then there is no need to further analyze the data.

Education

An analysis of Rosemont's general educational status (characteristics of school enrollment, years of schooling completed, and language spoken) and specific educational sources (e.g., public and private schools, both intra- and extracommunity) is presented in Table 12.8.

Major differences exist between the general educational status of CT 4104 and CT 4107. The status in CT 4104 is as follows:

- A small percentage of residents are high school graduates (28%), with the majority of persons enrolled in school attending elementary grades.
- Some 75% of the population has limited English proficiency.

In contrast, the CT 4107 data show that:

- A large percentage of residents are high school graduates (89%), and the majority of the persons who attend school are in college.
- Only 19% of the residents have limited English proficiency.

TABLE 12.8

Analysis of Educational Sources in Rosemont

Categories of Data	Summary Statements/ Measures	Inferences
Educational Status		
Years of schooling completed: % high school graduates		
CT 4104 28%		In CT 4104, only 28% of persons
CT 4107 89%		over age 25 are high school
Hampton 68%		graduates, compared to 89% in
		CT 4107 and 68% in Hampton
School enrollment: % elementary, % high school, % college		
CT 4104 59%, 23%, 4%		The majority of persons attend-
CT 4107 15%, 7%, 73%		ing school in CT 4104 are ele-
Hampton 48%, 23%, 19%		mentary grade students; in
		CT 4107, the majority of those
		attending school are in college
Language spoken: % of population with poor English proficiency		
Age 5–17 Age 18+		In CT 4104, some 75% of the
CT 4104 76% 74%		population has poor English
CT 4107 11% 19%		proficiency, compared to small
Hampton 21% 26%		percentages in CT 4107
Educational Sources		
Intracommunity		
Temple Elementary	Grades K to eighth	Mixed ethnicity, predominance
	Enrollment 924	of black children
	Ethnicity	
	42% black	
	33% Asian	
	18% Hispanic	
	5% white	
	Principal feels major	According to staff, major
	problems are	problems are
	Truancy	Truancy
	Academic failure	Academic failure (22%)
	Principal wants to stop	Inadequate parent–teacher
	bilingual classes	relationships
		English insufficiencies
		Stressed home environments with
		inadequate adult supervision

Data gap:
Explore the principal's statement about bilingual education. Why the opposition? What is the position and policy
  on bilingual education in Hampton Independent School District (HISD)?
What is the principal's perception of parental concerns?

	Teachers believe major impedi-	Same as above
	ments to student learning are	
	Inadequate parent–teacher	
	communication	
	Poor English proficiency	
	Stressed home environment	
	Inadequate adult supervision	

Categories of Data	Summary Statements/ Measures	Inferences
Data gap: Explore teachers' perceptions of bilingual education. What are teachers' perceptions of parental concerns?		
Temple Elementary	*Nurse believes* major health problems of youngsters are Poor hygiene Dental caries Prevalence of head lice Incomplete immunizations Lack of parent follow-through for needed medical care	Major student health problems are Inadequate hygiene Control of dental caries Control of head lice Parent follow-through with needed medical care Health education
Data gap: Document age, sex, ethnicity, and racial characteristics of children with specific health problems		
	Nurse believes more health teaching and screening would be possible with parent volunteers Present policy restricts nurse to clinic, permitting no classroom teaching	Same as above
Data gap: Document school policy regarding Recruitment and training of parent volunteers The nurse's presence and role in the clinic Explore nurse's attitude toward health education Discuss options for health programs for students, staff, and parents		
Temple Elementary	*Parents believe* Temple is a community strength but the present staff members are insensitive to ethnic and racial needs; attempts to discuss these concerns with Temple's staff have been frustrating	Parental concern and involvement are evident; however, attempts to discuss concerns with staff have been frustrating
Data gap: Identify officers and key people (committee chairs) of Temple's PTO. Are these officers/key people aware of ethnic and racial needs? Identify students' perceptions of their school. What activities do they enjoy? Are there afterschool activities? Who participates? What activities are needed?		
Busybee Day Care	One day care center in CT 4104; no facility in CT 4107	Inadequate day care facilities Parents leave children in crowded homes
Extracommunity Central Hampton High	Truancy and grade failure reversed with "Failproof" program Increased number of teenage pregnancies Decision by school board not to permit sex education classes Increased use of alcohol	Increased number of teenage pregnancies Increased use of alcohol among high school students Sex education classes not permitted in high school
Data gap: Number of pregnancies during last 3 to 5 years (for comparison) and age, grade level, racial, and ethnic characteristics of girls History and reason for HISD Board decision to stop sex education Document scope of alcohol use and characteristics of users		

With regard to specific educational sources, Temple Elementary is the primary educational resource in Rosemont. Temple has an enrollment of 924 students. The principal, teachers, nurse, and parents were interviewed during the assessment process. To summarize the situation at Temple, it has been concluded that:

- Problems of truancy exist, especially among Hispanic boys. There are large numbers of academic failures (22% of students last year).
- Large numbers of students have English–skills insufficiencies, further documented by general educational data.
- Inadequate working relationships exist between parents and teachers, compounded by the language barrier.
- Student health problems consist of:
  - Dental caries (62% of students)
  - Head lice, especially in grades kindergarten to second
  - Incomplete immunizations
  - Poor hygiene
  - Inadequate parental follow-through of needed medical care
  - Inadequate health-education program
- There is parental concern and involvement and a desire to communicate needs to staff.

One day care facility exists in Rosemont—the Busybee. This facility is extremely inadequate. As a result, parents are forced to leave children in conditions that may be crowded and undersupervised.

The major extracommunity educational facility is Central Hampton High. The major problems of Central Hampton High, according to the school nurse, include:

- Increased number of teenage pregnancies
- Lack of sex education classes
- Increased use of alcohol

Central Hampton has succeeded in reducing truancy and grade failure through a program called "Failproof."

Recreation

Recreational space and facilities are minimal. A sum of 5.6 acres of public recreational space is available for a population of 13,631 (combined populations of CT 4104 and CT 4107). The organized sports and recreational programs that are available through churches and associations require membership and usually charge a fee. There are no public recreational programs, and the few pieces of public recreational equipment that exist are in need of repair.

COMMUNITY NURSING DIAGNOSIS

The community's core and subsystems, its lines of defense and resistance, its stressors, and its degree of reaction comprise assessment parameters for the community nurse who views the community as partner. Analyzing data on these parameters with the community leads to the *community nursing diagnosis*. Note the similarities and differences between a nursing diagnosis of an individual and a community nursing diagnosis depicted in Table 12.9.

TABLE 12.9

Community Nursing Diagnoses

Community Response/ Concern/Problem (Actual or Potential)	Etiology Related to . . .	Documentation Signs and Symptoms as Manifested by . . .
Stress and anxiety of being criminally victimized	Increased episodes of thefts and burglaries Inadequate knowledge on the part of residents regarding self-protection measures	Police crime statistics of past 4 years Personal testimony of residents, especially gay men and the elderly
Potential for accidents (such as trauma and suffocation) as children and adults explore abandoned goods	Illegal dumping of machinery and appliances Abandonment of automobiles Nonenforcement of city ordinances	Parental concern for safety Observation of persons exploring abandoned goods
Potential for health problems associated with air pollution (such as initiation and exacerbation of respiratory conditions)	Increased air pollution Lack of knowledge regarding personal action required during an air stagnation advisory to decrease air pollution	Air Board reports of current air pollution levels Residents' complaints of eye irritation and increased number of respiratory conditions
Truancy and academic failure at Temple Elementary	Large number of students with poor English proficiency Stressed home environment in CT 4104, where 30% of homes are headed by females and 21% of families are below poverty level Inadequate communication links between parents and school personnel	Records at Temple Elementary
Stress within Rosemont between the homosexual and heterosexual populations	Differing lifestyles of gay men Lack of acceptance of gay male lifestyle	Lack of social programs for gay men in Westpark Church Resistance of older church members in South Main to existing program for gay men Large percentage of single males in CT 4107
Potential for inadequate coping of single parents, the elderly, and persons with sexually transmitted diseases (STDs)	Lack of support groups and programs for single parents, the elderly, and persons with STDs Inadequate resources at Third Street Clinic to offer programs although the need is recognized Inadequate resources at Hampton Health Center to offer programs although the needs is recognized	Health providers' perceptions of the Third Street Clinic Health providers' perceptions of the Rosemont Health Center High percentage of deaths owing to homicides and suicides in CT 4104
Unsafe working environment at Rosemont Health Center	Lack of orientation and inservice programs for staff Lack of procedure manuals and posted protocols for emergency care Lack of safety procedures	Visual assessment Perceptions of administration Perception of volunteer nurse

table continues on page 236

TABLE 12.9 (continued)

Community Response/ Concern/Problem (Actual or Potential)	Etiology Related to . . .	Documentation Signs and Symptoms as Manifested by . . .
Potential for inadequate cultural assimilation of Asian immigrants	Lack of programs to meet present needs Lack of staff at Indo-Chinese Refugee Program Increased need for programs Large Asian population in CT 4104 (19%) Large percentage of population in CT 4104 (75%) with poor English proficiency	Perceived needs of Asians in Rosemont
Incomplete immunization status of children at Temple Elementary	Inadequate communication between parents and school's staff Inaccessibility and unacceptability of Health Department's Sunvalley Clinic Inadequate income in CT 4104 to purchase immunizations	School health records at Temple Elementary
High infant, neonatal, and fetal mortality rate	Inadequate antepartum care at Sunvalley Clinic Lack of obstetric and family practitioners in Rosemont Lack of bilingual practitioners in Rosemont Inadequate income in CT 4104 to purchase essential medical care	Vital statistics
Potential for boredom and associated consequences (violence, vandalism)	Lack of public, no-fee recreational programs Minimal public recreational areas and equipment	A total of 5.6 acres of public recreational space in Rosemont Visual inspection of available land and equipment
High prevalence of pediculosis capitis among children at Temple Elementary	Crowded living conditions Knowledge deficit regarding transmission and treatment	Cases reported by school nurse at Temple Elementary

In the preceding pages, each subsystem of the Rosemont example has been analyzed in relation to its effect on the core (the people), and inferences have been drawn. The final task of analysis is the synthesis of the inference statements that include stressors and strengths into community nursing diagnoses.

A *diagnosis* is a statement that synthesizes assessment data. A diagnosis is a label that both *describes a situation* (or state) and *implies an etiology* (reason).

A *nursing diagnosis* limits the diagnostic process to those diagnoses that represent *human responses to actual or potential health problems that nurses are licensed to treat*. This stipulation is based on the American Nurses Association (ANA) Social Policy Statement (see Further Readings section at the end of the chapter). Although no standard format exists, most nursing diagnoses have three parts:

1. A description of the problem, response, or state
2. Identification of factors etiologically related to the problem
3. Signs and symptoms that are characteristic of the problem

A *community nursing diagnosis* focuses the diagnosis on a community—usually defined as a *group, population, or cluster of people with at least one common characteristic* (such as geographic location, occupation, ethnicity, or housing condition). To derive a community nursing diagnosis, community assessment data are analyzed and inferences are presented. Inference statements shape nursing diagnoses. Some inference statements form the descriptive part of the nursing diagnosis (i.e., they testify to a potential or actual community health problem or concern); for example:

- High IMR in Rosemont
- High prevalence of dental caries among children at Temple Elementary School in Rosemont

Other inference statements are *etiologic* and document the possible reasons for the health problem or concern. Etiologic statements are linked to the descriptive statements with a *"related to"* clause, for example:

- High infant mortality in Rosemont is related to
  - Inadequate resources at the health department's Sunvalley Clinic to meet antepartum care needs
  - Inaccessibility and unacceptability of present antepartum services at the Sunvalley Clinic
  - Lack of obstetric and family practitioners in Rosemont
  - Absence of nurse-midwives in the community
- High prevalence of dental caries among children at Temple Elementary School in Rosemont is related to
  - Lack of dental assessment and treatment at the Third Street Clinic
  - Lack of fluoride in Rosemont's drinking water
  - Low median household income in CT 4104 and associated limited economic resources for purchasing dental care
  - No dental hygiene education offered at Temple Elementary

Finally, the *signs and symptoms* of the community nursing diagnosis are the inference statements that document the duration or magnitude of the problem. Examples of documentation include record accounts, census reports, and vital statistics. This final piece of the community nursing diagnosis is linked to the first two parts with an *"as manifested by"* clause, for example:

- High IMR in Rosemont is related to
  - Inadequate resources at the health department's Sunvalley Clinic to meet antepartum care needs
  - Inaccessibility and unacceptability of present antepartum services at the Sunvalley Clinic
  - Lack of obstetric and family practitioners in Rosemont
- As manifested by
  - IMR in CT 4104 = 30.5; in CT 4107 = 17.3 (per 1,000 live births)
  - Specific data from clinic about lack of appropriate personnel
  - No city bus to Sunvalley Clinic
  - Clinic hours are 8 AM to 5 PM, Monday to Friday, not accessible to working people
  - Shortage of needed practitioners (include numbers if available)
  - No certified nurse-midwives live or work in the community
- High prevalence of dental caries among children at Temple Elementary School in Rosemont is related to
  - Lack of dental assessment and treatment at the Third Street Clinic
  - Lack of fluoride in Rosemont's drinking water
  - Low median household income in CT 4104 and associated limited economic resources for purchasing dental care

- No dental hygiene education offered at Temple Elementary
- As manifested by
  - No dental program at the Third Street Clinic
  - City of Hampton does not have naturally occurring fluoride in the water and does not add fluoride to the water supply
  - Median income is $28,247
  - No health-education programs are offered at Temple

Although a single problem is stated, the etiology and signs and symptoms may be multiple. Also notice that, although the health problem inference is drawn from the analysis of one subsystem (such as the health and social services subsystem or the educational subsystem), the etiologies may be, and usually are, drawn from several subsystems. For example, regarding the health problem of dental caries among children at Temple Elementary, etiologic inferences were derived from four subsystems: educational, health and social services, safety and transportation, and economic. This example sums up a most important lesson of community health nursing: *All community factors (subsystems) join to determine the health status of a community. No one subsystem is more important or crucial than any other in determining a community's health.*

The process of deriving community nursing diagnoses always remains the same. First, assessment data are categorized and studied for inferences that are descriptive of potential or actual health problems amenable to nursing interventions; next, associated inferences are identified that explain the derivation or continuation of the problem; and last, documentation is presented. Additional community nursing diagnoses for Rosemont are presented in Table 12.9. There is no particular order to the list, neither is the list conclusive. Determining the order of priority among community nursing diagnoses is part of program planning and depends on existing community goals and resources as well as the community's priorities. This important skill is discussed in Chapter 13.

There has been criticism that the diagnoses do not include the positive aspects of the community; however, as depicted in the model, the positives (lines of resistance or strengths) are part of the assessment and are considered in the statement of the degree of reaction (diagnosis). It is in the planning and intervention phases you will want to build on the community's strengths and you will have already identified what they are.

Deriving community nursing diagnoses requires critical decision making and astute study; it is a challenging and vital task. The completeness and validity of the diagnoses that have been derived will be tested during the next stage of the nursing process and will form the foundation of that stage—the planning of a health program.

T A K E   N O T E

This is an excellent time to share your assessment data with colleagues and people in the community to solicit their analysis. Because we all have opinions and values that color our perceptions, group critiquing and analysis of assessment data are ways to foster objectivity.

Summary

Critical analysis of the Rosemont community has been completed using the community assessment wheel as a guide. Subsequently, community nursing diagnoses were formulated, based on the inferences of the analyses. Although community nursing diagnoses are relatively new to practice, community health nurses have, since the profession's inception, derived inferences from assessment data and acted on those data. However, the terminology and format that have surrounded these informally produced inferences (diagnoses) have been inconsistent. There is considerable discussion, and some controversy, regarding the structure and terminology that would be optimal for community-focused nursing diagnoses. In your practice, you will be exposed to various formats for making community nursing diagnoses; evaluate and test the usefulness of each. It is only through collaboration and vigorous testing that a standard format will evolve. In the Further Readings list, there are additional sources to help you as you develop community nursing diagnoses.

Critical Thinking Questions

1. Using data from your community, develop a diagnosis that begins with "At risk for . . ."
   a. Include a clearly stated potential problem.
   b. List the possible etiologies (the "related to" statements).
   c. Include the data (and sources) that point to these "related to" statements.

2. Develop hypothetical information (etiologies and data) for the following community problem: "Potential for high-risk sexual behavior in high school teens."

3. Where would you obtain the necessary data for the problem in #2?

● R E F E R E N C E

U.S. Department of Health and Human Services, Office of Disease Prevention and Health Promotion. (1997). *Developing objectives for Healthy People 2010*. Washington, DC: U.S. Government Printing Office. http://www.healthypeople.gov.

■ F U R T H E R   R E A D I N G S

American Nurses Association. (2003). *Nursing's social policy statement*. Washington, DC: Author.
Best, A., Stokols, D., Green, L. W., Leischow, S., Holmes, B., & Buchholz, K. (2003). An integrative framework for community partnering to translate theory into effective health promotion strategy. *American Journal of Health Promotion*, 18(2), 168–176.
Racher, F. E., & Annis, R. C. (2005). Community partnerships: Translating research for community development. *The Canadian Journal of Nursing Research*, 37(1), 169–175.
Racher, F. E. & Annis, R. C. (2008). Community Health Action Model: Health promotion by the community. *Research and Theory for Nursing Practice*, 22(3), 182–191.
Reece, S. M. (1998). Community analysis for health planning strategies for primary care practitioners. *The Nurse Practitioner*, 23(10), 46–59.

Internet Resources can be found on the**Point**﹡ at http://thepoint.lww.com/Anderson6e.

Planning a Community Health Program

ELIZABETH T. ANDERSON AND JUDITH McFARLANE

LEARNING OBJECTIVES

This chapter covers the planning of nursing actions to promote community health.

After studying this chapter, you should be able to:

1. Validate community nursing diagnoses with your community.
2. Use principles of change theory to direct the planning process.
3. In partnership with the community, plan a community-based health program that includes:
   - Measurable goals and behavioral objectives
   - A sequence of actions and a time schedule for achieving goals
   - Resources needed to accomplish the plan
   - Potential obstacles to planned actions and revised actions
   - Revisions to the plan, as goals and objectives are achieved or changed
   - A recording of the plan in a concise, standardized, and retrievable form

Introduction

Once a community's health has been assessed, the data have been analyzed, and community nursing diagnoses have been derived, it is time to consider nursing interventions that will promote the community's health by formulating a community-based plan. Each of the three parts of the diagnosis statement—the descriptions of the actual or potential problem, its causes, and its signs and symptoms—directs planning efforts for the nurse. All three provide equally important information from which to plan. Figure 13.1 displays the process for deriving a community nursing diagnosis and summarizes how the parts of the diagnosis both describe the community assessment and give direction for program planning, intervention, and evaluation. Community-based plans are based on the nursing diagnoses and contain specific goals and interventions for achieving desired outcomes. Planning, like assessment and analysis, is a systematic process completed in partnership with the community.

Assessment

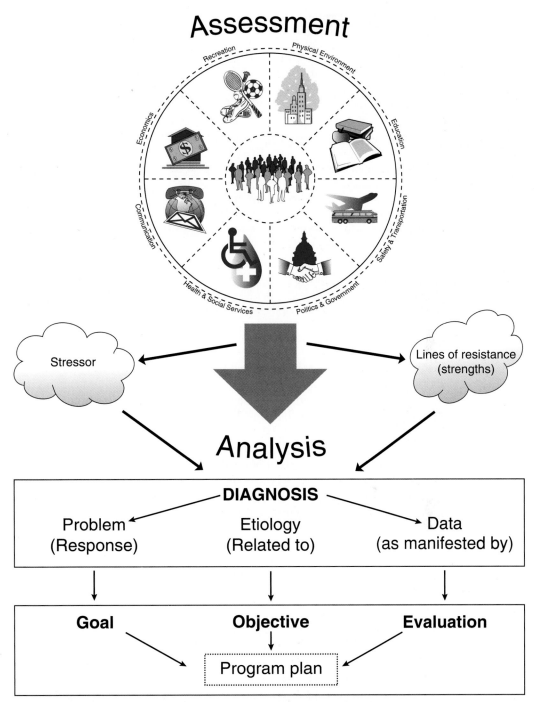

Figure 13.1 The process of program planning from the community nursing diagnosis.

In addition to forming a partnership with the community, the community health nurse must consider the influences of social, economic, environmental, and political issues. Many (if not all) community health issues are directly and profoundly affected by larger policy issues. For example, the high prevalence of dental caries among students at Temple Elementary is related as much to the lack of fluoride in Rosemont's drinking water as it is to the lack of dental hygiene education at the school. In turn,

> **T A K E   N O T E**
>
> Before proceeding, let's stop and consider the word *partnership* and its implications for community health nursing. Recall that a community is a social group determined by geographic boundaries and common values and interests. Community members function and interact within a particular social structure that both creates and exhibits behaviors and values. The normative behaviors and value systems of individuals, families, and the community that you have assessed may be very different from your own individual and family behaviors and values as well as the shared values of the community in which you reside. This difference creates a potential conflict. What may appear to you as a primary health problem of the community (e.g., the incomplete immunization status at Temple Elementary in Rosemont) may not hold the same importance for the community's residents. They may be far more concerned about the possibility of being criminally victimized. Hence, there is a real need to validate community nursing diagnoses with the community. There is one question to ask: Are the community nursing diagnoses of importance to community residents? Methods of validating community nursing diagnoses are presented in this chapter.

each etiologic antecedent is influenced by city, county, state, and national legislative actions and policies. None of the nursing diagnoses for Rosemont can be considered to be separate from the remaining diagnoses; all diagnoses document the health status of Rosemont and must be considered as a whole during the community-based planning.

Additional considerations of the nurse who is involved in community-based health planning are the health needs of populations at risk. Special at-risk groups reside in all communities: the homeless, the poor, people infected with HIV, pregnant women, infants, children, and the elderly are groups at increased risk for decreased health status. The health needs of at-risk groups must be considered as part of all community health plans.

Last, community-based planning involves an awareness and application of planned change—a process of well-thought-out actions to make something happen. Planned change is discussed in detail later in this chapter.

VALIDATING COMMUNITY NURSING DIAGNOSES

In reviewing the community nursing diagnoses for Rosemont (see Table 12.9), it can be seen that several diagnoses focus on the health status of children, and others focus on the health of special groups such as the Asian and gay male populations. Many diagnoses seem to affect all residents, such as the stress and anxiety of being criminally victimized. It may be helpful to stop and review your community nursing diagnoses and categorize them according to the population most affected. A categorization of Rosemont's diagnoses appears in Box 13.1.

Because several diagnoses focus on children and the age and dependency status of children place them at increased risk of decreased health status, a decision was made to begin the planning process by validating the diagnoses that focused on children.

BOX 13.1

COMMUNITY NURSING DIAGNOSIS FOR ROSEMONT BY POPULATION GROUP

Children
- Potential for accidents (e.g., trauma or suffocation as children explore abandoned machinery)

Specific to Children at Temple Elementary

- Truancy and academic failure
- Incomplete immunization status
- High prevalence of pediculosis capitis
- High prevalence of dental caries
- Lack of health-promotion information including nutrition, exercise, and safety

Infants
- High infant, neonatal, and fetal mortality rate

Gay Men
- Stress within Rosemont between the gay and heterosexual populations (especially the older heterosexuals)
- Potential for inadequate coping of people with sexually transmitted diseases

All Rosemont Residents
- Stress and anxiety of being criminally victimized
- Potential for health problems associated with air pollution
- At Rosemont Health Center, unsafe working environment

Validating your community nursing diagnoses with the community residents is an important step for establishing and maintaining the partnership. Equally important is the right of community leaders, organizations, and residents to confidentiality of privileged information and the right to choose not to participate in health planning. Communities have the right to identify their own health needs and to negotiate with the community health nurse with regard to interventions and specific programs. In turn, the community health nurse has the responsibility to provide or assist with the development of information needed for this process. The American Nurses Association's *Code of Ethics for Nurses With Interpretive Standards* (Fowler, 2008) provides a guide for the many human rights issues that the community health nurse encounters.

PLANNED CHANGE

We all experience change. As you read these words, your knowledge level is changing. Yet planned change differs from change that is not planned in that actions occur in a definite sequence, with each one serving as preparation for the next. Planned change is a well-thought-out effort designed to make something happen; all efforts are directed and targeted to produce change. (Many theorists have written about planned change; several works are listed at the end of this chapter.) An adaptation of Reinkemeyer's stages of planned change is presented in Box 13.2. The stages are like a recipe; it is helpful to follow them to produce the intended outcomes.

BOX 13.2

AN ADAPTATION OF REINKEMEYER'S STAGES OF PLANNED CHANGE

Stage 1   Identification and development of a felt need and desire for change
Stage 2   Development of a change relationship between the community health
              nurse and the community
Stage 3   Clarification or diagnosis of the community's problem, need, or objective
Stage 4   Examination of alternative routes and tentative goals and intentions of
              actions (planning)
Stage 5   Transformation of intentions into actual change (intervention)
Stage 6   Stabilization and evaluation
Stage 7   Termination of the relationship between the community health nurse and
              the community

Adapted from Reinkemeyer, A. (1970). Nursing's need: Commitment to an ideology & change. *Nursing Forum*, 9(4), 340–355.

One theorist, Kurt Lewin (1958), described three stages of planned change: unfreezing, moving, and refreezing, as shown in Box 13.3. During the unfreezing stage, the client system (in other words, the organization, community, or at-risk population) becomes aware of a problem and the need for change. Then the problem is diagnosed, and solutions to the problem are identified. From these alternative solutions, one is chosen that seems most appropriate for the situation. In the moving stage, the change actually occurs. The problem is clarified, and the program for solving the problem is planned in detail and begun. Finally, the refreezing stage consists of the accomplished changes becoming integrated into the values of the client system. In this stage, the idea is established and continues to be influential. Lewin also addressed forces that help or hinder change, labeling them the driving forces and the restraining forces, respectively. Using our own model, these may be the lines of resistance and the stressors.

Theories of planned change are important because they can be used to guide and direct the planning process.

BOX 13.3

LEWIN'S STAGES OF PLANNED CHANGE AND THEIR APPLICATION TO THE PLANNING PROCESS

Lewin's Stages of Planned Change	Application to the Planning Process
• Unfreezing	• Identification of a need for change
• Moving process	• Presence of a change agent
	• Identification of problems
	• Consideration of alternatives
	• Adaptation of plan to circumstances
• Refreezing	• Implementation of the plan
	• Stabilization of the situation

Lewin, K. (1958). Group decision and social change. In E. Maccoby (Ed.). *Readings in social psychology* (3rd ed.). New York: Holt, Rinehart and Winston.

APPLYING CHANGE THEORY TO COMMUNITY HEALTH PLANNING

To validate our nursing diagnoses and initiate the planning process, Reinkemeyer's stages of planned change have been chosen as a guide.

Stage 1: Identification and Development of a Felt Need and Desire for the Change

To initiate a felt need and desire for change within the Rosemont community, those organizations that reported actual or potential health concerns of children were contacted, and a meeting was suggested to report the findings of the Rosemont community assessment. Meetings were arranged with the staffs of Temple Elementary, the Third Street Clinic, and the YMCA Indo-Chinese Refugee Program. During the meetings, input from all staff members was sought regarding their observations and perceptions of child health needs as well as their desire to become involved in a planned program of health promotion.

Temple Elementary requested that the assessment data be shared with representatives of the Parent Teacher Organization (PTO) as well as with the school's newly formed parent–teacher liaison group. Both the Third Street Clinic and the YMCA Indo-Chinese Refugee Program requested a presentation to their community advisory boards.

Stage 2: Development of a Change Relationship between the Community Health Nurse and the Community

Both stages 1 and 2 were completed during the assessment presentations. All staff members were keenly aware of child health needs, and each organization desired to become involved in the planning process. To expedite planning, the Rosemont Health Promotion Council was formed. Each of the three organizations, Temple Elementary, the Third Street Clinic, and the YMCA Indo-Chinese Refugee Program, decided to send one staff member and one interested parent to the planning meetings. At this point, the community health nurse functioned as a change agent to guide and facilitate but not to direct the planning process. The council elected a chairperson and agreed on meeting dates. The purpose of the council was to coordinate interagency planning for a community-based health-promotion program.

Stage 3: Clarification or Diagnosis of the Community's Problem, Need, or Objective

The third stage is the time to validate the community nursing diagnoses. At the conclusion of each presentation, the community health nurse proposed a survey questionnaire to assess the target population's perception of their health concerns. Revisions were solicited from staff and community groups, and the final, agreed-on questionnaire is presented in Box 13.4. Notice that the questionnaire is directed to parents, yet the nursing diagnoses are focused on children. Some council participants believed two questionnaires were necessary—one for the parents and one for the children. What do you think? Because of the age of the children (some had not learned how to read) and the associated time and costs of two questionnaires, it was decided to use one questionnaire directed at the parents.

BOX   13.4

QUESTIONNAIRE TO VALIDATE COMMUNITY NURSING DIAGNOSIS

Dear Parent:

We are nursing students who are interested in learning more about what you think are the most important health needs of your family. Answering a few short questions will help us plan some information sessions for you about how to keep your family healthy. Please either place a √ in the appropriate box or fill in the line. Your participation is voluntary. All information is confidential, and you will not be identified in any way. If you have questions, please feel free to call us. Thank you.

Virginia Brown
Ricardo Guerrero
Ann Nguyen
Alice Washington

1. How many children do you have? _____
2. What are their ages? _____
3. If you have a baby, do you breast-feed?   Yes [   ]   No [   ]
4. If you have a baby, do you bottle-feed?   Yes [   ]   No [   ]
5. What other foods do you feed your baby? _____
6. What foods do you usually feed your children? _____
7. Would you like to know more about what to feed your baby and children to keep them healthy?   Yes [   ]   No [   ]
8. Would you like to know where you can take your children for health care, both when they are well and sick?   Yes [   ]   No [   ]
9. Check (√) the following common problems you would like to know more about.

   [   ] Vomiting   [   ] Worms
   [   ] Diarrhea   [   ] Fever
   [   ] Colds and allergies   [   ] Temper tantrums and angry behaviors
   [   ] Skin rashes   [   ] Refusal to do homework or go to school
   [   ] Cuts and falls   [   ] Poor school grades
   [   ] Head lice

10. Other concerns that you would like information about (this can include information for yourself, a friend, or a child):

    _____

    _____

11. Have you ever felt that you, a sibling, or another adult hurt your child when the child was punished?   Yes [   ]   No [   ]
12. Would you like to learn about ways to keep from hurting children when adults are angry?   Yes [   ]   No [   ]
13. Circle the best days and times for you to attend information sessions.

Monday	AM	PM		Friday	AM	PM
Tuesday	AM	PM		Saturday	AM	PM
Wednesday	AM	PM		Sunday	AM	PM
Thursday	AM	PM				

14. Circle the best place for you to attend information sessions.
    Temple Elementary
    Third Street Clinic
    YMCA
    Other (specify where)

Although the Rosemont questionnaire focuses on child health, the same format could be used to validate assessed health concerns of the elderly, well adults, teenagers, or pregnant women. The process of checking your assessed community data against the perceptions of the target population can be completed by a survey questionnaire (such as the one in Box 13.4) that can be mailed or conducted as an interview. Or you may choose to validate assessed data by interviewing community leaders and civic groups that are representative of the target population. The word *representative* is very important. For example, the Temple Elementary PTO would not be representative of parents in Rosemont because, as was noted during the assessment, most parents are not active in the organization.

Before we continue, a few words are needed about composing questionnaires. Everyone is confronted daily with people asking questions. Questionnaires arrive in the mail, and people call on the phone. Frequently, the interviewees learn neither the purpose of the questionnaire nor how the information will be used. When you draft a questionnaire, begin with introductory information that states who you are and what the purpose of the questionnaire is. Emphasize that participation is voluntary and that the information will be kept confidential. Sign your name and, if the questionnaire is to be mailed, include a phone number where you can be contacted. Write questions that can be answered quickly (the whole questionnaire should not take longer than 10 minutes to complete). Ideally, place all questions on one side of a standard 8½-inch by 11-inch piece of paper that, if it is to be mailed, can be refolded so that a return address shows. Before sharing the questionnaire with agencies or community residents, administer it informally to friends and family; any comments made (such as "What do you mean by ____?" or "I don't understand ____.") signal the need for rewriting and clarification.

Because Rosemont has a large population of Spanish- and Vietnamese-speaking residents, staff at Temple Elementary and the YMCA Indo-Chinese Refugee Program volunteered to translate the questionnaire into these languages. The questionnaire was then ready for distribution.

After several discussions by the Rosemont Health Promotion Council, it was decided to distribute the questionnaire from Temple Elementary by sending one form

T A K E   N O T E

How should the questionnaire be administered? Should the questionnaire be mailed to all households of children at Temple Elementary? Should the questionnaire be given to all adults who bring their children to the Third Street Clinic? Or should the questionnaire be used as an interview and given to a selected number of parents at Temple Elementary, or to clients at the Third Street Clinic, or to adults attending the YMCA Indo-Chinese Refugee Program? (Recall from research that people who have been randomly selected can be considered representative of the total population.) What would you recommend? Before making a decision, list each option and consider the benefits and drawbacks of each. Here is some information for your decision making: Mailed questionnaires have about a 50% return rate that can be increased somewhat with a reminder postcard or telephone call, whereas questionnaires administered as an interview potentially have a 100% return rate. However, interviews require interviewers and about 5 minutes per person per page of questionnaire, whereas mailed questionnaires require less labor but have the financial consideration of postage.

home with each child. The questionnaires were color-coded by language, and each child was given a questionnaire in the language that was spoken commonly at home.

Within 2 weeks, 410 of the 736 questionnaires had been returned. The results were tabulated and summarized by the community health nurse and the student nurses from the local university who were helping her. The summaries were then presented to the Rosemont Health Promotion Council. Examples of the summarized data are presented in Tables 13.1 through 13.4. Why do you think the information was presented by ethnicity? What differences do you notice between family

T A K E   N O T E

The Rosemont questionnaires were categorized by ethnicity (surmised from the language commonly spoken in the home). However, depending on the community, responses may be categorized by urban versus rural residence, age of respondents, or other meaningful variables. Once summarized, no preferred day and time emerged for the classes. However, a definite preference was shown for location, with all Vietnamese-speaking families preferring the YMCA location and Spanish-speaking clients preferring the Third Street Clinic.

TABLE 13.1

Family Composition by Ethnicity

	Hispanic		Vietnamese		Other*	
Number of Children	*N*	%	*N*	%	*N*	%
One	82	57	44	61	31	16
Two	12	8	3	4	112	58
Three	24	17	10	14	34	18
Four or more	26	18	15	21	17	8
Total	144	100	72	100	194	100

*Primarily white and black.

TABLE 13.2

Health Information Desired by Ethnicity

	Hispanic		Vietnamese		Other*	
	N	%	*N*	%	*N*	%
Vomiting	124	86	65	90	22	11
Diarrhea	134	93	71	98	34	18
Skin rashes	114	79	11	15	52	29
Cuts/falls	45	31	60	83	5	3
Colds/allergies	46	32	5	7	62	32
Head lice	24	17	10	14	74	38
Worms	85	59	70	97	10	5
Fever	132	92	69	96	93	48
Tantrums/angry behavior	10	7	4	5	175	90
School refusal	5	3	6	8	165	85
Poor grades	4	3	2	3	132	68
Total respondents	723		373		824	

*Primarily white and black.

TABLE 13.3

Percentage of Respondents Noting Other Concerns by Ethnicity

	Hispanic (%)	Vietnamese (%)	Other* (%)
Legal issues (child support, custody rights)	32	15	64
Finances/budgeting	23	26	51
Child-care programs	82	12	75
Adult health (weight reduction, birth control)	75	11	68
Employment	82	95	75
Crime prevention, especially prevention of rape and child molestation	88	84	89

*Primarily white and black.

TABLE 13.4

Percentage of Respondents Answering Yes to Questions 11 and 12 by Ethnicity

	Answered Yes		
	Hispanic (%)	Vietnamese (%)	Other (%)*
Question 11: Have you ever felt that you, a sibling, or another adult hurt your child when the child was punished?	89	92	94
Question 12: Would you like to learn about ways to keep from hurting children when adults are angry?	94	95	98

*Primarily white and black.

composition and ethnicity, health information desired and ethnicity, and further concerns and ethnicity? Of what importance are these ethnic differences for community health planning?

Stage 4: Examination of Alternative Routes and Tentative Goals and Intention of Actions (Planning)

Having validated the community nursing diagnoses, the Rosemont Health Promotion Council was anxious to establish a plan. Much discussion followed the presentation of the questionnaire results. Representatives from Temple Elementary focused on questions 9 and 10 and were eager to present a series of effective parenting seminars on discipline. Temple also felt the high percentage of white and black families who requested information about school phobias and poor grades–merited sessions on that topic. Temple's staff discussed how programs to meet the questionnaire needs were consistent with the school's goal of improved communication between teachers and parents as well as with the goals of their failproof program. In addition, recent state programs developed to prevent child abuse were proposed for presentation.

The staff of the Third Street Clinic focused on the families with infants and the associated desire for information on nutrition and the care of common health conditions. The Third Street Clinic had recently initiated a Healthy Baby Program, consisting of evening and Saturday well-child and prenatal clinics, as well as a total service day on Friday when clients could drop in without appointments for immunizations and screening tests for blood pressure, vision, and hearing. Informal counseling was also offered on Friday. The goal for the next 6 months was to invite various service providers, such as optometry and dental hygiene students as well as Medicare and State Employment Commission representatives, to use the clinic space for information sessions and services. After considering the results of the questionnaire, the staff began to discuss the possibility of offering health-promotion classes on Fridays that would focus on weight reduction, exercise and fitness, and information about common health conditions. The idea of inviting the police department to make presentations on crime prevention and legal rights was proposed and agreed on by everyone.

Representatives from the YMCA Indo-Chinese Refugee Program believed that, because of cultural taboos against discussing topics such as birth control in public, the information would be best accepted if offered at the YMCA by a respected member of the Vietnamese community. The YMCA was beginning a day care service for mothers of preschoolers, and staff members believed that some of the information on child care could become part of the new program as well as basic child health screening services of development, vision, and hearing. The YMCA representatives were equally concerned that Vietnamese refugees be culturally assimilated into the Rosemont community, and they wanted to plan interagency programs about crime prevention and legal rights that would bring the Vietnamese into more contact with other Rosemont residents. The suggestion was made that a program on crime prevention would bring not only residents of different cultures together but also residents of different lifestyles. Keenly aware of the tension and stress between the homosexual and heterosexual populations, a community awareness program on crime prevention that would involve all three agencies and all residents of Rosemont was suggested and approved.

TAKE NOTE

Notice that each agency is considering how information learned from the questionnaire can be assimilated into existing or planned programs. All agencies have budgets and a set number of staff members to deliver services. Agencies must be as cost-efficient as possible and will want to consider how to include new services (such as information desired by parents) into an existing program. Community health nurses can facilitate this process by becoming familiar with the organizational structure and purpose of each agency. When you establish a planned-change relationship with an agency, ask about their organizational structure (most agencies have an organizational chart with positions arranged according to authority). Decision making usually follows the organizational chart, with consent from all levels being required before major changes can be made or a new program can be begun. Learn the names of the staff members and their position on the organizational chart. (An organizational chart for the Third Street Clinic appears in Figure 13.2.) Ask for a statement of the agency's mission and goals. Ask if you can attend a board meeting and pertinent committee meetings. Your purpose is to learn as much as possible about the services and decision-making process of the agency to facilitate the planned-change nursing interventions.

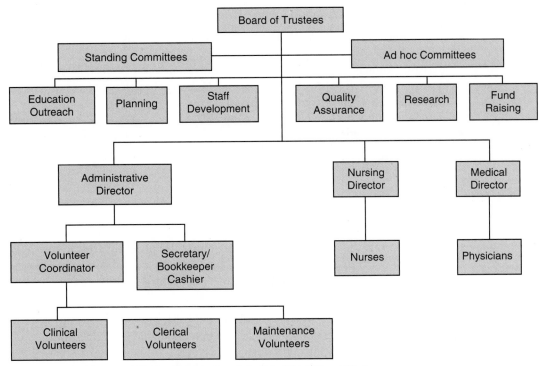

Figure 13.2 Organizational chart for Third Street Clinic.

COMMUNITY HEALTH GOAL

Now is the time to transform the ideas and proposals of each agency into a community-based goal and concrete intentions of action. After validating the nursing diagnoses with the community, the community-based goal was to provide health-promotion programs on issues desired by the community residents, using methods acceptable to cultural norms and offered in an accessible location at an affordable cost to the community.

This statement is very comprehensive and can be considered an umbrella goal for the Rosemont community under which each agency will have goals. Goals specific to Temple Elementary included:

- Reduce truancy 20% by the end of one school year
- Reduce grade failures 20% by the end of one school year
- Increase immunization levels to 95% within 1 year
- Improve communication between parents and teachers
- Increase parental knowledge on how to protect children from molestation

Goals for the Third Street Clinic that were congruent with the community goal included:

- Increased knowledge of community residents regarding crime prevention and legal rights
- Increased knowledge of parents regarding common health problems of children
- Increased knowledge and practice of effective parenting skills
- Increased percentage of adults who practice healthy lifestyle practices, including:
  - Exercise fitness
  - Weight control
  - Stress management

Goals for the YMCA Indo-Chinese Refugee Program included:

- 100% of children in the day care program screened for vision and hearing problems
- Increased knowledge and correct use of contraceptives
- Increased knowledge of parents regarding common health problems of children
- Increased rate of employed adults by 50%
- Increased rate of employed teenagers by 20%
- Increased knowledge of community residents regarding crime prevention and legal rights

PROGRAM ACTIVITIES

After formulation of goals, the next step is specifying the program activities. Program activities map out the actions necessary to deliver the program and thereby reach the goal(s). For example, one goal of the Third Street Clinic was increased knowledge of parents regarding health problems of children. Program activities for the goal might include:

- Third Street Clinic staff and the community health nurse will select topics that are congruent with the questionnaire results to be included in classes for parents on common health problems of children.
- Third Street Clinic staff and the community health nurse will select resources (such as audiovisual aids and pamphlets) for presentation on the selected topics.
- Third Street Clinic staff and the community health nurse will decide on a day, time, and presentation schedule that are congruent with the questionnaire results.

Each program activity deals with planning the program and is written as sequential steps, each step being required to reach the goal. In addition, each program activity needs a date of accomplishment (e.g., "By June 15, the Third Street Clinic staff and the community health nurse will . . .").

LEARNING OBJECTIVES

Once program activities have been established, learning objectives are written. Learning objectives are derived from a goal and describe the precise behavior or changes that will be required to achieve the goal. Whereas program activities map out the actions necessary to deliver the program, learning objectives specify what changes in knowledge, behaviors, or attitudes are expected as a result of program activities.

Learning objectives focus on the learner and state what changes the learner can expect as a result of participating in the program. For example, one topic selected for presentation during the classes on common health problems of children was fever assessment and home management. The learning objectives were as follows: After the class and practice session on fever assessment and management of the fever at home, each participant will be able to:

- Demonstrate how to take a rectal and axillary temperature
- Discuss common causes and dangers of fever during childhood
- State what constitutes a fever
- Explain at least three methods to reduce a fever
- Describe danger signs that require a medical assessment

BOX 13.5

EXAMPLES OF LESS PRECISE AND MORE PRECISE TERMS

Less Precise Terms (Many Interpretations)

To know	To appreciate
To understand	To be aware
To realize	To lower

More Precise Terms (Fewer Interpretations)

To identify	To compare and contrast
To discuss	To state
To list	To decrease by 20%

Both program and learning objectives can be written in sequential steps that are required to reach the goal, or each objective may have different aspects that, when combined, achieve the goal. Goals and objectives need to be measurable. To make statements measurable, use precise words. Examples of precise terms and less precise terms appear in Box 13.5.

In addition, strive for each goal and objective to include:

- A time frame for attaining the change (e.g., "By June 15 . . .")
- The direction and magnitude of the change (e.g., "Increase immunization levels to 95%")
- The method of measuring the change (e.g., "After the session, each participant will demonstrate _____")

Goals and subparts of the goals (objectives) help to clarify a program and establish the expected changes that will result from the program. Although much has been written on the mechanics of writing goals and objectives, little information exists on the collaborative relationship that must exist between the community health nurse and community agency(ies) before meaningful goals and objectives can result.

COLLABORATION

What is meant by a collaborative relationship? Recall from the initial community assessment data that the staff of Temple Elementary had voiced concerns about truancy and grade failure; these same concerns are their first two goals. However, when the nursing diagnoses were validated with the community, parents were more concerned about ways in which they could protect their children from molestation. Could the concerns of the parents and those of the Temple Elementary staff be addressed in the same program? If they could, what would be the program goal? The objectives? This process is an example of collaborative planning and is the essence of community health nursing. You may wonder how to establish collaborative planning and inform agencies about the usefulness of goals and objectives. Although you may be convinced of the value of planned change, how do you convince others, especially because planned change is not commonly practiced in agencies? Role modeling is probably the best strategy. After reviewing the community nursing diagnoses and validating data with an agency, propose goals and objectives that are congruent with the agency's purpose and organizational structure. Solicit input from the group and continue to revise the goals and objectives until a consensus is reached.

RESOURCES, CONSTRAINTS, AND REVISED PLANS

Once goals and objectives have been written, the next step is to identify available resources and any constraints to the plan. These are analogous to Lewin's driving and restraining forces. Last, revised plans are proposed to the planning group. Resources are all the available means for accomplishing a task, including staff and budget as well as physical space and equipment. Recall that part of your community assessment included the identification of strengths. As you consider resources, include those strengths that may facilitate meeting program goals and objectives. For program planning, it is important to identify the resources needed as well as the resources available. Constraints are obstacles that restrict or limit actions and can include a lack of staff, budget, physical space, and equipment. Constraints may be thought of as the difference between needs and resources. Revised plans are actions that are proposed based on the knowledge of resources and constraints.

Following much discussion and self-examination, each agency of the Rosemont Health Promotion Council formed program goals and objectives. Then, alongside each goal and objective, necessary resources were listed. For example, at the Third Street Clinic, the following resources and constraints were identified as crucial to the goal:

 GOAL *To increase the knowledge of parents regarding common health problems of children.*

Resources Needed

- Staff member to develop and assemble existing information on common health problems of children
- Staff member to present the information materials in English, Spanish, and Vietnamese
- Physical space and necessary equipment (e.g., thermometers and basins) to teach assessment and home care skills

Resources Available

- Staff members who speak English and Spanish
- Staff nurse knowledgeable about the care of children
- Physical space and some necessary equipment
- Staff interest and desire to offer information requested by parents

Constraints

It may be helpful to consider constraints as the mismatch between resources needed and resources available. Constraints at the Third Street Clinic include:

- No staff member who speaks Vietnamese
- Discomfort of staff because of inexperience in developing and adapting learning materials
- Time limitations
- Staff members' insecurity about their ability to perform group teaching (all previous teaching was performed on a one-on-one basis)
- Lack of resource material (e.g., audiovisual aids and brochures on care of common childhood problems)

TAKE NOTE

Universal constraints are staff and money—agencies never have enough. An additional constraint is resistance to change. All people are reluctant to change existing routines and patterns of behavior. Initially, change is uncomfortable, and, until new roles are learned, anxiety exists. Making people aware of the natural discomfort associated with change can help build rapport and establish a collaborative relationship.

When each agency had listed its program goals, objectives, and activities, along with resources and constraints, several alternative actions became apparent. For example, a constraint of the Third Street Clinic was lack of staff members who spoke Vietnamese. A similar constraint of the YMCA Indo-Chinese Refugee Program was lack of staff with necessary knowledge to offer classes on contraception or the care of children with common health problems. Therefore, the following revised plan was proposed:

REVISED PLAN **A bilingual (English–Vietnamese) staff member from the YMCA would attend the classes offered in English at the Third Street Clinic and then offer the classes in Vietnamese at the YMCA.**

Both the Third Street Clinic and the YMCA noted a lack of resource materials as a constraint to program implementation. Further assessment of community health resources by the community health nurse revealed that the Sunvalley Clinic, as part of the Hampton Health Department, had access to various audiovisual aids and printed materials on the subjects; however, all materials were in English.

REVISED PLAN **One Spanish- and English-speaking staff member from the Third Street Clinic and one Vietnamese- and English-speaking staff member from the YMCA would translate the materials into Spanish and Vietnamese free of charge with the provision that they be given copies of all the translated materials.**

REVISED PLAN **The community health nurse would provide instruction in basic principles of group teaching, including methods of presenting information. In addition, the community health nurse would participate in the development and adaptation of materials and the teaching of classes.**

For each constraint, a revised plan was proposed, discussed, and adopted. This is a period of intense collaboration between the community health nurse and community agencies, and only at the completion of this stage is the community ready for stage 5 of planned change—transformation of intentions into actual behavior change. This transformation of intentions is the actual program implementation (which is covered in the next chapter). However, before the plan is implemented, it must be recorded.

RECORDING

Community plans must be recorded in a standardized, systematic, and concise form that clearly communicates to others the purpose and actions of the plan as well as the rationale for revisions and deletions of actions. Discuss with each agency its present recording system and decide on a format and system for recording the plan. The format need not be elaborate, and a simple one such as that used at the Third Street Clinic would be adequate if agreed on by the agency.

Summary

Before concluding, let's review the learning objectives for this chapter and their application to community health nursing. The planning process begins with validation of the community nursing diagnoses—a process that establishes the community's perception and value of community health needs. Next, using theories of planned change, the community health nurse and the community form a collaborative partnership to establish program goals and objectives. Last, based on resources and constraints, plans are proposed, recorded, and adopted. Although only one example is offered here, the process of community health planning was the same for all eight programs that were developed by the Rosemont Health Promotion Council.

The next two chapters address stages 5 through 7 of planned change (transformation of intention into actual change [intervention]; stabilization and evaluation; and termination of the relationship between the community health nurse and the community). Stage 5 is implementation and stage 6 is related to evaluation. You will recognize that stage 7 may lead to further assessment, thereby bringing the process full circle.

Critical Thinking Questions

Using the data you generated for Critical Thinking question #2 in Chapter 12, develop a plan for the community diagnosis, "Potential for high-risk sexual behavior in high school teens."

1. What is the goal?

2. Name two objectives to reach the goal.

3. What actions do they require?

4. How will you evaluate the actions?

● REFERENCES

Fowler, M. (2008). *Code of ethics for nurses with interpretive statements*. Silver Spring, MD: American Nurses Association.

Lewin, K. (1958). Group decision and social change. In E. Maccoby (Ed.). *Readings in social psychology* (3rd ed.). New York: Holt, Rinehart and Winston.

Reinkemeyer, A. (1970). Nursing's need: Commitment to an ideology & change. *Nursing Forum, 9*(4), 340–355.

■ FURTHER READINGS

Campbell, M. K., Hudson, M. A., Resnicow, K., Blakeney, N., Paxton, A., et al. (2007). Church-based health promotion interventions: Evidence and lessons learned. *Annual Review of Public Health, 28*, 213–234.

Green, L. W., & Kreuter, M. W. (2005). *Health program planning: An educational and ecological approach*. Mountain View, CA: Mayfield/McGraw-Hill.

Hedley, M. R., Keller, H. H., Vanderkooy, P. D., & Kirkpatrick, S. I. (2002). Evergreen action nutrition: Lessons learned planning and implementing nutrition education for seniors using a community organization approach. *Journal of Nutrition for the Elderly*, 21(4), 61–73.

Hoyt, H. H., & Broom, B. L. (2002). School-based teen pregnancy prevention programs: A review of the literature. *Journal of School Nursing*, 18(1), 11–17.

Keller, H. H., Hedley, M. R., Wong, S. S., Vanderkooy, P., Tindale, J., et al. (2006). Community organized food and nutrition education: Participation, attitudes and nutritional risk in seniors. *The Journal of Nutrition, Health & Aging*, 10 (1), 15–20.

Kelly, P. J. (2005). Practical suggestions for community interventions using participatory action research. *Public Health Nursing*, 22(1), 65–73.

Li, Y., Cao, J., Lin, H., Li, D., & He, J. (2009). Community health needs assessment with precede-proceed model: A mixed methods study. *BMC Health Services Research*, 9(10), 181.

Lippitt, G. (1973). *Visualizing change: Model building and the change process*. La Jolla, CA: University Associates.

Paternite, C. E. (2005). School-based mental health programs and services: Overview and introduction to the special issue. *Journal of Abnormal Child Psychology*, 336, 657–663.

Peterson, J., Atwood, J. R., & Yates, B. (2002). Key elements for church-based health promotion programs: Outcome-based literature review. *Public Health Nursing*, 19(6), 401–411.

Rew, L., Chambers, K. B., & Kulkarni, S. (2002). Planning a sexual health promotion intervention with homeless adolescents. *Nursing Research*, 51(3), 168–174.

Thackery, R., Neiger, B. L., & Hanson, C. L. (2007). Developing a promotional strategy: Important questions for social marketing. *Health Promotion Practice*, 8(4), 332–336.

Weist, M. D. (2001). Toward a public mental health promotion and intervention system for youth. *Journal of School Health*, 71(3), 101–104.

Internet Resources can be found on the**Point** at http://thepoint.lww.com/Anderson6e.

Implementing a Community Health Program

Elizabeth T. Anderson and Judith McFarlane

LEARNING OBJECTIVES

Implementation is the action phase of the nursing process: it is the carrying out of the community-based plan. Implementation is necessary to achieve goals and objectives, but, more important, the implementation of nursing interventions acts to promote, maintain, or restore health; to prevent illness; and to effect rehabilitation.

This chapter discusses the process of implementing a community-based health program. Intervention strategies are presented, along with resources that are helpful in program implementation.

After studying this chapter, you should be able to:

1. Suggest strategies to the community for implementation of health programs.
2. List specific interventions for population-based nursing in partnership with the community:
   a. Implement planned programs
   b. Review and revise interventions based on community responses
   c. Use interventions to formulate and influence health and social policies that have an impact on the health of the community

Introduction

*O*nce goals and objectives have been agreed on and recorded during the planning stage, all that remains for implementation is to actually carry out the activities to meet those objectives. This probably seems straightforward and simple. Indeed, at this point, you will have spent considerable time assessing, analyzing, and planning a program. You will be ready and eager to begin. But this very eagerness (and the associated impatience of the intervention stage) is a danger. You must take time to consider how you can promote community ownership, a unified program, and a clear health focus.

This chapter focuses on the *process* of intervention and provides you with some general resources that may prove helpful in your community work. Many excellent examples of interventions in which community health nurses work as partners with the community are included in Part 3 of this text.

PROMOTING COMMUNITY OWNERSHIP

Essential to achieving the desired outcomes of the interventions is the active participation of the community. The meaning of partnership and collaboration was discussed in the preceding chapter, but the present concern is ownership. The people of the community need to feel a sense of ownership of the program or event, which can only come with their full participation in the decisions regarding planning as well as their assuming some responsibility for implementation. Herein lies a potential conflict. The profession of nursing is one of nurturing, sustaining, and caring for others. It is part of our profession to do for others what they would do for themselves if they were able. Indeed, most nurses interact professionally with people during an altered health state that requires nurses to do for others; but this is not true in community health nursing. Stepping into the community requires an attitude of doing *with* the people, not doing things *to* them or *for* them. When things are done to us or for us, our emotional commitment remains limited.

How might you ensure community ownership for a proposed program and planned interventions? How can you facilitate involvement? In Rosemont, the Rosemont Health Promotion Council coordinated interagency planning for a community-based health-promotion program. When the planning was completed, the council directed its attention to the coordination of activities for the program's implementation. The important point in this example is that a coordination group was already in place. Usually the planning committee can coordinate implementation.

When the Rosemont Health Promotion Council and designated staff in charge of program implementation reviewed the program objectives it became evident that resources had to be selected before the program could proceed. (Resources refer to audiovisual aids, pamphlets, and other material for presentation of the program.) Council and staff members began to ask where such materials could be obtained. What was available in Rosemont? What could you have suggested at this point?

Examining the initial assessment of Rosemont, it was noted that the United Way listed 42 private and publicly supported social service agencies located in Hampton or Jefferson County. The United Way listing included identifying information for each agency along with services and fees. Reviewing the list with the council and participating staff, the community health nurse suggested that selected agency representatives be invited to discuss programs and resources that they could make available, such as films and speakers. It was found that several agencies could provide relevant material. The March of Dimes was sponsoring a campaign in Hampton to increase public awareness of the importance of a healthy pregnancy for the birth of a healthy child. The Mental Health Association had developed teaching modules on effective parenting, and the police department and the Woman's Center were offering programs on crime prevention. All of these programs had recently received a brief description, including the names of their contact persons, in the *Hampton Herald*. At this point, it was decided to complete program and learning objectives for each of the health-promotion goals established by the Rosemont Council. Therefore, as various agency personnel discussed their program with the council, decisions could be made on the appropriateness of the material for the Rosemont community.

TAKE NOTE

Do not panic at this point and feel that you must be knowledgeable about all agencies and their programs in the community that you have assessed. At the implementation stage, do refer to your initial assessment and consider logically which service agencies may have resources helpful to the planned program(s). Then contact selected agencies, request information on their purpose and present programs, share with the agency your community-based program plans, and solicit recommendations with regard to materials and resources.

Box 14.1 lists voluntary organizations that have professional staff at the national and local levels and an affiliated or community linkage structure. These voluntary organizations have ongoing programs for a wide variety of health issues, and most acknowledge health promotion as a vital part of their mission. The list is not inclusive and is meant to serve only as a guide.

BOX 14.1

VOLUNTARY ORGANIZATIONS (A PARTIAL LISTING)

American Association of Retired Persons (http://www.aarp.org)
American Cancer Society (www.cancer.org)
American Heart Association (www.americanheart.org)
American Lung Association (www.lungusa.org)
American Red Cross (www.redcross.org)
Association of Junior Leagues, Inc. (www.ajli.org)
Boy Scouts of America (www.scouting.org)
Boys' Clubs of America, Inc. (www.bgca.org)
Cooperative Extension Service (www.csrees.usda.gov/extension)
Girl Scouts of America (www.girlscouts.org)
Girls' Clubs of America, Inc. (www.bgca.org)
March of Dimes (www.marchofdimes.com)
National Board of the YMCA of the USA (www.ymca.net)
National Board of the YWCA of the USA (www.ywca.org)
National Coalition of Hispanic Mental Health and Human Services Organizations (COSSHMO) (www.hispanichealth.org)
National Council on Alcoholism and Drug Dependence (www.ncadd.org)
National Health Council (www.nationalhealthcouncil.org)
National Kidney Foundation (www.kidney.org)
National Recreation and Parks Association (www.nrpa.org)
National Safety Council (www.nsc.org)
National Urban League (www.nul.org)
United Way of America (www.liveunited.org)

TABLE 14.1

Office of Disease Prevention and Health Promotion: Selected Programs and Initiatives

Program	Description	Contact
Healthy People	Launched in 1979; guides efforts to identify objectives for nation	http://www.health.gov/healthypeople
Healthfinder	A gateway web site to link consumers and professionals to health and human services information from the federal government. Reliable information via the Internet	http://www.healthfinder.gov
National Health Information Center	Central health information referral service for consumers and professionals	http://www.health.gov/nhic
Dietary Guidelines for Americans	Published with the U.S. Department of Agriculture; federally mandated nutrition education activities	http://www.health.gov/dietaryguidelines
Healthy Communities, Worksites, and Schools	With National Coalition for Healthier Cities and Communities, focuses on ways that communities can adapt the national Healthy People objectives for local use	http://odphp.osophs.dhhs.gov/pubs

Source: http://odphp.osophs.dhhs.gov/odphpfact.htm

In addition, the Office of Disease Prevention and Health Promotion (ODPHP), located within the Public Health Service (PHS; which, in turn, is located within the U.S. Department of Health and Human Services [DHHS]), publishes a tremendous amount of information that is designed to promote health and prevent disease among Americans. Special attention is given to facilitating the prevention activities of the five PHS agencies: the Alcohol, Drug Abuse, and Mental Health Administration; the Centers for Disease Control and Prevention (CDC); the Food and Drug Administration (FDA); the Health Resources and Services Administration (HRSA); and the National Institutes of Health (NIH). Several special programs, termed initiatives, are sponsored by ODPHP. A partial listing of the initiatives, services, and information available, along with web sites, is included in Table 14.1.

T A K E   N O T E

Several libraries are designated as government depositories and, therefore, have many government publications. The government also has bookstores located throughout the United States. The Further Readings list for this chapter contains several government publications and web sites that focus on disease prevention and health promotion. You will find the web sites easy to access and very informative.

Having discussed the importance of community participation and ownership of the program, the remaining issues to consider are a unified presentation of the program and an emphasis on health, not the program itself.

IMPLEMENTING A UNIFIED PROGRAM

Because of limited resources, staff constraints, and other situations beyond the control of the planners, many good programs are implemented in a piecemeal fashion that minimizes their impact. A unified program requires collaboration and coordination between the agency personnel who will implement the program and the program's recipients (the target population). Allowing plenty of time for publicizing the program (and how you perform the mechanics of publicity—the how, where, and to whom) can make a crucial difference in whether people attend and what the subsequent impact will be.

Coordinated Publicity

After a time and place have been selected (based on initial input from the survey questionnaires), how might you publicize a program? Public service announcements, notification in the newspapers, bulletin inserts for civic and religious associations, flyers sent home with school-age children, and posters and notices in community service buildings and local shopping centers are some of the methods to consider. The Rosemont Health Promotion Council decided to publicize the first program on child health by sending home a flyer with each child at Temple Elementary. The flyer thanked the parents for their participation during the survey and invited them to programs at the Third Street Clinic and the YMCA Indo-Chinese Refugee Center. Public service announcements were made on the radio, and feature articles about the Rosemont Health Promotion Council and upcoming programs appeared in the Vietnamese and Spanish newspapers as well as in the *Hampton Herald* and Rosemont Civic Association's newsletter. Posters were placed in local grocery stores, churches, and other gathering places (again, use your assessment to identify the best places). Because the parents on the Rosemont Health Promotion Council had expressed a concern that parents with young children might not be able to attend programs, arrangements were made for child care, and a separate health program for preschool and school-age children was planned during the adult programs. The program publicity was focused on health promotion for the whole family and not just on programs for selected family members.

Unified Goals: Healthy People

The idea of a health program based on unified goals and objectives is central to the Healthy People documents. In 1979, the first "health" initiative for the United States (Healthy People: The Surgeon General's Report on Health Promotion and Disease Prevention) promoted five goals. These broad goals focused on reducing mortality among targeted age groups—infants, children, adolescents, young adults, and adults—and on increasing the independence of older adults. These were the first "health" goals for the nation, and their target date was 1990 (U.S. Office of the Assistant Secretary for Health and Surgeon General, 1979).

Healthy People 2000 (U.S. Department of Health and Human Services, 1990) followed and was developed through broad collaborative efforts among government, voluntary organizations, professional organizations, businesses, and individuals. Three goals provided the framework:

1. Increase the span of healthy life for Americans;
2. Reduce health disparities among Americans; and
3. Achieve access to preventive services for all Americans.

In addition, organized under the approaches of health promotion, health protection, and preventive services, over 300 objectives were included under 22 priority areas.

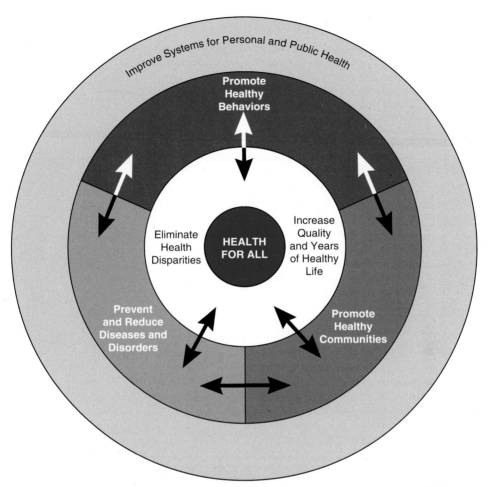

Figure 14.1   Healthy People 2010: Healthy people in healthy communities model. (U.S. Department of Health and Human Services. (1998). *Healthy People 2010 objectives: Draft for public comment*. Washington, DC: Author.)

Healthy People 2010 represents input from thousands of Americans. This new set of objectives, according to the introduction,

> . . . *will be distinguished from Healthy People 2000 by the broadened prevention science base; improved surveillance and data systems; a heightened awareness and demand for preventive health services and quality health care; and changes in demographics, science, technology and disease spread that will affect the public's health in the 21st century (U.S. Department of Health and Human Services, 1998, Introduction 1).*

Two broad goals (eliminate health disparities, and increase quality and years of healthy life) provide the framework and are incorporated into the model for Healthy People 2010 (Fig. 14.1).

General focus areas for the specific objectives are listed in Table 14.2. Each area represents a chapter in *Healthy People 2010* and can be readily accessed through the Internet (http://www.healthypeople.gov). Each chapter includes an overview of the area, issues of concern, trends, disparities, opportunities, progress, a summary of objectives, and links to related reports. In that these objectives are based on national data, as well as rigorous criteria (Table 14.3), they can be used as standards against

TABLE 14.2

General Focus Areas for 2010 Objectives for the Nation

1. Access to Quality Health Services
2. Arthritis, Osteoporosis, and Chronic Back Conditions and Disorders
3. Cancer
4. Chronic Kidney Disease
5. Diabetes
6. Disability and Secondary Conditions
7. Educational and Community-Based Programs
8. Environmental Health
9. Family Planning
10. Food Safety
11. Health Communication
12. Heart Disease and Stroke
13. HIV
14. Immunization and Infectious Diseases
15. Injury and Violence Prevention
16. Maternal, Infant, and Child Health
17. Medical Product Safety
18. Mental Health and Mental Illness
19. Nutrition and Overweight
20. Occupational Safety and Health
21. Oral Health
22. Physical Fitness
23. Public Health Infrastructure
24. Respiratory Diseases
25. Sexually Transmitted Diseases
26. Substance Abuse
27. Tobacco Use
28. Vision and Hearing

U.S. Department of Health and Human Services. (2006). *Healthy People 2010 objectives.* Washington, DC: Author. Retrieved August 26, 2006, from http://www.healthypeople.gov/Document/html/uih/uih_6.htm

TABLE 14.3

Criteria for Objectives Development

Objective Attribute	Notes
Important and understandable	Relate to 2010 framework and have broad audience
Prevention oriented	Should address health improvements that can be achieved through population-based and health-service intervention
Drive action	Including suggestion of steps that will achieve the proposed targets
Useful and relevant	Should be usable by states, localities, and private sector to target schools, communities, worksites, health practices, and other settings
Measurable	Should include a range of measures (health outcomes, behavioral and health-service interventions, and community capacity) directed toward improving health outcomes and quality of life
Build on Healthy People 2000 goals	To provide continuity and comparability
Scientifically supported	Based on scientific evidence

U.S. Department of Health and Human Services. (1998). *Healthy People 2010 objectives: Draft for public comment.* Washington, DC: Author.

which we can compare local data. They also provide excellent examples of clearly written, measurable objectives.

As pointed out in the Healthy People 2010 draft document:

Healthy People 2010 is the United States' contribution to the World Health Organization's (WHO) "Health for All" strategy. The U.S. effort will be characterized by intersectoral collaboration and community participation. Through national objectives, the United States provides models for world policy and strategies for population health improvement" (U.S. Department of Health and Human Services, 1998, Introduction 2).

The process for producing Healthy People 2020 has already begun and will include thousands of citizens' input. It will, no doubt, continue to promulgate the philosophy of Healthy People 2010 by challenging "individuals, communities, and professionals—indeed, all of us—to take specific steps to ensure that good health, as well as long life, are enjoyed by all" (http://www.healthypeople.gov, 2006).

T A K E N O T E

Are the goals and objectives for your community realistic in terms of the past and in relation to trends over time? Do the goals and objectives for your community-based program further the national goals and objectives? When the Rosemont Health Promotion Council reviewed its goals and objectives, each was found to be congruent with the national plan, as well as with Rosemont's state health department objectives for improved health.

MAINTAINING A HEALTH FOCUS

There is one remaining question to ask before initiating the program: Does it focus on health? This may seem to be a strange question. You might wonder, don't all community health programs focus on maintaining, restoring, or promoting health? Sometimes, the answer is no.

In Rosemont, the council and designated staff had become very involved in planning specific activities and information modules associated with the community health program. Several programs had been enlarged to include screening and health fairs; additional activities were suggested at each council meeting. The initial goal of promoting the health of Rosemont residents had seemingly changed to providing Rosemont residents with lots of activities and information about health. What had happened? Remember, we discussed the impatience and eagerness that are often associated with new programs. This situation is normal. Committees tend to overemphasize activities and knowledge and forget the initial reason for the program—to improve health. But it should be remembered that it is the sustained, day-to-day use of knowledge and lifestyle practices that improves health. Frequently, a program begins with enthusiastic momentum; media publicity attracts people to screening and information sessions—and then the program is over. Objectives are evaluated as having been achieved successfully, and another program is planned and implemented. But was there any real improvement in health? Did the participants change lifestyle practices? Will the changes be maintained and continued for a week? a month? a year? Most important, are the changed lifestyle or health practices supported by the surrounding environment and culture?

Environmental and Cultural Support

Many parents in Rosemont responded affirmatively to the survey questions about discipline. These parents believed that they or another person had hurt a child when the child was punished; the parents wanted to learn ways to keep from hurting children when adults were angry. The Rosemont Health Promotion Council responded with a series of programs on effective parenting that included information on various nonphysical strategies for disciplining youngsters, as well as role-playing and open discussion periods. However, as part of the community assessment, the community health nurse had recorded that the Hampton Independent School District (HISD) used physical punishment as a primary discipline method. Students at Temple Elementary were hit on the buttocks with a wide board that frequently left large bruises. The conflict between the effective parenting programs and punishment methods at Temple Elementary was obvious. What could be done? What would you suggest?

In Rosemont, part of the planned effective-parenting classes included discussion sessions on the difference between discipline and punishment and the importance of inquiring as to disciplinary and punitive procedures when parents left their children for supervision (e.g., at child care facilities and schools or with babysitters). Parents were asked to voice their feelings about the school district's policy on physical punishment. Although some parents were unaware of the school district's policy, most were aware of the punishment but believed the procedure could not be changed. After a discussion of parental rights and responsibilities, a group of parents made an appointment with the principal of Temple Elementary to discuss the situation. (After additional meetings with school board members, an open public hearing on public school discipline, and letters to state school board officials, the HISD changed the discipline policy to exclude physical punishment. The process took 2 years.)

Countless such incongruities exist between healthy lifestyles and environmental and cultural practices and policies. Here is one additional example: Recall that one community nursing diagnosis for children at Temple Elementary was a high prevalence of dental caries. During the effective-parenting discussions, several parents commented that their children were given hard candy as a reward for good behavior. When the nurse at Temple Elementary was contacted, it was verified that children exhibiting good behavior were given hard candy. This occurred on a daily basis.

TAKE NOTE

Identify the environmental and cultural practices and policies that are in conflict with the proposed community-based health program that resulted from your community assessment. What can be done to increase community awareness of these conflicts, and how can change begin? To focus on health and the maintenance of healthy lifestyles, all of the community must be involved.

Levels of Prevention

The best way to maintain a focus on health and not on the activities of the program is to use your nursing practice model as a guide. The nursing practice model built and described in Chapter 11 (see Fig. 11.1) defines intervention as primary, secondary, and tertiary levels of prevention. Do the programs proposed for Rosemont address these three levels of prevention?

Recall that *primary prevention* improves the health and well-being of the community, making it less vulnerable to stressors. Health-promotion programs are primary prevention, as are programs that focus on protection from specific diseases. Usually health promotion is nonspecific and directed toward raising the general health of the total community (e.g., teaching youngsters about nutritious foods or conducting adult exercise/fitness and stress-reduction sessions). Primary prevention can also be very specific, such as providing immunization against certain diseases. Additional primary prevention measures include the wearing of seat belts and the purification of public water supplies.

Secondary prevention begins after a disease or condition is present (although there may be no symptoms). Emphasis is on screening, early diagnosis, and treatment of possible stressors that may adversely affect the community's health. The tine test for tuberculosis, the Denver Developmental Screening Test for developmental delays, blood pressure assessments, breast self-examinations, and mammograms are secondary prevention interventions.

Tertiary prevention focuses on restoration and rehabilitation. Tertiary prevention programs act to return the community to an optimum level of functioning. Adequate shelters for battered women and counseling and therapy programs for sexually abused children are examples of tertiary prevention.

The distinction between prevention levels is not always clear. Is a program on the assessment of fever in children (and the prevention of febrile convulsions and dehydration through use of tepid baths and extra fluids) secondary or tertiary prevention? How would you classify an effective-parenting program? Support groups for single parents? A crime-prevention program? Sessions on stress reduction and physical fitness? Can some programs be primary, secondary, and tertiary depending on the needs of the people who attend? Certainly effective-parenting classes for the parent with a child who has a behavior problem will have a different purpose than classes designed for expectant parents of a first child. Likewise, the corporate executive who has been diagnosed with cardiovascular disease and placed on a low-cholesterol diet has very different nutritional learning needs from those of the senior citizen on a fixed income. Few programs pertain to only one level of prevention.

The important point is to evaluate your programs (the implementation phase of the nursing process) and ask if the nursing interventions are consistent with the nursing practice model. If the focus is prevention, are the programs directed toward prevention?

Levels of Practice

In addition to level of prevention, we need to consider the level of practice. This text promotes the community as partner; therefore, the level of practice is considered community- and systems-based. Individual-focused practice may also be incorporated into population-based nursing but is primarily aimed at one-on-one activity.

Specific interventions for population-based nursing practice have been identified by the Public Health Nursing Section of the Minnesota Department of Health (2001). The interventions are included in Box 14.2. Consider these interventions as you develop plans to address the problems identified in your community.

BOX 14.2

INTERVENTIONS FOR POPULATION-BASED NURSING PRACTICE

Community organizations
Coalition building
Collaboration
Counseling
Health teaching
Delegated functions
Case management
Advocacy

Referral and follow-up
Screening
Outreach
Disease and health event investigation
Surveillance
Policy development and enforcement
Social marketing

Minnesota Department of Health, Division of Community Health Services, Public Health Nursing Section. (2001). Public health interventions—Applications for public health nursing practice. Available at http://www.health.state.mn.us/divs/cfh/ophp/resources/docs/phinterventions_manual2001.pdf

---

TAKE NOTE

The model for population- and community-based practice is public health nursing. Now, many nurses consider their practice to be population- and community-based. We use the term *community health nurse* to incorporate these nurses. Criteria—cornerstones—for public health nursing are listed below to describe this specialty practice:

- Focuses on entire populations
- Reflects community priorities and needs
- Establishes caring relationships with the communities, families, individuals, and systems that comprise the population that community health nurses serve
- Is grounded in social justice, compassion, sensitivity to diversity, and respect for the worth of all people, especially the vulnerable
- Encompasses the mental, physical, emotional, social, spiritual, and environmental aspects of health
- Promotes health through strategies driven by epidemiologic evidence
- Collaborates with community resources to achieve those strategies, but can and will work alone if necessary
- Derives its authority from the Nurse Practice Act

Minnesota Department of Health (2004).

Summary

Having considered the importance of community ownership of the program, the need to offer a unified program, and maintain a focus on health, there remains one step in the process—evaluation. Before a program is implemented, the manner in which it is to be evaluated must be established. The following chapter explains why this final stage of the nursing process is essential before implementation.

Critical Thinking Questions

For the objectives you developed for the diagnosis, "Potential for high-risk sexual behavior in high school teens," in Chapter 13, identify one intervention.

1. What level of prevention does it represent? Give your rationale.

2. Is there an objective in Healthy People 2010 related to this intervention?

3. What is the health focus of this intervention?

● REFERENCES

Minnesota Department of Health, Public Health Nursing Section. (2004). Cornerstones of public health nursing. Retrieved August 26, 2006, from http://www.health.state.mn.us/divs/hpcd/chp/hpkit/text/hcheck_comm.htm

Minnesota Department of Health, Division of Community Health Services, Public Health Nursing Section. (2001). Public health interventions—Applications for public health nursing practice. Retrieved August 26, 2006, from http://www.health.state.mn.us/divs/cfh/ophp/resources/docs/phinterventions_manual2001.pdf

U.S. Department of Health and Human Services, Public Health Service. (1990). *Healthy People 2000: National health promotion and disease prevention objectives*. Washington, DC: U.S. Government Printing Office.

U.S. Office of the Assistant Secretary for Health and Surgeon General. (1979). *Healthy people: The surgeon general's report on health promotion and disease prevention*. Washington, DC: U.S. Government Printing Office.

■ FURTHER READINGS

Alvarez, R. A., Vasquez, E., Mayorga, C. C., Feaster, D. J., & Mitrani, V. B. (2006). Increasing minority research participation through community organization outreach. *Western Journal of Nursing Research*, 28(5), 561–563.

Brownstein, J. N., Chowdhury, F. M., Norris, S. L., Horsley, T., Jack, L. Jr., Zhang, X., et al. (2007). Effectiveness of community health workers in the care of people with hypertension. *American Journal of Preventive Medicine*, 32(5), 435–437.

Carter, K. F., Fournier, M., Grover, S., Kiehl, E. M., & Sims, K. M. (2005). Innovations in community-based nursing education: Transitioning faculty. *Journal of Professional Nursing*, 21(3), 167–174.

Fisher, J. W., & Peek, K. E. (2009). Collaborating for change: Creating a Women's Health Network. *Women's Health Issues*, 19(1), 3–7.

Flick, L. H., Reese, C., & Harris, A. (1996). Aggregate community-centered undergraduate community health nursing clinical experience. *Public Health Nursing*, 13(1), 36–41.

Flynn, B. C. (1998). Communicating with the public: Community-based nursing research and practice. *Public Health Nursing*, 15(3), 165–170.

Flynn, B. C. (1997). Partnerships in healthy cities and communities: A social commitment for advanced practice nurses. *Advanced Practice Nursing Quarterly*, 2(4), 1–6.

Graves, B. A. (2008). Integrative literature review: A review of literature related to geographical information systems, healthcare access, and health outcomes. *Perspectives in Health Information Management*, 5, 5–11.

Keller, L. O., Stroschein, S., Lia-Hoagberg, B., & Alfaro-Correa, A. (2004). Population-based public health interventions: Practice-based and evidence-supported. Part I. *Public Health Nursing*, 21(5), 453–468.

Keller, L. O., Strohschein, S., Schaffer, M. A., & Lia-Hoagberg, B. (2004). Population-based public health interventions: Innovations in practice, teaching, and management. Part II. *Public Health Nursing*, 21(5), 469–487.

Kim, S., & Crutchfield, C. (2004). An evaluation of substance abuse aftercare program for homeless women with children using confounding variable-control design. *Journal of Drug Education*, 34(3), 213–233.

Kuhajda, M. C., Cornell, C. E., Brownstein, J. N., Littleton, M. A., Stalker, V. G., et al. (2006). Training community health workers to reduce health disparities in Alabama's Black Belt: The Pine Apple Heart Disease and Stroke Project. *Family and Community Health*, 29(2), 89–102.

Lucey, P., & Maurana, C. A. (2007). Partnerships to address social determinants of health. *Nursing Economics*, 25(3), 179–182.

Pan American Health Organization. (2007). *Health in the Americas*. Washington, DC: Author.

Racher, F. E., & Annis, R. C. (2008). Community health action model: Health promotion by the community. *Research and Theory for Nursing Practice*, 22(3), 182–191.

Stephens, P. C., Sloboda, Z., Stephens, R. C., Teasdale, B., Grey, S. F., et al. (2009). Universal school-based substance abuse prevention programs: Modeling targeted mediators and outcomes for adolescent cigarette, alcohol and marijuana use. *Drug and Alcohol Dependence*, 102(1–3), 19–29.

Vasquez, E. P., Pitts, K., & Mejia, N. E. (2008). A model program: Neonatal nurse practitioners providing community health care for high-risk infants. *Neonatal Network*, 27(3), 163–169.

Wilson, K. M., & Satterfield, D. W. (2007). Where are we to be in these times? The place of chronic disease prevention in community health promotion. *Preventing Chronic Disease*, 4(3), A74.

Wolfe, T., & Kaye, G. (1995). *From the ground up: A workbook on coalition building and community development*. Amherst, MA: Tom Wolff & Associates.

Yoo, S., Butler, J., Elias, T. I., & Goodman, R. M. (2009). The 6-step model for community empowerment: Revisited in public housing communities for low-income senior citizens. *Health Promotion Practice*, 10(2), 262–275.

Internet Resources can be found on the **Point** at http://thepoint.lww.com/Anderson6e.

Evaluating a Community Health Program

ELIZABETH T. ANDERSON AND JUDITH McFARLANE

LEARNING OBJECTIVES

Evaluation is determining the worth (or value) of something. During the evaluation process, information is collected and analyzed to determine its significance and worth. Changes are appraised, and progress is documented. This chapter discusses evaluation and the nursing practices that are necessary to plan and implement it.

After studying this chapter, you should be able to:

1. Establish evaluation criteria that are timely and comprehensive.
2. Use baseline and current data to measure progress toward goals and objectives.
3. Validate observations, insights, and new data with colleagues and the community.
4. Revise priorities, goals, and interventions based on evaluation data.
5. Document and record evaluation results and revisions of the plan.
6. Participate in evaluation research with appropriate consultation.
7. Appreciate the complexity of program evaluation, as well as the multiple paradigms that affect its implementation.

Introduction

*T*he nurse evaluates the responses of the community to a health program to measure progress that is being made toward the program's goals and objectives. Evaluation data are also crucial for revision of the database and the community nursing diagnoses that were developed from analysis of the community assessment data.

Do you feel as though we are talking in circles? Evaluation is the "final" step of the nursing process, but it is linked to assessment, which is the first step. Nursing practice is cyclic as well as dynamic, and, for community-based interventions to be timely and relevant, the community database, nursing diagnoses, and health program plans must be evaluated routinely. The effectiveness of community nursing interventions depends on continuous reassessment of the community's health and on appropriate revisions of planned interventions.

Evaluation is important to nursing practice, but of equal importance is its crucial role in the functioning of health agencies. Staffing and funding are frequently based on evaluation findings, and existing programs are subject to termination unless evaluation evidence can be produced that answers the question: *What has been the program's impact on the health status of the community?* Recently there has been a growing focus on program evaluation; training programs on evaluation have become commonplace; and evaluation has become big business. Unfortunately, evaluation is sometimes practiced separately from program planning. It may even be tacked onto the end of a program just to satisfy funding sources or agency administration. The problems of such an approach are evident. Effective community health nursing requires an integrative approach to evaluation; it is a unique aspect of the field.

EVALUATION PRINCIPLES

Congruent with the theoretical foundations of working with the community as partner, we base our program evaluation on principles explicated by the W. K. Kellogg Foundation (1998). These principles are summarized below.

1. *Strengthen programs.* Our goal is health promotion and improving the self-reliance of the community. Evaluation assists in attaining this goal by providing an ongoing and systematic process for assessing the program, its impact, and its outcomes.
2. *Use multiple approaches.* In addition to multidisciplinary approaches, evaluation methods may be numerous and varied. No single approach is favored, but the method chosen must be congruent with the purposes of the program.
3. *Design evaluation to address real issues.* Community-based programs, rooted in the "real" community and based on an assessment of that community, must contain an evaluation to measure those criteria of importance to the community.
4. *Create a participatory process.* Just as the community members were part of assessment, analysis, planning, and implementation, so too they must be partners in evaluation.
5. *Allow for flexibility.* "Evaluation approaches must not be rigid and prescriptive, or it will be difficult to document the incremental, complex, and often subtle changes that occur" (W. K. Kellogg Foundation, 1998, p. 3).
6. *Build capacity.* The process of evaluation, in addition to measuring outcomes, should enhance the skills, knowledge, and attitudes of those engaged in it. This includes both professionals and nonprofessionals.

THE EVALUATION PROCESS

There is a burgeoning body of literature on evaluation (see Further Readings at the end of this chapter). Program or project evaluation has become a specialty, with entire departments and consulting firms focused on measurement and evaluation.

For our purposes (i.e., to provide an introduction to program evaluation), we will use a three-part model (Table 15.1). In this model, we look at the *process* of implementing the program, the program's *impact*, and the *outcome* of the program.

TABLE 15.1

A Model for Program Evaluation

	Process (Formative)	Impact (Summative; Short-Term Outcome)	Outcome (Long-Term Outcome)
Information to collect	Program implementation, including • Site response • Recipient response • Practitioner response • Competencies of personnel	Immediate effects of program on, for example: • Knowledge • Attitudes • Perceptions • Skills • Beliefs • Access to resources • Social support	Incidence and prevalence of risk factors, morbidity, and mortality
When to apply	Initial implementation of a program or when changes are made in a developed program (e.g., moved to a new site, provided to a different population)	To determine if factors that affect health—both within the individual and in the environment—have changed. For example, did the person's behavior change? Was the new policy implemented?	To measure if incidence and prevalence have been altered. For example, has the immunization rate of 2-year-olds increased? Did the rate of admissions for illnesses decrease? Did the industry filter its polluting smoke stack?

Adapted from Green, L. W., & Lewis, F. M. (1986). *Measurement and evaluation in health education and health promotion.* Palo Alto, CA: Mayfield.

Our focus in this text is on health promotion, and health-promotion programs are designed to "... influence target populations through planned activities (process) that may have immediate effects (impact) as well as more long-term effects (outcomes)" (Dignan & Carr, 1992, p. 153).

Process or formative evaluation answers the question: Are we doing what we said we would do? That is, did we deliver the program, provide a place to meet, include handouts at our meeting, and so forth? For example, when the first effective-parenting training program was offered in Rosemont from 8 PM to 9 PM, only five parents attended. They stated that the time was too late for them to return home and complete bedtime activities for their school-age children. As a result of this formative evaluation, the time was changed to 7 PM to 8 PM, and attendance increased to 20 parents. Some authors (Green & Lewis, 1986) make a distinction between formative and process evaluation by using processes to denote the evaluation conducted during the program, whereas formative may be applied (as the name implies) at formative or preprogram stages.

Impact (or summative) evaluation is concerned with the immediate impact of a program on a target group. If your program is aimed at changing a group's knowledge and behavior relating to sexually transmitted diseases (STDs), for instance, you might build in a test to find out what they learned and what their intent is about modifying behavior. In the case of effective-parenting classes, summative evaluation criteria might include parental self-reports of changes in their attitudes toward physical punishment and disciplinary practices before and following the program, any alteration in discipline policies at Temple Elementary, and change in the number of reported incidents of child abuse.

It is in the long-term outcome evaluation, however, that you find out if the changes had a lasting and real effect. That is, did the incidence of STDs drop in this group? Because we are getting closer to the cause–effect question, careful evaluative research is needed to determine the actual contribution of the program to the outcome being measured.

Before considering specific evaluation strategies, it is important to consider the "evaluability" of the program. To do this, review the program plan and ask yourself the following questions:

- Are program activities stated in precise words whose concepts can be measured?
- Has a time frame for attaining the change been included?
- Are the direction and magnitude of the change included?
- Has a method of measuring the change been included?
- Are the data that will be needed to measure the objectives available at a reasonable cost?
- Are the program activities that are designed to meet the objectives plausible?

If you find in your practice that any of these questions cannot be measured in one of your plans, review Chapter 13 and amend the plan to make it as concise and complete as possible.

COMPONENTS OF EVALUATION

Why collect evaluation data? To whom will the evaluation data be given, and for what purpose will they be used? What programs or activities will result from or be discontinued as a result of the evaluation? Before a strategy or method of evaluation can be selected, the reasons for and uses of the evaluation data must be established. An evaluation strategy appropriate for answering one type of evaluative question may not be useful for another. For example, if the Rosemont Health Promotion Council wanted to know the relevancy to community needs of a program on crime prevention, then questions would be asked of the participants concerning the usefulness and adequacy of the information that was given. Possible questions would cover a range of topics: Did the information make a difference as to how residents protect themselves from crime? What protection behaviors do the residents practice now that were not practiced before the program? Did the program answer the residents' questions? Did the program meet perceived needs? However, if the council wanted to know the outcome of the crime-prevention program (such as if the program decreased the incidence of crime experienced by the participants), then self-reports and community crime statistics would be monitored. Usually questions of evaluation focus on the areas of relevancy, progress, cost efficiency, effectiveness, and outcome.

Relevancy

Is there a need for the program? Relevancy determines the reasons for having a program or set of activities. Questions of relevancy may be more important for existing programs than for new programs. Frequently, a program, such as a blood pressure screening, is planned to meet an expressed community need. Then, the program continues for years without an evaluation of relevancy. The question should be asked routinely: Is the program still needed? Clearly, evaluation is necessary not just for new programs, but for all programs. A common constraint to beginning a new program is inadequate staff or budget. A remedy to that constraint can be a relevancy evaluation of existing programs. Staff and budgets from a program that is no longer needed can be redirected to the new program.

Progress

Are program activities following the intended plan? Are appropriate staff and materials available in the right quantity and at the right time to implement the program activities? Are expected numbers of clients participating in the scheduled program activities? Do the inputs and outputs meet some predetermined plan? Answers to these questions measure the progress of the program and are part of process or formative evaluation.

Cost Efficiency

What are the costs of a program? What are its benefits? Are program benefits sufficient for the costs incurred? Cost–efficiency evaluation measures the relationship between the results (benefits) of a program and the costs of presenting the program (such as staff salary and materials). Cost efficiency evaluates whether the results of a program could have been obtained less expensively through another approach. Cost–benefit analysis requires skills beyond the scope of this text, but references abound, particularly in economics and management literature.

Effectiveness (Impact)

Were program objectives met? Were the clients satisfied with the program? Were program providers satisfied with the activities and client involvement? Effectiveness focuses on formative evaluation as well as the immediate, short-term results.

Outcome

What are the long-term implications of the program? As a result of the program, what changes in behavior can be expected in 6 weeks, 6 months, or 6 years? Effectiveness measures the immediate results, whereas outcome evaluation measures whether the program activities changed the initial reason for the program. The fundamental question is this: Did the program meet its goal? (Was health improved?)

EVALUATION STRATEGIES: DATA COLLECTION AND ANALYSIS

Program "evaluation can be defined as the consistent, ongoing collection and analysis of information for use in decision making" (W. K. Kellogg Foundation, 1998, p. 14). As such, the choice of approach or method to collect the information is an important decision in itself and needs to be agreed on by all involved from the beginning. Realize that there is no one best approach to evaluation, but whichever approach is chosen needs to fit the questions you wish to answer.

Four key points need to be considered as you decide which method of data collection to use:

1. What resources are available for the evaluation tasks?
2. Is the method sensitive to the respondents/participants of the program?
3. How credible will your evaluation be as a result of this method?
4. What is the importance of the data to be collected? To the overall program? To participants? (W. K. Kellogg Foundation, 1998).

Consider, too, that there are several frameworks or paradigms that may inform your choices. A summary of five such paradigms is included as Table 15.2.

Taking the key points and paradigms into consideration, let us review the various methods of data collection.

TABLE 15.2

Paradigms for Evaluation

	Natural Science Research Model	Interpretivism/ Constructivism	Feminist Methods	Participatory Evaluation	Theory-Based
Roots	Western "science"; European, white, male	Anthropology	Feminist research, power analysis	Education, community organization, public health, anthropology	Application in comprehensive community programs
Key points	Control of variables	Study through ongoing and in-depth contact with those involved	Women, girls, and minorities historically left out; conventional methods are seriously flawed	Create a more egalitarian process, make process more relevant to all, democratizing	Every social program is based on a theory—the key to understanding what is important is through identifying the theory
Approach	Hypothetico-deductive methodology, statistics	In-depth observations, interviewing	Contextual, inclusive, experiential, involved, socially relevant	Practical, useful, empowering	Developing a program logic model—or picture—to describe what works
Purpose	To explain what happened and show causal relationships between outcomes and "treatments"	To understand the targets of the program and the program's meaning to them	To include the feminine voice in all aspects of evaluation, being open to all voices	Actively engage all in process, capacity building	Revealing what works in comprehensive, community-based programs

From Minkler (1997); W. K. Kellogg Foundation. (1998). *Evaluation handbook.* Battle Creek, MI: Author.

Case Study

A case study looks inside a program to determine its adequacy to meet stated needs. The case-study method provides insight into an entire program and, unlike many forms of evaluation, can be started at any time during the program. The data collected during a case study include observation of program activity, reports prepared by the program, unstructured conversations with program personnel, statistical summaries of program activities, structured or unstructured interview data, and information collected through questionnaires. Subjective data and objective data can both be collected. Subjective data include information collected primarily through observations of participants or program staff. Objective data are collected from the organization or program documents or structured questionnaires and interviews. The distinction between subjective and objective is not readily perceptible. All questionnaires, regardless of how carefully written, have a subjective component, and, likewise, "objective" records or documents are all written by people and, therefore, introduce a subjective factor. It is best to have a mix of both objective and subjective data.

Techniques of the case study method include observation and interviews, nominal group, and Delphi technique.

Observation and Interviews

Observation is one method of collecting data for a case study. Observation can be participatory or nonparticipatory. The participant observer assumes a working role in the agency or organization and collects data about the program while working within the group. The nonparticipant observer remains an "outsider," does not assume a working role within the agency, and reviews and examines the program for designated periods.

The types of observations that are made are determined by the questions that have been asked about the program. For example, if the question is one of relevancy, the observer would concentrate on the who, what, why, and when of the program. Who is using the services? Record the demographics of age, ethnicity, geographic location, educational level, and employment status. What services are the participants receiving? (For example, what services are offered in the well-child clinic? Immunizations? Physicals? Health teaching? Screening? How often are the services offered, and what are the ages of the children who use the services?) Why is the population using the offered services? (Availability? Affordability? No other options?) Lastly, when are the services accessed? (Do people come at appointed times or only when they are ill? Or do people tend to cluster at opening and closing times?)

Some data can be collected from agency records; other information can be collected by informal conversations with the participants—both the professional health care providers and the clients. When interviewing, always have a checklist of topics you want to consider, arranged in a logical sequence, along with the who, what, why, and when questions. Informal conversations, sometimes referred to as "unstructured interviews," afford the opportunity to explore with the participants their perceptions of the program. The results of unstructured interviews provide specific areas from which a "structured" interview can be developed. Recall from Chapter 13 that an interview is administered by an interviewer, whereas a questionnaire is self-administered. Observations and interviews share the problem of selective perception.

Selective Perception
Selective perception is the natural tendency of everyone to consciously classify into categories the behaviors or statements of others. These categories have been

established by our cultural values, learning, and life experiences. To a certain extent, this process is desirable because it limits the number of observations that need conscious consideration and permits the rapid and effective handling of information. For example, if it was observed that a client waited 1 hour for a scheduled appointment, most people, based on the common orientation to time, would classify that observation as a negative aspect of the clinic's functioning.

Herein lies the major problem of selective perception. Statements and behaviors are classified according to the selective perception of the observer, which may be completely different from the selective perception of the client or other health care providers. The most dangerous effect of selective perception in program evaluation is when the observer has a preconception that a program will be successful or unsuccessful. This can produce a self-fulfilling prophecy because the biased observer may unconsciously record only data that support the preconceived belief. Both selective perception and self-fulfilling prophecy are sources of subjective data. Perhaps the most important point is that you should be aware of the problem of selective perception and share your observation and interview data with a mixed group of clients and health care providers. Ask the group for categorization and summation implications.

Interactiveness

Interactiveness is an additional event to be aware of during all observations. When an observer, whether participant or nonparticipant, observes and records program activities, the person's presence affects and shapes the activities observed. Productivity may increase because staff members are aware of being observed or because they are concerned about client satisfaction or dissatisfaction. All evaluation strategies can have an interactive component, but perhaps the interactive consideration is strongest in case studies because of the presence of an observer.

Nominal Group

Both the nominal group and Delphi technique are based on the belief that the people in a program are the most knowledgeable sources on its relevancy. The nominal group technique uses a structured group meeting, during which all individuals are given a judgmental task, such as to list the functions of the program, problems of the program, or needed changes in the program. Each member is asked to write a response on paper and to not discuss it with other people. At the end of 5 to 10 minutes, all members present their ideas, and each idea is recorded (without discussion), so everyone can see all the suggestions. Once all ideas have been presented, a discussion begins, during which ideas are clarified and evaluated. After the discussion, the group votes to determine the order in which to address different areas. The nominal group technique allows all individuals to present their ideas before the entire group. Involving the entire group both decreases selective perception and promotes individual cooperation with the group's decisions because people believe they have been involved in the decision-making process.

Delphi Technique

The Delphi technique tends to be used in large survey studies but is also useful as a case-study method. It involves a series of questionnaires and feedback reports to a designated panel of respondents. An initial questionnaire is distributed by mail to a preselected group (this could be all nursing staff members, a group of clients, or program administrators). Independently, respondents express their thoughts through the questionnaire and return it. Based on the responses of the group, a feedback report and a revised version of the questionnaire are sent to the respondents. Using the feedback information, the respondents evaluate their first answers and complete the questionnaire again. The process continues for a predetermined number of feedback rounds.

Usefulness to Evaluation

The case-study method of program evaluation can help answer questions of *relevance*. Questioning clients and health care providers helps to explore perceptions of how well the program is meeting its defined goals and to ascertain problem areas and possible solutions. The case-study method would not point to any one solution but rather would offer several possible choices.

Questions of *progress* can also be addressed through the case-study method. The extent to which a program is meeting predetermined standards of service indicates progress. Because the case study provides an examination of the program, much can be learned if program activities are already in place.

Cost *efficiency* of the program is difficult to evaluate using a case-study method. First, to evaluate if the program could have been offered more economically, a comparable program must exist; and, second, the case-study method is designed to look at only one program. The method is not formatted to look at two programs and compare them. However, judgments can be made as to the operating efficiency of the program. These judgments must be based on the experience and knowledge of the evaluator and cannot be based on comparisons with other operating programs.

Effectiveness determines if the program has produced what it intended to produce immediately after the program, as opposed to the outcome, which measures long-term consequences. Although the case-study method may determine aspects of effectiveness, such as whether the aims of the program have been met in the short run, it is very difficult to measure long-term consequences unless the case-study method is conducted over a long period that allows a retrospective view of the program.

Surveys

A survey is a method of collecting information and can be used to collect evaluation information. Surveys are usually completed by self-administered questionnaires (the process used in Rosemont to determine community perception of health information needs) or by personal interviews. Surveys are formulated to describe (*descriptive* surveys) or to analyze relationships (*analytic* surveys). (Actually, most surveys can be used both to describe and to analyze.)

Surveys can be used to describe the need for a program, the actual operations of a program, or a program's effects. Along with the descriptive information, questions of analysis can be answered through a survey. For example, a survey could be used to *describe* the composition of the groups that attend crime-prevention or weight-reduction classes, as well as to *analyze* the relationship between descriptive data of sex, for instance, and weight-reduction success.

Surveys are usually performed for summative (impact) evaluation. Did the program accomplish what it was proposed to do? Was the program perceived as successful by clients? By personnel? If the program was considered successful, what parts were most helpful? Least helpful? What should be changed? Left unchanged? The questions asked by the survey are determined by the initial list of questions about program evaluation.

Like the case-study method, the answers on surveys come from the perceptions, values, and belief systems of the respondents. The response given to questions of program usefulness by the nurse who planned and implemented the program may be very different from the answers of the participants. Awareness of perception bias can direct evaluation efforts to consider the perceptions of all persons (providers, clients, and management) involved in program implementation.

Reliability and Validity

Surveys that are used for program evaluation must be concerned with the *reliability* and *validity* of the information collected. Reliability deals with the repeatability, or reproducibility, of the data (i.e., if the same questions were asked of the same people 1 week later, would the same responses be recorded?). Validity is the correctness of the information. If questions are written to evaluate knowledge, and the answers of the respondents reflect behaviors, then the questions are not valid because they do not measure what they claim to measure.

Usefulness to Evaluation

Surveys can be very valuable to answer questions of *relevance*, or the need for proposed or existing programs, especially if the perceptions of clients, providers, and management are solicited. In a similar fashion, surveys can measure *progress*. People critiquing surveys as an evaluation strategy may be concerned with the subjectivity of the survey—indeed, individual perception affects every response to every question. However, most decisions are based on subjective judgments, not objective reality. It is important to understand whose subjective impression is being used as a basis for judgment; it is imperative for community health nurses to ensure that clients' perceptions are represented alongside those of health care providers and managers.

Cost efficiency, effectiveness, and outcome are difficult to measure using a survey. Although a survey can measure the perceived efficiency of the program or ideas on alternative ways of operating to make the program more cost-efficient, these perceptions are formed only in the context of the existing program. There is no other comparison program against which recorded perceptions can be measured. A survey can provide information on the characteristics of program activities that are perceived by the respondents to have caused changes in their health status, but these impressions are reported in the absence of any comparison group. A comparison group is especially important with regard to effectiveness and impact because it is impossible to tell if an alternative program (or no program at all) might have been more or less effective in accomplishing the same objectives.

TAKE NOTE

You may be wondering if a comparison group is so important and if perceptions cloud the evaluation with subjective impressions, then why use surveys at all? Two pluses exist in surveys: a great deal of information for program evaluation can be obtained, especially about the activities of the program from the perception of several groups; and important evaluation data can be inferred if the instrument (questionnaire or interview schedule) is reliable and valid.

Experimental Design

Completed correctly, an experimental design study can provide an answer to the crucial questions: Did the program make a difference? Are health behaviors, knowledge, and attitudes changed as a result of the program activities? Is the community healthier because of the programs offered by the Rosemont Health Promotion Council? However, the problem with experimental studies in program evaluation is that they require selective implementation, meaning that people who participate are selected through a process such as random assignment to a control group and an experimental group. For many ethical, political, and community health reasons, selective implementation is difficult to complete and is sometimes impossible. Despite these problems, the experimental study remains the best method to evaluate summative effects (outcomes) of a program and the only way to produce quantified information on whether the program made a difference.

T A K E   N O T E

Reviewing the steps of the research process at this point may be of help to you in understanding the examples to follow. Indeed, each issue—such as a theoretical framework, sampling, reliability, and validity—must be addressed if an experimental design is proposed for evaluation.

The following designs are the most feasible and appropriate to health care settings. Apply the research process to each design.

Pretest–Posttest One-Group Design

The pretest–posttest design applied to one group is illustrated in Table 15.3. Two observations are made, the first at Time 1 and the second at Time 2. The observation can be the prevalence of a health state (e.g., the percentage of adults in Rosemont who exercise regularly, the teenage pregnancy rate, cases of child abuse, and so on), knowledge scores, or other important community health facts. Between Time 1 and Time 2, an experiment is introduced. The experiment may be a planned program aimed at a target group, such as teen sexuality classes, or with a community-wide focus, like a crime-prevention program. The evaluation of the program is measured by considering the difference between the health state at Time 1 and the health state after the program at Time 2.

If the experiment in Table 15.3 was teen sexuality classes for 10th-grade girls at Hampton High School, Time 1 was a teen pregnancy rate of 5 per 100, and Time 2 (1 year later) was a teen pregnancy rate of 3 per 100 among the girls taking the classes, then would you agree that the teen sexuality program was responsible for the decrease in teenage pregnancies? What other information do you need to know in order to decide? (Are there other factors that could account for the decrease in the teen pregnancy rate? Perhaps family-planning programs have been focused on teenagers, or maybe local churches and social service agencies have sponsored teen sexuality programs. Teen access to and the use of contraceptive methods may have increased, or laws regarding teen access to contraceptive methods may have changed.) None of these factors can be eliminated as unassociated with the decrease

TABLE 15.3

Pretest–Posttest One-Group Design

	Time 1		Time 2
Experimental group	Observation 1	Experiment	Observation 2

TABLE 15.4

Pretest–Posttest Two-Group Design

	Time 1		Time 2
Experimental group	Observation 1	Experiment	Observation 2
Control group	Observation 1		Observation 2

in the teen pregnancy rate. To eliminate other possible explanations for program effectiveness, a control group must be added.

Pretest–Posttest Two-Group Design

A pretest–posttest with a control group design is illustrated in Table 15.4. The design has both an experimental group and a control group. At Time 1, an observation is made of both the experimental and control groups. Between Time 1 and Time 2, an experiment is introduced with the experimental group. At Time 2, second observations are made on both the experimental and control groups. Program evaluation is the difference between Observations 1 and 2 for the experimental group when compared to the comparison group (which has been selected to be as similar as possible to the experimental group). Will the pretest–posttest with a control group design eliminate the effect of outside factors that occurred simultaneously with the experiment and that might account for the change between Observation 1 and Observation 2, the very problem that plagued the pretest–posttest one-group design? The answer is yes, if the experimental and control groups are similar.

To explain, let us return to Rosemont and the idea of a teen sexuality class for 10th-grade students at Hampton High School. If 10th-grade students, similar in social, economic, and geographic characteristics, were randomly selected and then randomly assigned to the experimental or control group, then it could be assumed that any other factors that influenced the experimental group would also affect the control group. However, frequently, the decision is made that all students must be given the same program, thereby eliminating a comparison group. At the Rosemont Health Promotion Council, when the information was received that all 10th graders must be given a teen sexuality program that had been proposed by the school nurse as a response to an increasing number of teen pregnancies, the suggestion was made that perhaps another high school could be used as a control group. How would you respond to that suggestion? Perhaps another high school class of 10th graders could be used, if the students were similar in social, economic, and geographic characteristics to the students at Hampton High (an unlikely situation).

Another possibility mentioned by the Rosemont Health Promotion Council was to offer the program in one school year to one half of the Hampton High 10th graders (using the other half as a control) and then in the following year to offer the program to the remaining students. This method would ensure that all students would be given the program but would also allow for an experimental pretest–posttest design for evaluation.

A third method that was suggested to ensure an experimental design was to give the control group sexuality education and give the experimental group sexuality education plus assertiveness training. The assertiveness training would differentiate the groups and allow an experimental design. All the suggestions were discussed with school officials, and it was decided to offer a traditional sex education class to half the 10th-grade students (the control group); the remaining students (the experimental group) would get the traditional sex education material but would also receive classes on assertiveness training and values clarification. This design will not allow for the evaluation of traditional sex education classes versus no information, but it will provide all students with the health information (an ethical compromise) and allow for the evaluation of a traditional program on sexuality versus that traditional program plus assertiveness and values clarification information (an approach to reduce teenage pregnancies that is supported in the literature).

> ### T A K E   N O T E
>
> Notice that the decision to offer information on assertiveness and values clarification as part of teen sexuality classes was based on documentation from the literature. Rosemont is not the first community to offer health-promotion programs. Many communities have assessed the health status and perceived health needs of the residents and have followed up with planned and implemented programs that have been evaluated, with the results reported in the literature. One contribution that the community health nurse can make is to review and synthesize the results of similar programs and present this information to the community for use in decision making. After the program topics have been decided, you should begin a literature review to study the ways in which other communities have addressed and evaluated similar programs.

Usefulness to Evaluation

An experimental design can yield data on whether a program has produced the desired *outcomes* when compared to the absence of such a program or, alternatively, whether one program strategy has produced better results with regard to the desired outcomes than some other strategy. However, the experimental design is not useful for the evaluation of program progress or program cost efficiency.

Monitoring (Process)

Monitoring measures the difference between the program plan and what has actually happened. Monitoring focuses on the sequence of activities of the program, specifically, how the program is to be implemented (the activities), by whom (the personnel and other resources), and when (the timing of activities). Monitoring is usually done with a chart, and, although there are several different styles of charts, all arrange activities in a sequence and specify the time allotted to complete each task. Figure 15.1 shows an example of a monitoring chart.

Monitoring Charts

To construct a monitoring chart for your program plan, information is needed on the *inputs* (resources necessary to carry out the program such as personnel, equipment, and finances), the *process* (the program activities, their sequencing, and timing), and *outputs* (the expected results of the program, including immediate and long-term health effects). It is helpful to make a list of inputs, processes, and outputs.

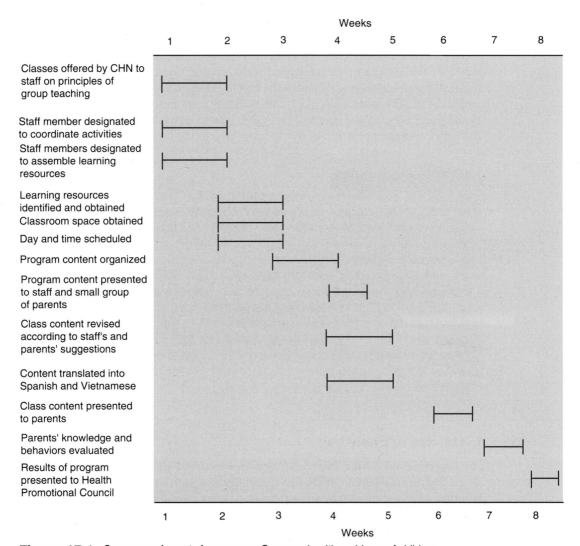

Figure 15.1 Sequence of events for program: Common health problems of children.

You have already recorded this information as part of your program plan. Refer to Chapter 13 and note that resources, program activities, and learning objectives were listed for the proposed class on common health problems of children. Resources are the same as inputs; program activities correspond to processes; and learning objectives designate expected outputs. So all that remains is to place the data into a chart for monitoring.

Figure 15.1 lists the inputs, processes, and outputs for the proposed program in Rosemont, along with a time sequence for beginning and completing each event.

It is difficult to decide on the amount of time that will be needed to complete any task. After assessing the organizational structure and management methods of the agency, you can determine the approximate amounts of time that will be needed to complete the activities of the program. Monitoring charts are easy to formulate and provide useful information for measuring program evaluation if the chart is realistic. The Further Readings list at the end of this chapter includes references to several other types of monitoring charts, including the Gantt, Program Evaluation and Review Technique (PERT), and Critical Path Method (CPM). These provide a slightly different variation of the basic time-sequencing, activities-monitoring chart that appears in Figure 15.1.

Usefulness to Evaluation

A monitoring chart measures progress and can be used to evaluate whether a program is on schedule and within budget. Perhaps no other evaluation method is as perfectly suited to *process evaluation* as the monitoring chart. In addition, monitoring can provide information on the *cost efficiency* of the program by measuring the average cost of the resources required per client served. The effectiveness of the program can be measured by monitoring the chart if the chart records outputs achieved. Monitoring charts cannot determine program relevance or the long-term impact of a program, however.

Cost–Benefit and Cost–Effectiveness Analyses

Much has been written and discussed about the escalating cost of health care services and ways that cost can be reduced. The turmoil over health care reform in the United States and the intense debate regarding the pros and cons of various alternative approaches to health care delivery were testimony to the need to contain cost and yet increase access and maintain quality. Every program has a dollar price both in terms of the resources needed to offer the program (e.g., personnel and equipment) and the dollar benefits to be gained from improved health (such as increased worker productivity).

Two of the most common methods of analyzing the economic costs and benefits of a program are cost–benefit analysis (CBA) and cost–effectiveness analysis (CEA). Both CBA and CEA are formal analytic techniques that list all costs (direct and indirect) and consequences (negative and positive) of a particular program. The distinction between CBA and CEA is based on the value that is placed on the consequences of a program. In CBA, consequences or benefits of a program are valued in terms of dollars; this makes it possible to compare different projects, because all measurement is made in dollars. Therefore, the worth of a project can be judged by asking if dollar benefits exceed dollar costs and, if so, by how much. In contrast, CEA does not place a dollar value on either the consequences or the costs of a project. Another outcome is used for programs whose benefits or costs are difficult to measure (e.g., how could a dollar value be placed on each suicide prevented by a primary prevention program to decrease teenage suicide?). Therefore, CEA, unlike CBA, does not determine if total benefits exceed total costs.

However, CEA can be used to compare programs with similar goals and objectives (e.g., two different primary prevention approaches to decrease the incidence of teenage suicide share the same benefits, so only costs need be compared—a CEA). A CEA can also be used if the costs of alternative programs are the same or if only a given amount of money exists and the objective is to select the program with the greatest benefits (not measured in dollar terms). The decision is obvious; select the program that produces the most effectiveness (i.e., the most benefits per dollar spent or the least cost for each unit [individual, family, or community] benefited).

The choice between CBA and CEA depends on the type of questions and programs considered. Neither technique is superior to the other. Both techniques can be used in planning for future programs or as an evaluation strategy of present or past programs. The actual procedures for completing a CBA or CEA are beyond the scope of this book; however, several references that include the procedural steps are listed in the Further Readings list. Obviously, both CBA and CEA are strategies for measuring program cost efficiency and do not address the issues of relevancy, progress, effectiveness, or impact.

Summary

Several methods of evaluation have been presented and discussed. No one method will evaluate the components of relevancy, progress, cost efficiency, effectiveness, and outcome equally well. It is important to be knowledgeable about different methods of program evaluation and to discuss the benefits and limitations of each with the community as the program is being planned and before program implementation occurs. Table 15.5 presents a summary table of appropriate evaluation methods for program components. Once evaluation methods are selected, the methods (case study, experimental design, or monitoring charts) become part of the program plan.

You may be wondering which evaluation methods were used to evaluate the health-promotion programs in Rosemont. A variety was used. To evaluate the relevancy of the health-promotion programs (crime-prevention and effective-parenting classes), nominal group meetings were scheduled, and both health care providers and consumers attended. In addition, the use of rates and demographics of the participants using the health-promotion programs was assessed, as were the participants' perceptions of the value of the information. Program progress was evaluated with monitoring charts such as the one presented in Figure 15.1. The effectiveness and impact of individual programs were evaluated with knowledge, attitude, and behavioral intent surveys (i.e., questionnaires, interviews, and tests) given to participants before the program, immediately after the program, and at predetermined follow-up times (6 weeks and 3 months after the program). As often as was feasible, an evaluation research design was followed, such as a one-group

TABLE 15.5

Examination of the Appropriateness of Different Evaluation Methods for Program Components

Components	Method			
	Case Study	**Survey**	**Experimental**	**Monitoring**
Relevancy	Yes	Yes	No	No
Progress	Yes	Yes	No	Yes
Cost-efficiency	No	No	Yes	Yes
Cost-effectiveness	Some	No	Yes	Some
Impact	No	No	Yes	No

pretest–posttest. Additional measures of effectiveness and impact were community statistics on crime, child abuse, and teenage pregnancies before as compared to after the program, as well as health policy changes that affected the residents of Rosemont (e.g., access of minors to contraceptives, disciplinary practices in the public schools, and financial eligibility requirements for health services). CEA was completed on several of the programs.

You are ready now for program implementation and the reinitiation of the nursing process; namely, assessment of the program's effects. As you implement the planned program, data will be added to the community assessment profile, which will demand addition, deletion, and revision of the community nursing diagnoses and the associated program plans and interventions. Let us take a final look at the community-as-partner model (see Fig. 10.4) and ask: Will the planned programs assist the community to attain, regain, maintain, and promote health? Strengthen the community's ability to resist stressors? Enhance the community's competence and self-reliance?

T A K E   N O T E

It is fitting that the final chapter of this section on the application of the nursing process in community health nursing ends with questions. Community health nursing is the constant questioning, prodding, probing, and pondering of the health status of a population. Although individual and family health are always important, the uniqueness of our field is the application of nursing techniques to the health of a community. Each community is unique and special. No other community is quite like the one in which you are practicing community health nursing. We have enjoyed sharing the uniqueness of Rosemont with you and the application of the nursing process to community health nursing.

Critical Thinking Questions

Describe an evaluation plan for your intervention chosen in Chapter 14:

1. Which program evaluation type (process, impact, outcome) will you use? Why?
2. What method will you use? Provide rationale.
3. Who will be involved in the evaluation?
4. How will you collect data that are sensitive to your target audience?
5. How credible will your evaluation be? Describe your rationale.

● R E F E R E N C E S

Dignan, M. B., & Carr, P. A. (1992). *Program planning for health education and promotion* (2nd ed.). Philadelphia, PA: Lea & Febiger.

Green, L. W., & Lewis, F. M. (1986). *Measurement and evaluation in health education and health promotion*. Palo Alto, CA: Mayfield.

Minkler, M. (Ed.). (1997). *Community organizing and community building for health*. New Brunswick, NJ: Rutgers University Press.

W. K. Kellogg Foundation. (1998). *Evaluation handbook*. Battle Creek, MI: Author.

■ FURTHER READINGS

Aronson, R. E., Wallis, A. B., O'Campo, P. J., Whitehead, T. L., & Schafer, P. (2007). Ethnographi-cally informed community evaluation: A framework and approach for evaluating community-based initiatives. *Maternal and Child Health Journal*, 11(2), 97–109.

Fatar, K. H. (2007). Enhancing new students' perceptions of nursing using a Healthy People 2010 group project. *The Journal of Nursing Education*, 46(2), 96.

Felix, H. C., White, M., McCullough, H. A., Morgan, J., & Stewart, M. K. (2004). Issues in assessing satisfaction: Findings of the Arkansas Medicaid family planning demonstration waiver evaluation. *Journal of Public Health Management and Practice*, 10(6), 533–538.

Fetterman, D. M. (Ed.), (2001). *Foundations of empowerment evaluation*. Thousand Oaks, CA: Sage.

Issel, L. M. (2008). *Health program planning and evaluation: A practical, systematic approach for community health* (2nd ed.). Sudbury, MA: Jones and Bartlett.

Kegler, M. C., Norton, B. L., & Aronson, R. E. (2008). Strengthening community leadership: Evaluation findings from the California Health Cities and Communities Program. *Health Promotion Practice*, 9(2), 170–179.

Loue, S. (2006). Preventing HIV, eliminating disparities among Hispanics in the United States. *Journal of Immigrant and Minority Health*, 8(4), 313–318.

Minkler, M. (Ed.), (2004). *Community organizing and community building for health* (2nd. ed.). New Brunswick, NJ: Rutgers University Press.

Minkler, M., & Wallerstein, N. (2008). *Community based participatory research for health: From Process to Outcomes* (2nd ed.). San Francisco, CA: Jossey-Bass.

Mulroy, D. A., & Lauber, H. (2004). A user-friendly approach to program evaluation and effective community interventions for families at risk of homelessness. *Social Work*, 49(4), 573–586.

Mulroy, E. A. (2008). University community partnerships that promote evidence-based macro practice. *Journal of Evidence-Based Social Work*, 5(3–4), 497–517.

Rew, L., Hoke, M. M., Horner, S. D., & Walker, L. (2009). Development of a dynamic model to guide health disparities research. *Nursing Outlook*, 57(3), 132–142.

Rossi, P. H., Lipsey, M. W., & Freeman, H. E. (2004). *Evaluation: A systematic approach* (7th ed.). Thousand Oaks, CA: Sage.

Roy, K., Haddix, A. C., Ikeda, R. M., Curry, C. W., Truman, B. I., et al. (2009). Monitoring progress toward CDC's health protection goals: Health outcome measures by life stage. *Public Health Reports*, 124(2), 304–316.

Internet Resources can be found on the**Point** at http://thepoint.lww.com/Anderson6e.

Practicing With Diverse Communities

Promoting Healthy Partnerships With Schools

Nina M. Fredland

LEARNING OBJECTIVES

After studying this chapter, you should be able to:

1. Design programs that are specific to the specialized school setting at the primary, secondary, and tertiary levels of prevention.
2. Design culturally relevant, developmentally appropriate programs that are appealing to school-aged youth and are congruent with the goals of Healthy People 2020.
3. Implement creative programs that nurture healthy relationships and model healthy behavior to school-aged children, their parents, school faculty, and staff.
4. Utilize the community resources of the school's geographic community, and involve the local residents in program planning and implementation.
5. Identify strategies that influence the school climate and are designed to reduce bullying, sexual bullying/harassment, and violence in the school setting.

Introduction

*M*ost health care professionals would agree that a major goal for the 21st century would be to create a nation of children who are optimally well so they can lead long, happy, productive lives. This goal is congruent with the overarching goals of the Healthy People 2020:

1. Eliminate preventable disease, disability, injury, and premature death.
2. Achieve health equity, eliminate disparities, and improve the health of all groups.
3. Create social and physical environments that promote good health for all.
4. Promote healthy development and healthy behaviors across every stage of life. (http://www.healthypeople.gov/HP2020/advisory/PhaseI/summary.htm#_Toc211942896).

How do we as nurses achieve this goal? This chapter focuses on strategies and partnerships within the community setting of the school. The school nurse or the public health nurse, depending on the community, is ideally situated to provide health care to school-aged children. Nurses with advanced preparation in child health, such as pediatric nurse practitioners and family nurse practitioners, are also well prepared to initiate partnerships with schools. An ideal model is one in which the school nurse or public health nurse collaborates with the advanced practice nurse. In this way, health promotion, disease prevention, and health maintenance are important components included within the delivery of health care. School-aged children are a captive audience, and their parents/guardians are closely connected to the school community. This situation makes the school community an ideal center for health-promotion activities for the entire family.

The health of our nation's children has been an area of concern for some time. Casual observations at any school reveal a high percentage of overweight children, youngsters easily fatigued while running around the playground, and children choosing nonnutritious snacks. Obviously, these children are at a disadvantage; their health is compromised. One has only to observe adult role models to understand why children are making unhealthy choices. Therefore, health-education approaches must be comprehensive and include the children as well as all groups of individuals involved in their care and nurturing. For the purposes of this chapter, these key adults, together with the children and adolescents they serve, are referred to as the school community. The school community encompasses:

- School-aged children and adolescents
- Parents and guardians
- School personnel (faculty, staff, and administrators)
- Neighborhood residents, businesses, and service agencies

Healthy People 2020, scheduled to be launched in 2010, builds on the 11 priority areas of Healthy People 2010 for health education for school-aged children/adolescents: unintentional injury, violence, suicide, tobacco use and addiction, alcohol and other drug use, unintended pregnancy, HIV/AIDS and sexually transmitted infection, unhealthy dietary patterns, inadequate physical activity, and environmental health. For regular updates on the collaborative campaign and for details as they evolve subscribe to Healthy People Listserv (http://www.healthypeople.gov/HP2020/).

In addition to promoting optimal health and preventing illness through the education of all members of the school community, school health programs must strive to identify and resolve existing health problems. Therefore, comprehensive school health programs should focus on delivering health services mandated by state laws and the individual school system as well as on health education. Additionally, both internal and external environmental issues are critical areas of assessment and intervention for school nurses.

DELIVERING HEALTH SERVICES FOR HEALTH PROMOTION

Each state mandates certain requirements to maintain the health of school-aged children. Vision and hearing screening programs are required. Measurements of height, weight, and blood pressure are also usually part of these health services. Spinal, nutritional, dental, and developmental screening may also be required in the school setting. To find out about requirements in your state, contact your local state health department. The following list outlines some common state requirements:

Vision: Screen all new students within 120 days of enrollment. Screen students in kindergarten, 1st, 3rd, 5th, 7th, and 9th grades by May of each school year.

Hearing: Screen all new students within 120 days of enrollment. Screen students in kindergarten, 1st, 3rd, 5th, 7th, and 9th grades by May of each school year.

Spinal: Screen all 6th- and 9th-grade students.

Certification is required to perform vision and hearing screening. Certification training is available through state health departments or through individuals the state has designated with this authority. To find out how to receive certification training, contact your state health department. Certification for registered nurses is not usually required for spinal screening, yet ancillary personnel or volunteer assistants are required to have attended an approved educational program. Therefore, it is important that student nurses be taught a thorough procedure for assessing spinal deformities as part of their health assessment curriculum. Recent controversy has argued that due to limited resources and a low yield related to identifying spinal deformities that actually progress to require surgical intervention, school-based spinal screening is unnecessary. Some states have moved to eliminate this requirement. Nurses and many orthopedic physicians would agree that the potential to prevent severe cardiac and respiratory complications in even a few children is worth the effort. Therefore, nurses should adopt a holistic approach, using the preferred terminology of "spinal screening" and not "scoliosis screening," which focuses on only one condition and medicalizes the entire process. Spinal screening, a more positive term, is an opportunity to assess a child's overall health as well as the condition of the spine.

When screenings are conducted privately and confidentially, the nurse can assess for many things, such as nutritional status, dermatological conditions, bruising, etc. During the process, the nurse has an opportunity to engage the child in health-related conversation. This may be a follow-up to a previous visit to the health room. A question such as, "What did you have for breakfast this morning?" can lead to a discussion reinforcing the importance of a nutritious breakfast. What barriers might prevent the child from eating a healthy breakfast, and what self-responsibility measures can the child take toward the goal of getting adequate nutrition in the morning? A few simple suggestions can empower even a very young child, and this health education can occur within the context of "spinal screening."

Immunizations are required by state law to be current and on file before or on the first day of school, although a school district can establish a short grace period, usually 30 days. Immunization requirements must be strictly supported by the school administration. Each state sets a standard for immunizations; a school district can increase the requirements but must include the minimum standard. For example, tuberculosis (TB) screening for school-aged children may not be required by state law; however, school districts can set a higher standard and require new students to have an approved skin test for TB screening at the time of initial enrollment. Furthermore, school districts can require school personnel to be tested biennially. The Centers for Disease Control and Prevention (CDC) is the best source for recommended immunization schedules for children and adults. It would be helpful to familiarize yourself with the CDC website (http://www.cdc.gov) and the current recommended immunization schedule for school-aged children because these requirements change frequently.

Although most parents are vigilant about immunizing their children in a timely manner, some parents question the need or safety of some vaccines. They may have concerns about immunizing in general or they may have specific questions related to select vaccines, the combinant forms, or the recommended timing. Nurses in school settings are well positioned to respond to such concerns, and provide parents and guardians with accurate information to make informed choices about immunizing their children. The CDC provides reliable information in both English and Spanish to help health care professionals and consumers to better understand vaccine issues and maintain "herd immunity." These resources can be easily accessed at www.cdc.gov/vaccines or 800-CDC-INFO (232-4636).

In addition to conducting mass screening programs, a nurse in the school setting identifies and monitors existing health problems, both acute and chronic, such as common respiratory infections and asthma. The school nurse is a referral agent and case manager, and offers education within the scope of nursing practice.

HEALTH EDUCATION FOR HEALTH PROMOTION

Major issues affecting children in the United States can be categorized under headings of nutrition; interpersonal violence; substance abuse; mental health issues; safety; sexuality; and environmental hazards such as lead, asbestos, and air pollution. Specific topics from which you might select health-education programs are listed in Box 16.1. Some of these topics are more appropriate for children, parents, or teachers. As you are thinking of the topic, consider the audience you are targeting. For example, healthy food choices might be geared toward easy recipes that children can prepare. There are a number of cookbooks written with children in mind; a favorite is the American Heart Association's *Children's Help Your Heart Cookbook*. Alternatively, have students compile their own cookbook with simple healthy recipes. This activity can be conducted at grade level or as a schoolwide fundraiser. Box 16.1 is not exhaustive; it is designed to promote ideas. Consider how you might assess interest for any of the programs.

Health-Promotion Programs for School-Aged Children

Programs for children and adolescents in the school setting must be age-appropriate. Obviously, breast self-examination and testicular self-examination are not appropriate material for elementary school children. It is critical to assess the developmental and maturity level of the children before deciding on the educational content of a program or a strategy. Even if you think you know how to relate to a certain age group, each class is different. The children may be in a very young class for their grade level, or they may be a very advanced group. The students may or may not be well socialized. Several may have attention deficit disorder or exhibit hyperactivity. Students are sometimes mainstreamed despite having considerable behavioral issues that can affect the class group dynamics.

Important information is gained from observing the student population before planning programs. Always visit the classroom and observe how the students and teacher interact. Classroom management skills are essential. It is difficult to manage the classroom successfully when the nurse's contact with the youngsters is only occasional. Relying on the regular classroom teacher for assistance always works best. Unfortunately, the amount of time that classroom teachers have to

HEALTH EDUCATION PROGRAM IDEAS

Nutrition
Healthy food choices
Healthy recipes for busy families
Healthy lunches children can prepare
Disordered eating (such as anorexia, bulimia, and compulsive eating)

Violence
Domestic violence—effects on children and sources of help for the whole family
Discipline versus child abuse
Anger management/impulse control
Bullying behaviors
Dating violence
Date rape/acquaintance rape
Gang behavior
Signs of child abuse/incest

Substance Use
Cigarettes and chewing tobacco
Underage drinking
Illicit drugs (marijuana, crack, cocaine, inhalants, speed, ecstasy, heroin, and so forth)

Mental Health Issues
Self-esteem
Attention deficit disorder/hyperactivity disorder
Depression
Suicide

Personal Safety
"Latchkey" kids
Problem-solving/decision-making skills

Recreational Safety
Bicycles, in-line skates, sports
Vehicle safety (seat belts, booster seats, riding in open vehicles)
Water safety (swimming, boating, skiing)

Sexuality
Personal hygiene
Teenage pregnancy
Teen parenting
Sexually transmitted diseases

Environmental
Internal (air, water, space)
External (pollution, noise)
Psychological (grade stress, parent–child discord, parent–teacher and teacher–teacher
  conflicts, peer harassment)

Societal Influences
Changing family structure
Peer pressure
Media influences (video games, films, television)

devote to programs beyond the prescribed curriculum is limited. They may not feel that they can assist with programs beyond the prescribed curriculum duties. Therefore, it is critical to involve key people such as the teachers, counselors, school nurses, and parents from the very beginning of the planning phase of health programs. Outlining their expectations will contribute to the overall success of the program and help them become vested in the outcomes of the project. Such an approach is usually well received by students, administrators, teachers, and parents.

Another consideration is marketing your program. It may be a great idea, but if no one attends or follows through, it will be a waste of time and resources. Use flyers, bulletin boards, and public address announcements to reach your audiences. Try various strategies to pique interest. For example, brightly colored signs and charts; guessing games; poster contests; door-decorating competitions; and age-appropriate, healthy food rewards (e.g., juice bars, fruit) are a few suggestions. Involving the students in the promotion of the program is ideal. The following are examples of health-promotion programs for school-aged children:

- Red Ribbon Week
- Breast self-examination/Testicular self-examination (teens)
- Muscle Mover Club, Triathlon, or Walk-a-Thon/Swim to Bermuda
- Monthly health bulletin board
- Make a cookbook
- Pet responsibility
- Arts-based interventions

The following sections discuss some of these health-promotion programs.

Red Ribbon Week

Red Ribbon Week occurs in October each year to celebrate being drug free. The Red Ribbon Campaign was established in 1988 by the U.S. Congress. The goal was to increase the awareness of the dangers associated with the use of tobacco, alcohol, and other drugs. Since then, Red Ribbon Week has become standard in many schools. The Internet has many examples of how different schools across the nation celebrate the week. A sample agenda for a week's program focusing on drug abuse prevention, which can be incorporated into the curriculum of an elementary school, appears in Box 16.2. Each student recites a promise to stay away from drugs and wears a red ribbon for the week.

The community should be involved in the program along with the students. Parents can be invited to some programs. The parents' organization can be asked to decorate the school with red ribbons. Community leaders (e.g., church, civic, and police) can judge contests. The police and fire departments can facilitate a parade route and provide security. Media coverage, such as local newspapers and radio and television stations, is an important strategy that schools should use. (Often, worthwhile events are not covered by the media simply because media personnel have not been notified.) Older students and campus leaders can influence younger students by positive peer pressure, such as wearing their ribbons, participating in all activities, and having a major role in organizing and implementing the activities.

It is very important to give clear messages to young people, particularly on the subject of drugs. The nurse should select speakers very carefully. Recovering drug abusers should not be used to speak to groups of students who are not users. It is

SAMPLE AGENDA FOR RED RIBBON WEEK

Monday Flag ceremony and recital of the drug-free pledge by student body.
PLEDGE:
I pledge to be drug free and support the ___(state)___
Red Ribbon Campaign by taking a stand against
alcohol and drug abuse

_____
Signature
http://www.tcada.state.tx.us/Redribbon/redpledge.pdf

Designate a place for pledge signing for the students, faculty/staff.
Display the pledge cards in a central location.
Have a group of children, parents, and school staff deliver the signed
  pledge cards to an official person in city government (e.g., the mayor).
Red ribbons are delivered to all classes by 5th graders (or oldest students
  in school). Each student wears a red ribbon.
Decorate school grounds with red ribbons.

Tuesday	Wear red to school day
	Drug-free poster contest in art classes
Wednesday	Classroom door-decorating contest
	Display finished posters in halls
Thursday	Drug prevention programs per grade levels
Friday	Judging posters and doors
	Assembly and drug-free pep rally
	Motivational speaker
	Drug-free songs and cheers
	Announce contest winters
Saturday/Sunday	Community parade

For more ideas check out the many red ribbon week web sites. Search
via www.google.com and insert the words red ribbon week.
http://www.imdrugfree.com is a good one!

also risky to choose high-profile role models, such as well-known sports or media individuals, who may be positive nondrug users one day but may appear in the news media at a later time for using drugs or for violent behavior. Consider asking the students to give 1-minute talks on why they are not going to use drugs. Have a poem or "smart saying" contest. Get the speech club involved.

Muscle Mover Club, Triathlon, or Walk-a-Thon

The Muscle Mover Club encourages physical activity by rewarding aerobic exercise, such as walking, running, swimming, and biking. Each child receives a badge and adds stickers for city blocks or track laps completed. Healthy competition can be encouraged by racing to a goal either individually or as a classroom. Another strategy is to include parents by having them sign off on triathlon or walk-a-thon mileage sheets. Encourage parents to do the activity with their children. A parent/teacher bulletin board recognizing athletic achievement, such as running a 5-mile race or marathon, highlights adults leading healthy lifestyles. Children are very proud to have their parents and teachers value their achievements. They are also delighted when healthy behaviors their parents engage in are acknowledged and appreciated by their teachers and school administrators. In addition to health promotion, these strategies reinforce positive adult role modeling, which is so important in a child's formative years.

Health-Promotion Programs for Parents

The following are ideas for healthy partnerships with parents:

- Parent information sessions
- Parent peer groups
- Late breakfast meetings; "second cup of coffee meeting"
- Grandparents' day
- Breast cancer awareness
- Parents' nutrition committee

The most difficult part of planning health-promotion activities that include parents is timing. Most parents are employed and have very little flexibility in their work schedules. Breakfast meetings that are short and occur as children are brought to school may be well attended. Issues must appeal to parents, and it is always a good idea to conduct a "needs assessment" before deciding on topics. In this way, you can include important health information as well as meet parental expectations.

Programs to Promote Healthy Habits

Childhood overweight/obesity is a major health challenge facing the nation. Effective ways of treating and managing pediatric obesity have yet to be documented in the research literature (Robinson, 2008). According to the World Health Organization (WHO), this global problem affects more than 1 billion adults, with approximately 300 million considered "clinically obese" (WHO, 2009). In the United States, one out of three children are considered overweight or obese (Robinson, 2008). Statistics indexing childhood obesity have been stable from 2003 to 2006 (Ogden, Carroll, & Flegal, 2008). However, it is difficult to determine whether this is a true plateau, and efforts to improve school meals and increase physical activity are beginning to pay off (Ebbeling & Ludwig, 2008). What is known is that we continue to have many children who are overweight or obese. Government, media, communities, schools, and families must continue their efforts to sustain healthy nutrition and support safe, active environments.

Excess weight is recognized as a potential risk factor for chronic conditions and has been associated with heart disease, hypertension and stroke, type 2 diabetes, and some types of cancer (http://www.cdc.gov/obesity/causes/health.html, December 4, 2009). In fact, adolescents who are obese are likely to become obese adults (http://www.surgeongeneral.gov/obesityprevention/factsheet/index.html, December 4, 2009). In addition, to chronic disease risks, there is the more immediate concern of social discrimination. This experience could lead to mental health problems such as poor self-esteem or depression. Some children become targets of bullies because of their weight (Robinson, 2006).

Therefore, it has become essential that school health programs focus on healthy eating and physical activity to promote healthy weight. It is much more effective to address unhealthy childhood weight gain at the primary prevention level than to treat it once it has occurred. There is evidence that school health programs implemented without concurrent family interventions and societal campaigns against overweight/obesity may be ineffective (Muller, Danielzik, & Pust, 2005). This finding

HEALTHY HABITS, HEALTHY KIDS! (AN EVENING FOR PARENTS)

Agenda
Register, sign up for door prizes, complete survey related to nutritional knowledge
Welcome and panel introductions
Healthy Habits, Healthy Kids overview
Effects of cholesterol, sugar, and salt on our daily diet
Making sense of food labels
Making good choices in the grocery store
Making good choices in the restaurant
Making your family recipes healthy
Healthy heart discussion
Door prizes awarded

is understandable because the determinants of excess weight are also related to socioeconomic factors and living in an environment that permits easy access to food and encourages inactivity. However, programs in the school setting can be effective if enhanced by national efforts and simultaneous family interventions.

Box 16.3 provides an example of an agenda for a parent information session on nutrition. Marketing strategies for this evening program include: credit for parent volunteer service hours, a cooking demonstration with samples, and prizes such as a 1-year subscription to a parenting magazine or a healthy fruit or vegetable basket. Always try to involve the community merchants in the donation of prizes. Perhaps the local grocery store will donate a fruit or vegetable basket, or the beauty salon will donate a free hair styling. The more involved community businesses are in school activities, the better the community health nurse can promote the health of all citizens.

Parent Peer Groups

Establishing a parent peer group in which parents agree to certain rules of behavior for the children or teens, such as curfews and party rules, is helpful to parents and school personnel. Parents can agree not to allow drinking of alcohol, use of tobacco, or drugs at their house. Parents in the group can then feel comfortable when their children/teens are in the company of peers whose parents ascribe to the same rules. A consistent approach sets limits for youth while providing an atmosphere of positive peer pressure. Parents also feel comfortable consulting with each other and form a support system.

Grandparents' Day

Grandparents' Day is a day in which the school actively involves grandparents, many of whom may not have been in an educational setting for a long time. Activities of the day can include classroom visitation, a healthy lunch, and blood-pressure screening. Seventh-grade (or higher grade) students can be taught to measure blood pressure in science, physical education, biology, math, or health class. Nurses can work with the respective teacher and conduct the practice sessions together. Youth take the elders' blood pressure under the supervision of a health professional such as a community health nurse, parent volunteers who are nurses, or other trained adults. This activity provides a service for the elderly guests and also increases the students' awareness of the importance of preventing heart disease and monitoring blood pressure. If elevated blood pressures are noted, have a referral plan complete with name and phone numbers of clinics, the local health department, or private medical care providers to which the person with an elevated blood pressure can be referred if he or she does not have a primary health care provider. Also follow up on elevated blood pressure measures and offer all participants written information on elevated blood pressure and its association with poor health.

Mother–Daughter and Father–Son Programs

Cancer-prevention programs for mothers and daughters can promote breast self-examination and mammography. Culturally appropriate programs can be designed to attract women of various ethnic backgrounds. For example, if it is not culturally acceptable to discuss breast matters in public meetings, perhaps you can involve the local worship centers or other culturally acceptable agencies where the information could be hosted. (Those centers may also be able to provide bilingual presentations for women not fluent in English.)

Equally important is awareness for fathers and sons about testicular cancer and the correct technique for testicular self-examination. Perhaps mother–daughter talks can be scheduled at the same time as father–son talks. This program can be fun for the whole family, regardless of age, and, again, can involve the whole community. Girl Scout and Boy Scout troops or Future Farmers of America clubs might be interested in sponsoring a family awareness day because they are usually interested in hosting activities for the entire family.

HEALTH-PROMOTION STRATEGIES FOR THE SCHOOL

The following are ideas for health-promotion strategies that can be used with groups such as teachers or staff in the school setting:

- Blood pressure screening on the same day each month
- Cancer awareness programs
- Stuffing payroll envelopes with health-promotion material
- Healthy heart lunches, such as salad day once a week
- Referral and resource information
- TB skin testing

Again, this list is not exhaustive, but is meant to generate ideas for viable strategies. Have an in-service day to assess the school climate and create a more social school atmosphere. Many other health issues for members of the school community are particular to the school environment. The following sections discuss some specific health-promotion strategies.

Nutrition Awareness

If the school meal program is not healthy, form an ad hoc committee to study the problem. The committee should consist of students, parents, the public health/school nurse, cafeteria personnel, representatives of the faculty and administration, and a dietitian, if available. (Hint: Seek consultation from parents. Frequently, a professional dietitian is among the parents.) Action steps would include the following:

1. Conduct a survey to assess parental interest and areas of concern. What would parents like to see happen? What are they willing to do to make change happen?
2. Conduct a survey to assess student opinion and food preferences.

BOX 16.4

PLATE WASTE STUDY

1. Recruit parent volunteers, cafeteria staff, and teachers to help you.
2. Choose at least two days of the week to conduct the study.
3. Place volunteers next to the tray return and trash containers.
4. Record types and amount of food put into the trash.
5. Look into lunch bags for types of discarded, uneaten food.
6. Record all information (perhaps onto form with different food types).
7. You now have important information, such as nutritious food waste and the amount of soft drinks and candy consumed (from the wrappers).
8. Write a one-page report.
9. Give the report to parents, staff, and students.
10. Present the results to school administration along with suggestions to decrease food waste.

3. Do a plate waste study to determine what children are actually eating (Box 16.4).
4. Form a committee, remembering to include the students.
5. Based on what you learned in steps 1, 2, and 3, identify other options to evaluate the present menu, such as hiring a nutritionist to study the present food service. You may also want to organize a committee to visit other schools to sample food, look at menus, and talk to those students about satisfaction.
6. Make recommendations to the school administration.
7. Make a presentation to the school board.
8. Pilot alternatives.

Antibullying and Bullying Prevention Programs

Bullying has become a topic of much concern in the United States. Research has focused on trying to understand the phenomenon. The word *bully* or *boele* can be traced to Dutch roots; however, the most common definition, first articulated by Olweus, includes three elements: aggression, repetition, and a power imbalance (Fredland, 2008). Repetition and power inequality are central to the concept of bullying. Two main types of bullying behavior are described in the literature: direct bullying and relational bullying (Woods & White, 2005). Different characteristics of behavior can be identified within each type. For example, there are pure bullies and pure victims as well as a mixed type (i.e., one who is a victim of bullying but also behaves as a bully). In addition, there are always neutral individuals or bystanders who watch the behavior but do not intervene in any way. The silent onlooker or bystander exemplifies indirect bullying behavior. Girls are said to engage more than boys in indirect bullying behavior. This latter, more subtle form of bullying may be just as devastating to childhood development. Both direct and indirect bullying must be addressed with age-appropriate, effective intervention programs.

A number of antibullying programs have been implemented; however, more information is needed to ascertain what interventions work best to prevent bullying behavior and to curtail instances of bullying when they do occur. What is known is that the problem is a public event (i.e., bullying usually occurs in the presence of others). Solutions must target the bullies, those bullied, children who fall into the category of bully-victims, and the bystanders. Most bullying takes place on or near school grounds in classrooms, hallways, bathrooms, and playgrounds during school hours and after dismissal while the children are still on school property. Bullying also can take place on school buses. Nansel et al. (2001) in a landmark study in the United States reported that 29% of 6th to 10th graders were involved in some form of bullying behavior. Olweus (1994) reported that students with a bullying history were four times more likely to engage in criminal behavior in their twenties. Bullying may escalate to dating violence and later adult intimate partner violence.

Bullying has also been associated with a variety of physical, psychosomatic, and mental health effects such as colds, poor appetite, and fear of going to school. Although more research is needed to truly understand the effects of bullying on health, school nurses should consider bullying a contributory factor when children come to the school clinic complaining of sore throat, colds, respiratory problems, and gastrointestinal ailments (Wolke, Woods, Bloomfield, & Karstadt, 2001). Bullying behaviors have been linked to physical and psychological symptoms in a comparative cross sectional survey of 28 countries (Due et al., 2005). Students, aged 11, 13, and 15, who had been bullied weekly were almost twice as likely to experience headaches, stomachaches, and sleeping problems compared with students who were not bullied. These youth were also two to four times as likely to admit feeling "low," "lonely," "irritable," and "nervous" when compared with the students who were not bullied. Violent youth frequently admit to perceived feelings of loneliness and being disliked by classmates (Thomas & Smith, 2004). Improving school connectedness and individual social skills may reduce negative behaviors and symptomology and should be studied further. For these reasons, it is important to address bullying behavior in its early stage with young students. Students should be encouraged to know what their personal boundaries are and to articulate when someone is crossing the line. Standing up for themselves and learning to be an active bystander when others are being victimized nurtures healthy social development.

Changing the school atmosphere to promote prosocial behavior and to not accept antisocial behavior such as bullying and other forms of aggression may be the most important strategy. A systemic, rather than an individualistic, approach is important to guard against glorifying or passively accepting the bullying behavior. A multifaceted, multicomponent approach that includes students, administration, teachers, staff, and parents is necessary. Legal actions have been taken against school personnel and school districts that failed to intervene in situations of "hostile and abusive learning environments." Federal law requires schools to have a sexual harassment policy (Cavendish, 2001). Check on your school policy. Perhaps you could be involved in developing and implementing an antibullying policy.

There are a number of ways a nurse working in a school setting can address the problem of bullying. The following sections suggest ways to implement a prevention program modeled after Olweus' Bullying Prevention Program at the primary, secondary, and tertiary levels of intervention (Olweus, 2001).

Primary Prevention

A core component of any antibullying intervention program is the awareness and involvement of key adults in the school community. Implementing primary prevention may include the following steps:

1. Conduct a teacher/staff in-service program to educate the members of the school community about the problem of bullying.
   a. Discuss the prevalence of bullying in the United States.
   b. Discuss the various roles that are pertinent to the bullying issue, such as the bully, the victim, the bully-victim, and the bystander role.

2. Determine if bullying/sexual harassment policies are in place in the school system.
   a. If no policies exist, assist school administration to develop a school policy for handling bullying/peer sexual harassment situations.
   b. If a policy exists, formulate a plan to increase awareness.
3. Have a parent meeting to discuss preventing school violence and explain that addressing and stopping bullying is an important component of violence prevention. (Parents are very concerned about this issue due to media coverage about school shootings and the threat of terrorism. With careful planning, you could get a sizeable turnout.)
4. Formulate a coordinating group of teachers, staff, school nurse, administration, parents, community members, and students.

Secondary Prevention

Screen for bullying behaviors to determine the prevalence of both victimization and perpetration of bullying. An assessment of school climate (i.e., tolerance of such behaviors and bystander attitudes) is also indicated.

Schoolwide/classroom measures include:

1. Assess for bullying behaviors using a student questionnaire such as the Peer Relations Questionnaire available at http://www.kenrigby.net/prq-child.pdf.
2. Having a school conference day to disseminate the results of the survey and launch a multicomponent plan to tackle the problem.
3. Implementing effective adult supervision during recess, lunchtime, and classroom/bathroom breaks. Monitoring hallways and other congregating areas, especially before and after school, should be part of the plan.
4. Teacher–student discussion groups to reinforce antibullying messages and contribute to changing the school culture. In other words, students must believe that the adults in the school community will not tolerate bullying behavior and that victims can comfortably report such behavior.
5. Developing classroom rules based on respect.

In addition to schoolwide and classroom measures, the problem of bullying must be addressed on an individual level. Special consideration must be given to how to handle bullies and their victims. Individual measures include:

1. Separate counseling of bullies and victims.
2. Involve parents of bullies and victims in the discussions.
3. Develop individual care plans for students, both bullies and victims, addressing physical, mental, and behavioral health needs.
4. Make referrals to health care providers as appropriate.

Tertiary Prevention

Once the policy and plans have been implemented, it is necessary to monitor the progress, particularly the school climate and bystander behavior. A maintenance program aimed at reducing the prevalence of future bullying is crucial and includes the following:

1. Have regular meetings of the coordinating committee.
2. Formally assess for bullying behaviors on an annual basis.
3. Continue school meetings and teacher–student discussion groups.
4. Encourage parental involvement in a variety of school activities.

BOX 16.5

SUGGESTED RESOURCES FOR BULLYING PREVENTION PROGRAMS

Olweus, D., Limber, S., & Mihalic, S.F. (1999). *Blueprints for violence prevention, book nine: Bullying Prevention Program.* Boulder, CO: Center for the Study and Prevention of Violence.

Steps to Respect: A research based bullying prevention program. Available at http://www.cfchildren.org/programs/str/research/, accessed December 4, 2009.

Take Action to Stop Bullying. Available at http://www.olweus.org/public/index.page, accessed December 4, 2009.

For more information about bullying prevention programs, the resources listed in Box 16.5 are suggested.

HEALTH-PROMOTION STRATEGIES FOR THE COMMUNITY

Involving the neighboring community in health-promotion programs can benefit school-aged children and their families, as well as members of the surrounding community. Health-promotion strategies involving the community may include the following:

- Involve the elderly in school activities such as reading programs, mentoring, and monitoring lunch hour
- Collaborate with the local civic association
- Establish a drug-free zone
- Have a community parade celebrating being drug free
- Establish a safe traffic pattern
- Publicize a smoke-free environment for all who work at or visit the campus
- Contact radio and television stations and newspapers and ask them to report health-promotion events
- Plan immunization programs
- Provide school-based family clinics
- Use the community forum to address neighborhood alcohol availability/consumption
- Collaborate with local law enforcement to conduct a gun safety awareness program, including handgun issues

Summary

This chapter focused on health-promotion strategies that are congruent with the *Healthy People Initiative* and that can be implemented in the school setting to achieve the goal of optimum wellness for school-aged children. We have reviewed the components of health services, health education, and environmental issues. Suggestions regarding ways to incorporate groups associated with the school children, such as parents, teachers, staff, and the neighboring community, in health-promotion efforts have been outlined. Community resources specific to the school setting have been included in this chapter. Now, we hope you will have fun promoting healthy partnerships with schools.

Critical Thinking Questions

1. Bullying at school is an increasingly common problem that can affect a child's physical and psychological health. As part of your community assessment, it is important to ascertain whether the school climate hinders bullying behaviors or promotes them. Pick a school in your geographic area. Does the school have an antibullying policy? If yes, how was it formed? Explain the policy and how it is implemented.

2. Some schools have adopted a zero-tolerance policy related to bullying. What are the advantages and disadvantages (if any) of having a zero-tolerance policy against bullying in the schools? What are the pros and cons of such a policy from the school administration perspective and from the student perspective? Discuss the impact of expulsion on students, the school, the community, and society.

3. Do antibullying policies tend to curtail deviant behaviors or lump relatively minor incidents, such as name calling, in with more serious aggressive behaviors? Does such a policy tend to trivialize sexual harassment? Discuss a legal situation that involves bullying or sexual harassment in the school setting. (Consult the literature for real case scenarios.)

4. Examples of several advocacy campaigns related to clean air and the prevention of respiratory conditions are listed below. Check out the American Lung Association website (http://www.lungusa.org) for information about these campaigns. Pick one and develop an action plan for the school community. Be sure to note applicable federal regulations.

   What is the State of Your Air?

   Make 2009 the Year FDA Gets Control Over Tobacco Products

   American Lung Association Offers Parents Seven "Back to School" Tips for Kids with Asthma

   Sign the Kids with Asthma Bill of Rights

   Survey Finds that Mothers See Influenza as a Serious Health Threat, But Often Don't Get Their Families Vaccinated

5. To date, schools are not required to report student injuries to the Department of Education (Kaldahl & Blair, 2005). Frequently, injury and violence prevention programs are sporadic and limited in scope. Do you think injuries should be reported? What are the advantages and disadvantages of reporting injuries? Develop a standardized checklist that can be used for schools to inspect environmental hazards. How might such a list be customized to individual schools?

6. School violence is an increasingly distressing phenomenon. What are the warning signs that might identify a student with problems? What schoolwide steps can be implemented to address the issue of school violence?

● References

Cavendish, R. S. C. (2001). Bullying and sexual harassment in the school setting. *The Journal of School Nursing, 17*(1), 25–31.

Centers for Disease control and Prevention. Overweight and obesity. Retrieved December 4, 2009 from http://www.cdc.gov/obesity/causes/health.html

Due, P., Holstein, B., Lynch, J., Diderichsen, F., Gabhain, S., Scheidt, P., et al. (2005). Bullying and symptoms among school-aged children: International comparative cross sectional study in 28 countries. *European Journal of Public Health, 15*(2), 128–132.

Ebbeling, C. B., & Ludwig, D. S. (2008). Tracking pediatric obesity: An index of uncertainty? *Journal of the American Medical Association, 299*(20), 2442–2443.

Fredland, N. (2008). Sexual bullying: Addressing the gap between bullying and dating violence. *Advances in Nursing Science, 31*(2), 95–11.

Kaldahl, M. A., & Blair, E. H. (2005). Student injury rates in public schools. *Journal of School Health, 75*(1), 38–40.

Muller, M. J., Danielzik, S., & Pust, S. (2005). School- and family-based interventions to prevent overweight in children. *Proceedings of the Nutrition Society, 64,* 249–254.

Nansel, T. R., Overpeck, M., Pilla, R. S., Ruan, W. J., Simons-Morton, B., & Scheidt, P. (2001). Bullying behaviors among US youth: Prevalence and association with psychosocial adjustment. *Journal of the American Medical Association, 285*(16), 2094–2100.

Ogden, C. L., Carroll, M. D., & Flegal, K. M. (2008). High body mass index for age among US children and adolescents, 2003–2006. *Journal of the American Medical Association, 299*(20), 2401–2405.

Olweus, D. (1994). Annotation: Bullying at school: Basic facts and effects of a school based intervention program. *Journal of Child Psychology and Psychiatry, 53*(7), 1171–1190.

Olweus, D. (2001). Bullying at school: Tackling the problem. Research Center for Health Promotion, University of Bergen, Norway. Retrieved August 10, 2005, from http://virtual.clemson.edu/groups/ncrj/pdfs/bullying_fact_sheet2.pdf

Robinson, S. (2006). The victimization of obese adolescents. *Journal of School Nursing, 22*(4), 201–206.

Robinson, S. (2008). Treating pediatric obesity generating the evidence. *Archives of Pediatric and Adolescent Medicine, 162*(2), 1191–1192.

Thomas, S. P., & Smith, H. (2004). School connectedness, anger behaviors, and relationships of violent and nonviolent American youth. *Perspectives in Psychiatric Care, 40*(4), 135–148.

U.S. Department of Health and Human Services, Office of Disease Prevention and Health Promotion. Healthy People 2010. Retrieved August 10, 2005, from http://www.healthypeople.gov

U.S. Department of Health and Human Services. The Surgeon General's Call to Action to Prevent and Decrease Overweight and Obesity. Retrieved December 4, 2009, from http://www.surgeongeneral.gov/obesityprevention/factsheet/index.html

Wolke, D., Woods, S., Bloomfield, L., & Karstadt, L. (2001). Bullying involvement in primary school and common health problems. *Archives of Disease in Childhood, 85*(3), 197–201.

Woods, S., & White, E. (2005). The association between bullying behavior, arousal levels and behavior problems. *Journal of Adolescence, 28,* 381–395.

World Health Organization. Global strategy on diet, physical activity and health. Retrieved December 4, 2009, from http://www.who.int/dietphysicalactivity/publications/facts/obesity/en/

■ FURTHER READINGS

Journals

Journal of School Health—Official monthly journal of the American School Health Association focusing on health issues from pre-K to 12th grade.
Journal of School Nursing—Bimonthly publication
NASN School Nurse—The official clinical bimonthly publication of the National Association of School Nurses

Books and Articles

Crowley, A. A., Gains, R. M., & Pellico, L. H. (2005). A model vision and hearing screening program. *American Journal of Nursing, 105*(6), 52–55.

Felton, G., Saunders, R. P., Ward, D. S., Dishman, R. K., Dowda, M., & Pate, R. R. (2005). Promoting physical activity in girls: A case study of one school's success. *Journal of School Health, 75*(2), 57–62.

Fredland, N. (2008). Nurturing hostile environments: The problem of school violence. *Family and Community Health, 31*(1S), s32–s41.

Great Resources

Guidelines/health manuals/continuing education programs for school nurses developed by local school districts
State and local health department guidelines and laws
State associations for school nurses. Websites: access through state associations
Volunteer agencies such as the American Heart Association, American Lung Association, American Cancer Society, and American Diabetes Association.

Internet Resources can be found on the**Point** at http://thepoint.lww.com/Anderson6e.

Promoting Healthy Partnerships With Faith Communities

NINA M. FREDLAND

LEARNING OBJECTIVES

After studying this chapter, you should be able to:

1. Define a faith community.
2. Relate the goals of the *Healthy People Initiative* to the faith-based movement.
3. Discuss the roles of the nurse in promoting the health of faith communities.
4. Design and implement health-promotion programs in partnership with faith communities.
5. Identify potential sources of collaboration, funding, and resources to assist the faith community nurse in planning and implementing health programs.

Introduction

*I*n the face of the changing health care environment, congregations of worshipers are increasingly forming partnerships with nursing for health-promotion programs. This movement of nursing in faith communities is based on the principles of holistic nursing that recognize the dynamic relationship between spirituality and health of mind and body throughout the life span (Solari-Twadell, 1999). Factors such as an increasing concern for disparities in health care; access to health care and insurance coverage; dissatisfaction with the disease-focused medical model; recent emphasis on bioethics as evidenced by institutions devoted to the interface of medicine and health; and church-based 12-step and meal programs have historically contributed to the movement (Evans, 1999). Other influencing components are self-responsibility for health care, increasing autonomous roles in nursing, increasing lay ministry responsibilities in faith-based communities, and limited health care system resources. Congregational nursing, parish nursing, faith-based organizations (FBOs), and faith community nursing are descriptive terms found in the literature and apply equally to the concept of nursing in faith communities. Faith community nursing refers to "a model of care that uses nurses based within faith communities (e.g., churches, synagogues, etc.) to provide health services to the other members of those communities, including health-promotion and disease prevention programs, chronic disease management, and culturally sensitive services" (McGinnis, 2009, p. 173). For the purposes of this chapter, faith community will be used to describe the setting, and the term *faith community nurses* (FCNs) will denote nurses working in such settings. People in these faith communities are referred to as "participants."

Although faith community nursing programs have been in existence for some time, attention has focused on these types of programs as alternative methods of delivering services, through the establishment of the White House Office of Faith-Based and Community Initiatives (Executive Order 13199, 2001). Recently, the administration has called for an expansion of the Office, renaming it the White House Office of Faith-Based and Neighborhood Partnerships (Amendments to Executive Order 13199, 2009). Faith communities and secular initiatives will be eligible to apply for support from this Office. Priority areas are now focused on (1) economic recovery and easing poverty through community groups; (2) addressing issues related to women, children, and pregnant teens; (3) supporting responsible fatherhood through financially rewarding employment opportunities, and (4) fostering global interfaith communication (http://www.whitehouse.gov/the_press_office/ObamaAnnounces WhiteHouseOfficeofFaith-basedandNeighborhoodPartnerships/). Clearly, the notion of delivering health care through faith communities has been acknowledged and encouraged. The understanding that healthy people are interrelated with healthy communities has been affirmed by the Healthy People Initiative (HP).

Healthy People 2020, scheduled to be launched in 2010, expands the HP 2010 goals. These goals are consistent with the philosophy of faith community nursing. The goals are (1) to eliminate preventable disease, disability, injury, and premature death; (2) to achieve health equity, eliminate disparities, and improve the health of all groups; (3) to create social and physical environments that promote good health for all; and, (4) to promote healthy development and healthy behaviors across every stage of life (Internet site: Retrieved February 20, 2009, from http://www. healthypeople.gov/HP2020/advisory/PhaseI/summary.htm#_Toc211942896).

In sum, faith community programs fit the vision of the White House initiative and meet the objectives of the grass roots initiative of Healthy People. A community-planning guide, entitled *Healthy People in Healthy Communities* is available on the Internet at http://www.healthypeople.gov/publications/healthycommunities2001/ healthycom01hk.pdf. Use the leading health indicators (Box 17.1) as a model for planning health programs.

BOX 17.1

HEALTHY PEOPLE LEADING HEALTH INDICATORS

Physical activity
Overweight and obesity
Tobacco use
Substance abuse
Responsible sexual behavior
Mental health
Injury and violence
Environmental quality
Immunizations
Access to health care

(Available: http://www.healthypeople.gov/LHI/lhiwhat.htm)

INITIATING HEALTHY PARTNERSHIPS WITH FAITH COMMUNITIES

The role of the nurse with faith communities is dictated as always by the needs of the people and includes, but is not limited to, health educator, health counselor, referral agent, advocate, facilitator, and liaison between the dimensions of spirituality and health (Watts, 2007). Frequently, FCNs are licensed professional nurses, with varied educational backgrounds and areas of expertise, who share their nursing skills as a means to give something back to their community of spiritual support. Frequently, the professional nurses donate their time and expertise as well as their own equipment (e.g., stethoscopes or sphygmomanometers). In some settings, however, the faith community may employ the nurses. Some are advanced practice nurses specializing in critical care, trauma, or ambulatory care, or are nurse practitioners with adult and family certification. Some are professional nurses in home health rehabilitation, nursing homes, and acute care. Other volunteers are retired professional nurses. This group of FCNs is rich with varied experiences. As the nursing workforce ages along with the baby boomer generation creative ways to maintain an adequate cadre of nurses to meet the health needs of the population are needed. It will be important to restructure health care delivery by innovative opportunities to keep the most experienced nurses in the workforce (McGinnis, 2009). Older nurses are likely to want or need more flexibility in their schedules and work situations that are less physically demanding. Faith communities are ideal settings to gain from the vast experiences of this group of nurses, who may be able to contribute in new and important ways.

From the very beginning, faith community nursing has embodied the holistic approach to health care with an understanding of the dynamic relationship of human needs (physical, psychological, spiritual, emotional, social, and economic) to a person's health (Solari-Twadell, 1999). Nurses in faith communities are recognized members of the ministerial team. Home health care and invasive treatment procedures are usually not in this nursing practice; however, these procedures could be included should the faith community and the nurse so agree. Nursing within faith communities is not intended to compete with public or private health service organizations. Rather, faith community programs are ways to increase access to the health care system and reduce health care costs for individuals and society in general.

Research has documented that health care costs may rise more from delayed access to care rather than overuse or misuse of the health care system by the worried well (Rydholm, 2006). FCNs can intervene by encouraging participants in faith communities to seek care earlier. Infected wounds, confusion related to medications, allergic reactions, shortness of breath, ignoring dental decay, and urinary tract infections are just a few examples of instances where conditions could deteriorate and end up costing much more to resolve. FCNs through health counseling/education, advocacy for the vulnerable, referrals, brokering for services, and providing resources can prevent the exacerbation of many conditions.

If nursing with FBOs is based on a model such as the community nursing assessment, intervention, and evaluation model presented in this textbook, then the continuous growth and evaluation of programs are ensured. Assessments (monthly screenings), annual surveys, and analysis of the components of participants' needs dictate what intervention programs need to be implemented (e.g., healthy eating classes, exercise classes, walking clubs, or diabetes management instruction). These programs are implemented in a timely fashion that is most supportive of the participants. Evaluations of the programs lead us to expand or to minimize programs, depending on their effectiveness. Effectiveness is measured by the number of

BOX 17.2

TOOL FOR ASSESSING EDUCATIONAL NEEDS OF FAITH COMMUNITIES

Anonymous Demographic Data: Include age group, sex, language preference
Program Timing Preferences: Time of day, day of week, time of year
Topics faith community members are interested in:

- CPR Skills
- Cancer Prevention
- Cardiovascular Risk Factors
- Community Safety
- Diabetes Education
- Domestic Violence
- End-of-Life Issues
- Exercise
- First Aid
- HIV+ Information

- Navigating Managed Care
- Nutrition for Youngsters
- Parenting and Child Care Issues
- Retirement Issues
- Screening Programs
- Sexuality
- Stress Management
- Warning Signs: Stroke/Heart Attack
- Weight Management
- Other

participants in the individual programs, as well as individual goal accomplishment and overall satisfaction with the health outcomes (e.g., weight loss, increased feelings of fitness, decreased fatigue, better perceived control of stress with lowered blood pressure, and actual control and direction of one's lifestyle choices).

The following are some strategies for identifying faith community needs:

- Distribute an educational needs survey to various groups within the faith community, such as the women's auxiliary, the young mothers' support group, the young adult group, the elder group, the men's organization, and the non-English-speaking community. A helpful tool appears in Box 17.2.
- Attend meetings for the different groups.
- Form focus groups to discuss options to increase health or join an initiative already in progress, such as prayer groups or faith renewal groups.
- Provide a suggestion box.
- Form an ad hoc committee to study the health ministry and include key people such as clergy, lay ministers, school principal, social and health agency personnel, and so forth. Be sure that both formal and informal leaders are included.
- Remember to only make decisions with input from the faith community.

The educational needs survey in Box 17.2 could be distributed at worship meetings to maximize the number of people reached. Of course, the survey should be available in all appropriate languages. It is helpful to have pencils available so that surveys can be completed and collected at this time. After the information has been gathered and synthesized, concerns and topics are prioritized. If an English version and non-English version are used, respective priorities are noted.

HEALTH–PROMOTION PROGRAMS FOR FAITH COMMUNITIES

After assessing the community's educational preferences, the nurse plans intervention programs based on the results. Here is a list of classes that may be of interest to faith community members:

- Exercise group
- Nutrition classes

- Cardiopulmonary resuscitation (CPR) and emergency cardiovascular care
- Positive parenting
- AIDS/HIV information sessions
- Planning for a healthy retirement
- Immunization program
- Health fair
- Stress-reduction and coping strategies
- Emergency preparedness

Walking Programs

If the community is interested in an exercise group, suggest a walking map. A walking map is a self-directed exercise tool that is popular particularly with the elderly. These maps have mileage-marked routes in each neighborhood. Many participants may be trying to begin an exercise program but do not know where to begin. Such maps can be helpful in starting and continuing a daily exercise program that contributes to the feeling of good health and, more important, can prevent or control high blood pressure. Physical activity is important to maintain physical and psychological health. In addition to the effects on blood pressure, it is associated with reducing the risks of developing diabetes, colon cancer, and even dying from cardiovascular disease. To construct a walking map, follow the instructions outlined in Box 17.3.

Nutrition Programs

The Healthy Heart Club combines nutrition and education in a monthly gathering at lunchtime. This nursing action can be geared to adults, teens, or children. It is designed to teach the basics of eating a balanced diet, how to shop wisely for healthy food, and how to make good choices in restaurants. This is a good opportunity to introduce the new, reengineered food guidance system, MyPyramid. In an attempt to address the national problem of overweight and obesity, the U.S. Department of Agriculture (USDA) developed *The 2005 Dietary Guidelines for Americans*. These guidelines individualize the approach to healthy eating, incorporate physical activity

BOX 17.3

INSTRUCTIONS FOR CREATING A WALKING MAP

- Design a 1-mile map around the worship center.
- Extend the map to include shopping malls, a recreational park, or neighborhood school yards.
- Make sure the area is safe and accessible.
- Indicate 1/4-mile markers, such as a retail store, a "no parking" sign, a mailbox, and so forth.
- Provide an opportunity for participants to learn how to do warm-up and cool-down exercises.
- Teach target heart rates and how to monitor pulses.
- Provide a mechanism for people to meet and become walking buddies, such as a kickoff party, convening at the worship center, or meeting at a nearby mall.
- Provide for ongoing encouragement and follow-up.

BOX 17.4

HEALTHY HEART CLUB ACTIVITIES

- Gather in the faith community center at a convenient time once a month.
- See if a faith community member who is a dietitian is available; this tends to attract people to the session.
- Identify content to be explored, such as healthy food recognition and preparation, economic purchases, eating out, and celebrating with healthy food choices.
- Assist class in personalizing their healthy eating and activity plan using the http://www.MyPyramid.gov website technology.
- Include cooking demonstrations with healthy nonalcoholic drink or smoothie recipes that can be made in a blender and then sampled by participants.
- Initiate recipe sharing that includes multicultural traditions; this is always popular for the young and old alike.
- Offer tips on how to maintain favorite tastes in family recipes and still eat healthy (e.g., substitution of 1% milk for full cream milk, egg substitute for eggs, or oil for lard).
- Schedule field trips to ethnic restaurants and grocers.

into the guidelines, and use interactive technology. This simple concept can be personalized by visiting the website http://mypyramid.gov/. Many tips and resources are available through this Internet link. Box 17.4 offers a plan for Healthy Heart Club activities.

This heart-healthy eating idea can be expanded to include children. Try starting a "Healthy Tots" or "Kids' Club" focusing on healthy food choices for healthy kids. How about serving chicken or tuna salad in an ice cream cone? Toss a banana, a peach (without the pit), some orange juice, and plain yogurt in a blender. Serve it over crushed ice. Challenge the children to come up with their own healthy, fruity concoction. Finally, celebrate with a heart-healthy party. Box 17.5 shows a healthy lifestyle program for children that reinforces the notion that healthy choices can be incorporated into celebrations. (Tip: MyPyramid can be personalized for anyone over age 2.)

BOX 17.5

PEAR AND APPLE PARTY TIME ACTIVITY FOR KIDS

- Pick a time when children are assembled (perhaps after the worship service).
- Equipment you will need: pears, apples, toothpicks, little plates, napkins, a chalkboard (for tallying votes), cutting board, and knife.
- Have a variety of apples on hand (Red Delicious, Jonathan, McIntosh, Granny Smith, Golden Delicious).
- Have a variety of pears on hand (Anjou, Bosc, Comice).
- Cut the apples and pears into cubes.
- Have children taste each kind.
- Take a vote on what kind of apple and pear they liked most.
- Tally the votes on a scoreboard.
- Decorate the apple and pear with the most votes.
- Take a picture of everyone (and the pears and apples, of course).
- Celebrate and enjoy!

Emergency First Aid Programs

CPR training and emergency cardiovascular care classes are other healthy lifestyle primary prevention activities. The American Heart Association (AHA) offers these related classes: CPR for Friends and Family, Heartsaver First Aid, CPR, and Heartsaver Automatic External Defibrillator (AED). Many public facilities now have an AED in a prominent area. Faith communities should consider purchasing an AED. A fundraiser can be dedicated for the purchase of an AED, or a local business may want to donate one.

The AHA (2001) strongly encourages businesses and organizations to install these units in their facilities and train a cadre of responders in both CPR and the use of AEDs. Together these strategies can significantly reduce death from sudden cardiac arrest. Each year, 310,000 people die out-of-hospital and in emergency departments from unexpected cardiac deaths (http://www.americanheart.org/downloadable/heart/1200082005246HS_Stats%202008.final.pdf). Of these deaths 60% are treated by emergency responders (EMS), but only 27.4% receive bystander CPR, and only 2% receive defibrillation by a lay person. Because emergency medical personnel are not always able to respond immediately, public access to defibrillators (PAD) potentially could save many more lives. The AHA has a guide to help establish PAD programs. FBOs are a logical place to conduct community training programs. Instructions on how to establish a PAD program can be found on the AHA website at http://www.americanheart.org/downloadable/heartsmart/10957146338164Cpadoverview.pdf. The FCN can implement a program related to heart disease. Most often you can arrange for an instructor to come to the faith community if enough participants are interested, or participants can find a nearby class through the AHA website. This instruction is usually highly valued and can be an annual event. Because CPR for community groups is an awareness session instead of a certification program, it is less difficult to conduct. However, it still provides people with valuable information and skills should they be faced with a life-threatening situation. Attendees gain confidence in their ability to recognize warning signs and initiate life-saving measures that perhaps can save loved ones. This training can include children over age 10 and teens as well. Check out the website at http://www.americanheart.org.

Health Fairs

If a faith community undertakes the project of a health fair, timing is very important. One theory is that it should have its own special time of year; another view is that it can coincide with an annual bazaar or fundraiser. Because the community usually supports the annual fundraiser, a captive audience is present. On the other hand, sometimes people would rather take health more seriously and not try to focus on fun and games and screening or health-education activities at the same time. Also, if immunizations are provided, sometimes this is an unpleasant association for children who set out for a fun time. Both situations can work with proper planning and marketing, depending on the commitment and support of the faith community. Box 17.6 lists steps to consider when setting up a health fair. This outline is not meant to be exhaustive but to provide ideas and some direction. Although the faith community is a church, synagogue, mosque, or temple, it is important to include the greater community in its health ministry. A health fair is a wonderful opportunity to open the boundaries of the faith community.

BOX 17.6

Organizing a Health Fair for a Faith Community

- Contact the clergy and lay council.
- Set the date (try to allow at least 6 to 8 weeks to prepare).
- Decide what health-promotion areas to cover, depending on the audience (adults only, families, elders).
- Invite identified organizations to participate.
- Invite health care providers, health service vendors, and community resources from the geographic area.
- Solicit prizes from local merchants.
- Offer incentives for attendance, such as door prizes and coupons for free services (e.g., mammograms, heart scans).
- Collaborate with other professionals, such as a dental school, pharmacy school, or optometrist.
- Offer free immunizations.
- Have a women's health booth, a men's health booth, a teen's health booth, and a children's health booth.
- Include screening stations, such as vision, hearing, blood glucose, blood pressure, lead, tuberculosis skin testing, depression, HIV testing, and counseling.
- Have a plan for referral and follow-up.
- It may be a good idea to have an HIV-positive ministry booth providing information about HIV, as well as providers from treatment centers.
- Have stations that focus on environmental health, including booths on mosquito control and water safety. People from rural areas can bring in water samples for testing.
- A home safety booth sponsored by the utility company and/or fire department can address indoor air quality, electrical hazards, and gas appliances.
- A Crime Watch booth sponsored by the police can address self-defense and home security.
- Set up computers for health risk appraisal programs.
- Assign booth areas considering flow pattern. Provide for privacy if breast self-examination is demonstrated or skin cancer checks are done.
- Invite the media.
- Include fun activities, such as craft booths for the children and adults.

Tip: Visit the Family and Consumer Services website for a Health Fair Planning Guide that offers national resources for health fairs at http://fcs.tamu.edu/health/health_fair_planning_guide/national_resources.php.

Additional Programming Considerations

Additional health-promotion strategies for faith communities include:

- Blood pressure screening
- Glucose screening
- Vision and glaucoma testing
- Bereavement program
- Weight-management programs—how about "Weigh to go!" for a title?
- Smoking cessation programs
- Diabetic education classes
- Caregiver support groups
- Asthmatic support group
- Respite care programs

Involving nursing volunteers from the community ensures that the multicultural diversity of the community can be mirrored in the nursing team. The problem of language is thereby mitigated by the volunteers, who speak the same language as the participants. Cultural practices that contribute to healthy lifestyle (e.g., Vietnamese and Chinese cultures' heavy use of vegetables in the diet) are emphasized at social and educational activities. Importance is placed on cultural recognition and adaptation of health-supporting behaviors.

Economic factors as well as cultural factors are essential concerns of problem identification and solution. The faith community is a microcosm of the larger economic pattern of the city. Services should be accessible to all members of the faith community as appropriate. The affluence of the community will affect the type of programs that can be implemented. It is an accepted fact that families with more discretionary income are more able to engage in health-promotion activities. This fact will impact the overall health of the community. Economics also influences how members of the community access health services. The faith community for an increasing number of participants may be the only consistent source of health care.

ESTABLISHING A LASTING PARTNERSHIP WITH FAITH COMMUNITIES

Now that background information and program strategies have been explored, let us focus on the essential elements of establishing a nursing partnership with an FBO. Building a healthy community will take time, careful planning, and a great deal of organization. The Healthy People Initiative suggests a formula for this process, MAP-IT (Internet site: http://www.healthypeople.gov/Publications/HealthyCommunities2001/healthycom01hk.pdf). MAP-IT stands for Mobilize, Assess, Plan, Implement, and Track (Box 17.7). These are essential

BOX 17.7

MAP-IT STRATEGY FOR CREATING A HEALTHY COMMUNITY

MOBILIZE	individuals that care about the faith community's health into a coalition.
ASSESS	the areas of greatest need in your community, and the resources and strengths you can tap into to address those areas of need.
PLAN	your approach: Start with a vision of where you want to be as a community; then add strategies and action steps to help you achieve that vision.
IMPLEMENT	your plan using concrete action steps that can be monitored and will make a difference.
TRACK	your progress over time.

Healthy People in Healthy Communities. A Community Planning Guide Using Healthy People 2010. Office of Disease Prevention and Health Promotion. Office of Public Health and Science. US Department of Health and Human Services. Available at: http://www.healthypeople.gov/Publications/HealthyCommunities2001/default.htm

components the nurse working with a faith community should follow. Here are some suggestions:

- Obtain support from the clergy and administration.
- Identify a core of health professionals willing to participate. Ideally, they will be participants in the faith community.
- Establish a marketing system.
- Find a school of nursing or a community college to assist you in developing the ministry.
- Identify sponsor support through faith community members and neighborhood establishments. (Local businesses are usually supportive because they recognize that their clients are of the faith community.)
- Acquire supplies, such as cotton swabs, rubber gloves, stethoscopes, blood pressure cuffs, glucose meters, and so forth, from various sources.
- Recruit additional volunteer health professionals to participate.
- Have a team meeting and plan nursing actions. Probably the first action would be to conduct a needs assessment. Be sure it is conducted in languages that reflect the constituency.

It is acceptable to start small or to have volunteers who are only able to give a little time. The nature of the ministry is that it builds on itself as time and community needs dictate. A successful marketing strategy is critical to starting and maintaining an active program. Several approaches can be implemented. Depending on resources and community contacts, some approaches may be more feasible than others. Local newspapers, radio and television spots, and civic association bulletins are possibilities. Posting on the faith community marquee or other community billboards is usually a very effective way of notifying the community about activities. Another effective strategy is pulpit announcements during or immediately after regularly scheduled services. Surveys completed at this time usually yield excellent response. A nurse column in the faith community's weekly bulletin announcing scheduled health-screening activities and health-education programs can be a regular feature. Catchy names such as "Positively Healthy Choices," "Nurse's Notes," or "Here's to Healthy Choices" will focus attention on the health information, which should be published in all languages commonly spoken. Remember to partner with nearby or affiliated schools, community stores, and fast-food restaurants. Ask to market the faith community "nursing news" and events in their flyers and newsletters and on their marquees.

Partnerships between faith communities and schools of nursing though challenging can be mutually beneficial (Otterness, Gehrke, & Sener, 2007). FCNs should consult with nursing faculty at area community colleges or universities to assist with establishing health-promotion programs and health services. Faculty members may be willing to assist with the writing of a needs assessment survey. Then, the faith community can be assessed annually with a tool, an invaluable part of the process. Graduate student nurses can be lead players in the community assessment. They can work with lay members of the faith community and guide the actual assessment. Student help would be a tremendous asset to the FCNs because, most often, they are volunteering and such needs assessments can be very time consuming. Reciprocally, the students would have an opportunity to gain cultural awareness and competence and hone critical thinking and communications skills, while participating in a valuable and realistic clinical experience. Another benefit to colleges is the opportunity for sharing research data. Government funding sources are available to pilot projects that address health and social issues. Partnerships between university academics and faith communities should explore such funding opportunities.

Health care provider systems (hospitals, HMOs, PPOs) have come to realize the importance of collaborating with faith community health programs as a valuable model. Frequently, faith communities will sign agreements of support with health-management systems such as hospitals, private clinics, or group medical practices. The collaborator may be a local public health department who partners with the faith community. Activities may include sharing information among health care professionals, disseminating information to the community at large, setting community health goals, sponsoring community health activities, conducting community assessments, coordinating and delivering direct services to community clients, and implementing specific state health agendas (Zahner & Corrado, 2004). The collaborating health care system can be a referral option for faith community participants. Fast-food restaurants, retail shops, businesses, colleges and universities, as well as civic and public service organizations (e.g., Lions Clubs, women's organizations, League of Women Voters), as well as national and local foundations, such as the March of Dimes, may be receptive to being a sponsor, thus providing needed money for supplies, brochures, and other essential items. Because space on faith community property is usually limited, the program is totally portable. Many volunteers bring their own equipment (e.g., stethoscopes and sphygmomanometers). Representatives from drug companies and medical supply companies who are members of the faith community may supply the program with other needed equipment.

An example of how important this program is concerns a "healthy-feeling" parishioner who, because of his spouse's urging, had his blood pressure and glucose checked. The results were abnormal for age and gender. He was given the written test results, counseled, and referred to a health provider of his choice. A month later, the spouse reported that her husband was recuperating splendidly from coronary bypass surgery and learning to manage his newly diagnosed diabetes.

Registered nurses, who are the diabetic management experts, and the nurse practitioners, with the support of the sponsor agent, can be the usual blood glucose screeners. Participants feel comforted and assured when their screening data are within normal range. The participants who regulate their Type 2 diabetes without monitoring at home, usually because of limited income, can use the screening program for self-management evaluation and further education.

Classes that are age or content specific are popular and well attended. For example, a nurse with a background in men's health issues can speak to the men's organization. A male nurse can make a particular contribution speaking to the group about testicular self-examination, prostate and colon cancer, and penile erection issues. Nurses also have an opportunity to discuss domestic violence and abuse. Presentations focus on defining abusive situations, identifying community resources available to victims and perpetrators of abuse, and especially teaching skills for relationships without violence. A special meeting of teen or youth groups should address the subject of dating violence.

A goal should be to establish the faith community nursing program as a valuable ministry. Visibility is key to gaining rapport with participants and credibility for health programs. FCNs should seek opportunities to support other ministries of the faith community in diverse ways such as assisting with emergencies at services, providing health coverage during retreats or scout outings, organizing back-to-school immunization programs, creating multilanguage health literature displays, and offering to speak at meetings.

Role of Faith Communities during Extraordinary Circumstances

Churches, synagogues, and other places of worship have historically been recognized as focal points of care during natural disasters, large-scale accidents, and terrorist attacks. A faith community with a nurse ministry system in place could provide immediate holistic care and quickly coordinate services with federal agencies. Since the tragedy of September 11th, 2001, our nation realizes how important it is to have extensive community-based emergency plans in place. Faith communities can be part of the short- and long-term plans to deliver health services to communities suffering from injuries and traumatic stress. Community Education Response Teams (CERT) work with professional responders should a disaster occur. Check out the CERT website to find out more about how to organize a CERT team at https://www.citizencorps.gov/cert/index.shtm.

Closing the Gap on Health Disparities

Faith communities are ideal places to deliver health services to minority populations and thus contribute to closing the gap between majority and minority populations in relation to health disparities. For a variety of reasons, minority groups often fall through the cracks when it comes to health care. These same groups are often socially connected through a faith community. By valuing the environmental context, participants who worship together and share common interests and beliefs are more likely to accept behaviors that enhance physical and mental health (Drayton-Brooks & White, 2004.)

AN EMERGING MODEL

Nursing in faith communities has made great strides in recent years; yet it is still in the development phase. It has an enormous potential to grow and evolve into an enhanced health care delivery system especially in this era of economic uncertainty, high unemployment rates, and limited health care resources. Nurses are singularly well equipped to use their multifaceted skills and their extensive body of knowledge to improve the health status of individuals, families, and communities in a changing health care arena.

Through the expansion of the nurse role—specifically the nurse practitioner role—more services can be brought to the faith community. Faith community nursing can be expanded to include primary care services across the life span. Annual faith community surveys can expand to the wider neighborhood. Nursing students can assist with this activity. Analyzing databases to identify community assets as well as problem focuses will provide important information for prioritizing programs.

One of the most crucial steps will be acquiring physical space for the nurse ministry to provide services. Clergy and administrative personnel, who are supportive of the program and eager for it to advance, will see this as a necessity. If renovation plans are under way, space for the nurse ministry should be incorporated. Although the program can be entirely mobile, it is more practical to have a designated space for storage and to render services. To maintain focus, ensure quality, and preserve the volunteer and multicultural components of the faith community, both short- and long-term goals are required. Identify a variety of health-promotion strategies and health-education needs to be addressed in the future. Then set realistic, short-term goals that focus on the specific areas identified, such as enhancing diabetic education, restructuring the weight-management classes, or offering stress-reduction methods (e.g., aromatherapy, realistic relaxation techniques, caregiver support). Because members of the team are often managing careers, professional commitments, and family and personal responsibilities, limiting the focus at the beginning stage of development is the best strategy to ensure continued success of the program.

An important aspect to working with faith communities is related to the delivery of culturally competent care. Cultural competence is very important in terms of religious beliefs. It is likely that the FCNs will be of the same faith as participants. However, public health nurses may be employed by a collaborating sponsor such as a public health department and may not share the same religious beliefs. Therefore, nurses working with faith communities should educate themselves in the values and beliefs of the members of the faith community. They should also recognize that there are often a number of variations within each faith.

Summary

Partnerships between local health departments and FBOs potentially can do much to deliver services and reduce health disparities experienced by vulnerable groups (Zahner & Corrado, 2004). More exploration is needed to determine how these collaborations can work best. Information is emerging related to the cost-effectiveness of such partnerships. This type of articulation between health departments and faith communities should be explored and developed further. Public health nurses and other providers should pursue this opportunity.

The practice model of nursing partnerships with faith communities described in this chapter is still evolving. Nurses need to be proactive in this era of continuous health care reform. We must participate in and help shape future decision making for health care delivery. This nurse ministry, whether volunteer or reimbursed service, is a cost-effective enhancement of health care delivery systems. Nursing partnerships with faith communities are part of the solution.

Critical Thinking Questions

1. Several members of the faith community have come to you to voice concerns and frustrations associated with balancing care-giving duties for elderly family members and maintaining their own family integrity. Often, these responsibilities are overwhelming and impact the woman in the family to the greatest extent. As the FCN, you decide to create a support system for this group.

    a. How would you begin to address the concerns of the faith community members? What methods could you use to identify specific issues? What strategies could be implemented to educate, support, and alleviate some of the extra burden care giving creates? How would you advocate to make needed services available through the faith community? Who should be included in the planning and decision-making phases?

    b. Visit the Internet and identify sources available to address this issue. How would you incorporate this information in your plan?

2. Faith communities have belief systems that may reflect commonalities as well as differences. It is important to consider how different processes influence health outcomes. Pick two faith communities and explain how their belief system may affect their health choices, including access to care. What specific methods would you use to identify concerns?

3. Several residents from the retirement home within the geographic area of your faith community have learned about PAD (public access to defibrillator) programs. They are interested in obtaining an AED (automated external

defibrillator) for the premises. Make a case for implementing such a program at the retirement home. How would you go about gaining approval? What requirements would be necessary? Plan an educational approach for implementation of the unit.

● REFERENCES

Amendments to Executive Order 13199 and Establishment of the President's Advisory Council for Faith-Based and Neighborhood Partnerships retrieved February 20, 2009 from http://www.whitehouse.gov/the_press_office/ObamaAnnouncesWhiteHouseOfficeofFaith-basedandNeighborhoodPartnerships/

American Heart Association (2001). The case for Public Access Defibrillation (PAD Programs). Retrieved February 20, 2009 from http://www.americanheart.org/downloadable/heartsmart/10957141855334Apadcase.pdf

Drayton-Brooks, S., & White, N. (2004). Health promoting behaviors among African American women with faith-based support. *The ABNF Journal*, September/October, 84–90.

Evans, A. R. (1999). *The healing church: Practical programs for health ministries*. Cleveland, OH: United Church Press.

Executive Order 13199 (2001). Establishment of the white house office of faith-based and community initiatives. *Federal Register*, 66, 84599.

McGinnis, S. L. (2009). The emerging role of faith community nurses in prevention and management of chronic disease. *Policy, Politics, & Nursing Practice*, 9, 173–180.

Otterness, N., Gehrke, P., & Sener, I. M. (2007). Partnerships between nursing education and faith communities: Benefits and challenges. *Journal of Nursing Education*, 46(1), 39–44.

Rydholm, L. (2006). Wanda Alexander builds bridges to better care. *Creative Nursing*, 12(2), 10–12.

Solari-Twadell, P. (1999). The emerging practice of parish nursing. In P. Solari-Twadell & M. McDermott (Eds.), *Parish nursing: Promoting whole person health within faith communities* (pp. 3–24). Thousand Oaks, CA: Sage.

U.S. Department of Health and Human Services and Department of Agriculture. Dietary Guidelines for Americans, 2005. Retrieved December 5, 2009 from http://www.health.gov/dietaryguidelines

U.S. Department of Health and Human Services, Office of Disease Prevention and Health Promotion. (2001). Healthy People in Healthy Communities. A Community Planning Guide Using HealthyPeople 2010. Retrieved February 20, 2009 from http://www.healthypeople.gov/Publications/HealthyCommunities2001/default.htm

Watts, J.M. (2007). Faith Community Nursing. *Virginia Nurses Today*, 15(1), 11.

Zahner, S. J., & Corrado, S. M. (2004). Local health department partnerships with faith-based organizations. *Journal of Public Health Management*, 10(3), 258–265.

■ FURTHER READINGS

American Nurses Association (2005). *Faith community nursing: Scope and standards of practice*. Silver Spring, MD: ANA.

Fowler, M. (2008). *Guide to the code of ethics for nurses: Interpretation and application*. Silver Spring, MD: ANA.

Smucker, C. J., & Weinberg, L. *Faith community nursing: Developing a quality practice*. Silver Spring, MD: ANA.

Journals

Creative Nursing Journal, quarterly; based on values, issues, experiences, and collaboration, nurses are encouraged to think creatively and take risks

Journal of Holistic Nursing, quarterly; integrates holistic health concepts of body, mind, emotions and spirit within the context of a changing environment

International Journal for Human Caring; published three times a year and focuses on the knowledge of care and care giving within the discipline of nursing and in collaboration with other disciplines

Internet Resources can be found on the**Point** at http://thepoint.lww.com/Anderson6e.

Promoting Healthy Partnerships With Marginalized Groups

NINA M. FREDLAND

LEARNING OBJECTIVES

After studying this chapter, you should be able to:

1. Discuss what it means for a group to be "marginalized," "vulnerable," or "disadvantaged."
2. Identify groups that society has marginalized.
3. Discuss commonalities of marginalized groups.
4. Discuss barriers to health care specific to marginalized groups.
5. Adapt a program for a vulnerable or marginalized population, such as the homeless, migrants, or persons with chronic disabilities.

Introduction

*N*urses throughout history and in modern times have been concerned about "vulnerable populations" (Nyamathi, Koniak-Griffin, & Greengold, 2007). Public health nurses particularly are committed to remain focused on the health needs of populations who, for various reasons, have been relegated to the margins of society. These groups may be impoverished, discriminated against, or functionally impaired in some way.

The word *marginalize* means to treat someone or something as if he or she is of no consequence or is unimportant. Marginalization conveys a process in which individuals in certain groups seem not to matter or to be of little concern to the rest of society, thus falling beyond the margins (Vasas, 2005). To marginalize or be marginalized may be more accurate terminology than the concept of vulnerability, which may imply a degree of "blaming the victim." "Vulnerable" stems from the Latin word *vulnare*, which means "to wound." This terminology implies that the wounded or the "less than perfect" are not particularly valued and easily marginalized. By using the terminology of marginalization instead, the emphasis is societal.

Flaskerud and Winslow define vulnerable populations as "social groups who experience limited resources and consequent high relative risk for morbidity and premature mortality" (Flaskerud & Winslow, 1998, p. 69). Vulnerable groups in a review of five decades of nursing research included people of color; the poor; and those individuals marginalized by sexual preference, immigrant/refugee status, and religious beliefs (Flaskerud et al., 2002). The National Institute for Nursing Research (NINR), in keeping with national and international recognition that health is negatively affected by factors of race, ethnicity, gender, economic disadvantage, geography, and culture, has adopted a strategic plan focused on reducing health disparities. NINR supports research designed to increase understanding of the determinants of health disparities and culturally appropriate strategies and interventions to reduce and eliminate health disparities in underserved and vulnerable populations (NINR, 2006). Health disparities seem to disproportionally affect ethnic minority populations to a greater degree than nonethnic minority populations, especially in conjunction with economic disadvantage. African Americans and Hispanics in the United States frequently experience worse health than the majority white populace (Stone, 2002). In addition, poor whites have below-average health. Vulnerable groups, including minorities, women, children, and those with disabilities, are more susceptible to infectious diseases, especially HIV/AIDS and sexually transmitted infections (STIs) (Peragallo & Gonzalez, 2007). The World Health Organization (WHO, 2008) in its latest report advocates making health disparities more visible so that any given society can create objectives and mobilize resources for change. Although progress has been made in some nations, others are falling behind. Therefore, focusing on the health disparities, rather than on ethnicity, is a more productive approach. National agendas, therefore, should have action plans to identify and monitor health disparities among all groups and increase awareness when these inequities exist in marginalized or vulnerable groups. The U.S. government addressed health disparities by establishing the Healthy People Initiative, the Office of Minority Health, and the National Institutes of Health's National Center on Minority Health and Health Disparities (Stone, 2002). An overarching goal for HP 2020, scheduled to be launched in 2010, directly applies to the issue of health disparity. The goal is "to achieve health equity, eliminate disparities, and improve the health of all groups" (US Department of Health and Human Services (HHS), Phase I Report, 2008).

WHO ARE THE MARGINALIZED?

Individuals or groups who live on the fringes or margins of society lack key resources and are most often underserved or not served at all, particularly in health care systems. Included among marginalized groups are the homeless, immigrants, migrants, and those with chronic disabilities. Furthermore, gender, ethnicity or race, education or income, geographic location, or sexual preference may account for group differences that lead to marginalization and subsequent health inequities (Healthy People, 2010, 2000). The comprehensive report by the Institute of Medicine (2002) in its review of more than 100 studies found that minorities were less likely to obtain health care than were whites. The review also documented inequities related to cancer, heart disease, diabetes, HIV/AIDS, and mental illness.

Persons With Disabilities

The American Disabilities Act (ADA) Public Law 101-336 enacted July 26, 1990, by the 101st Congress ensures that persons with disabilities are not discriminated against in employment opportunities and public services, including public accommodations, recreation, and transportation. The ADA Amendments Act of 2008, effective January 1, 2009, ascribes to the basic ADA definition: "an impairment that substantially limits one or more major life activities, a record of such impairment, or being regarded as having such impairment" (The U.S. Equal Employment

Opportunity Commission, ADA amendment, 2009). However, the amendment revises the regulations defining "substantially limits" and amends the definition of the term "disability" by expanding the list of activities specifically identified, such as walking. For example, reading, bending, and communicating are now identified. Bodily functions (immune system, bowel/bladder, etc.) are now also identified as potential disabilities. The notion is that the definition of disability should be interpreted in a broad sense. (See the Internet site for a full report of these important changes at http://www.eeoc.gov/ada/amendments_notice.html.)

Nurses should assess for disability because it may not always be obvious. Two simple questions can begin the conversation: (1) Are you limited in any way in activities because of physical, mental, or emotional problems? (2) Do you now have any health problem that requires you to use special equipment, such as a cane, a wheelchair, a special bed, or a special telephone? (CDC, Disability and Health, 2006).

The ADA home page provides information and technical assistance related to the provision and spirit of the law at http://www.ada.gov/. Another useful resource is the ADA information line 800-514-0301 (voice) or 800-514-0383 (TTY). The Department of Justice (DOJ), Civil Rights Division, Disability Section ensures that all persons with disabilities have equal opportunity through implementation of the ADA (http://www.usdoj.gov/crt/drs/drshome.htm). The DOJ website maintains information related to legal assistance and offers a *Guide to Disabilities Rights and Laws*.

Because the definition of disability is evolving, it is difficult to report the prevalence of persons with disabilities in general. It depends on how the data are collected and for what purpose. For example, the limitation may relate to a sensory, physical, mental, self-care, or a work disability. The National Center for Health Statistics (NCHS) reports that 34.4 million (11.8%) of noninstitutionalized individuals have a limitation in usual activities due to a chronic condition (http://www.cdc.gov/nchs/fastats/disable.htm). For specific disability information, the reader is directed to the U.S. Census Bureau disability main page at http://www.census.gov/hhes/www/disability/disability.html.

Homelessness

Individuals who make up the U.S. homeless population are among the most marginalized and vulnerable to disabilities and disease, and represent up to 10% of all individuals living in poverty (National Coalition for the Homeless, 2009c).

The economic crisis, foreclosures, the collapse of the housing market, job shortages, and devastating natural events have affected individuals who are homeless and those at-risk for homelessness despite efforts over the last decade to end homelessness (National Coalition for the Homeless, 2009b). Affordable housing, defined as housing that costs no more than 30% of income, exceeds the means of many families, rendering them at-risk of becoming homeless (Cunningham, 2009).

According to the Stewart B. McKinney Act, 42 USC 11301, et seq. (National Coalition for the Homeless, 2009a), the definition of a homeless person is one who "lacks a fixed, regular, and adequate night-time residence." Those people whose primary night residence is a supervised temporary shelter, an institution that provides temporary shelter for those intended to be institutionalized, or a public place not intended for sleeping would be considered homeless under the McKinney Act, 42 USC 11302. Homeless people who live in shelters, abandoned buildings, or other public areas are considered literally homeless. The McKinney definition is consistent with the literally homeless view including those people who face imminent eviction (i.e., within 1 week). Marginally homeless people live doubled up in places they do not own or rent and consider their situation to be temporary. These people may be an illness, an accident, or a paycheck away from eviction and usually depend on utility assistance. When hospitalized, they often have no place to go after discharge.

It is extremely difficult to assess accurately the prevalence of homelessness in the United States at any given point in time. Between 2.3 and 3.5 million people are estimated to experience homelessness annually (National Coalition for the Homeless, 2009c) including over 1.35 million children from 600,000 families (Institute for Children in Poverty, National Data on Family Homelessness, 2008). Some individuals are not counted because they may be doubled up in temporary housing, living in cars, abandoned buildings, and on the street). Two alarming trends are that homeless youth and young adults seem to be homeless longer, and elders who have had relatively stable housing over their life span are now finding themselves homeless (Cunningham, 2009). Twenty-three percent of the homeless are over 50 years old. Single individuals continue to be the largest group of homeless, comprising 76% of the national homeless population (67.5% male) (U.S. Conference of Mayors, 2007). However, families with children are growing rapidly, comprising 23% of the homeless population (U.S. Conference of Mayors, 2007).

Veterans have historically numbered among the homeless. Recent estimates, reported by the Office of Veteran Affairs, found that between 130,000 and 200,000 veterans will be without housing on any given night (National Coalition for the Homeless, 2009d). Many veterans are currently paying too much for housing, and many have sustained psychological trauma and/or traumatic brain injury, making them at-risk for future homelessness (Cunningham, 2009).

Demographics of the homeless have changed, especially in recent years. The alcoholic or illicit drug user is no longer the typical homeless person. Demographic profiles of homeless persons show that women with children comprise an exceedingly large portion of this marginalized group. The lack of affordable housing continues to be one of the primary causes of homelessness in the United States, with many Americans paying close to 50% of their disposable income for housing (Cunningham, 2009). Short-term solutions such as sheltering are not the ultimate answer. A multifaceted approach that focuses on affordable housing and resources that help people who are homeless or at-risk for homelessness deal with the complex issues that affect their lives, whether they stem from abuse, unemployment, or the sequelae of war or natural disasters, is essential. In light of this continuing public health problem, nurses must explore how effective, healthy partnerships with people who are homeless or at-risk can be initiated and sustained.

HEALTH-PROMOTION STRATEGIES FOR PEOPLE WHO ARE HOMELESS

Primary Prevention

Primary prevention measures to prevent people who are at-risk for homelessness from becoming homeless are the first steps in health promotion for this population. Short-term solutions must be coupled with strategies to assess and care for the health needs of those vulnerable in our society. Affordable housing is crucial if the goal is to keep people in their homes. Some short-term measures are

Emergency financial assistance—Frequently, utility companies have an emergency fund that can be used to prevent utilities, such as water and electricity, from being discontinued. To find out if such an emergency fund exists, call the local utilities and ask. Inform at-risk homeless people how to apply for this assistance, and advise them of the information they will need to have handy when they call.

Legal assistance, such as consultation or mediation to prevent eviction—Is there a volunteer group of lawyers in the community? Find out where no-cost or sliding-scale legal assistance is available. Call the organization and learn about waiting time for an appointment, required documentation, and so forth.

Financial advisement—Free financial counseling programs are available in most communities. These programs can help inform people about money management. If instituted early enough, this strategy can effectively prevent homelessness.

It is important that people at-risk for homelessness not be disconnected from the social support that they currently have. Sometimes, a small, one-time loan (i.e., money that is paid back) or grant (i.e., money that is not paid back) is all that is needed to pay the rent, thus preventing homelessness. Some state welfare programs have added a "one-time" emergency financial grant for housing and basic needs (water, electricity) in lieu of ongoing welfare assistance. Inquire about present assistance programs in your community. Such emergency financial aid for rent, security deposits, utility bills, and moving expenses can maintain an at-risk person in his or her residence during a critical period until a paycheck is received. However, with unemployment on the rise, many will need more than short-term or a one-time type of assistance.

Secondary Prevention

Secondary prevention focuses on people who no longer have stable housing. Begin by listing all their perceived needs. It is helpful to categorize needs as housing needs, health care, or employment. Health care needs must be addressed first. Identify the barriers homeless people encounter in receiving health care and how these barriers might be eliminated. Many times, homeless people cannot access the health care system because they do not have a permanent address or adequate identification forms, such as a valid driver's license. Perhaps the person is a military veteran entitled to health care and other benefits, such as financial support associated with a disability. Frequently, waiting at hospitals and clinics for health care can interfere with obtaining shelter for the night. Often there are a limited number of beds at homeless shelters, and, once the beds are filled, no additional people are admitted.

To promote the health of persons who are homeless, assess and evaluate community resources for serving this population. How many shelter beds are available? Are there shelters for families? for teens? for pregnant women? for people with special dietary needs (e.g., diabetics or those with lactose intolerance)? Are emergency shelters available on a "walk-in" basis? What is available in terms of social and psychological support? Once in a shelter, rehabilitation may be necessary for medical or substantive problems such as alcohol or drug addictions. Is a counselor available to the shelter, and is a nurse or physician available for emergency medical needs?

The ultimate goal is exiting homelessness and counteracting the effects of being homeless. To reverse homelessness, transitional housing is important. Transitional housing needs to be free or very low cost. Frequently, homeless people are allowed to live in such housing units for extended periods of time to save up to afford permanent housing. In addition to shelter, social support is usually available (and always essential) at transitional housing.

A common concern for homeless people is following medication and treatment regimens. The following is a list of common conditions that require your constant awareness as you promote healthy partnerships with homeless people:

- Frequently, medications cannot be easily refrigerated.
- It is difficult to follow special dietary restrictions when meals are eaten at a shelter. Food is often very salty, high in fat, with limited fruits and vegetables. It is important for nurses to learn about food served at shelters and day centers. Ask if you might stay for a meal.
- Food may not be allowed in the sleeping areas at the shelter, so taking medication along with food may not be possible.
- Sometimes, medicine is swapped or sold for cash or people are assaulted for the medicine. Counsel those in the shelter as to where medicines may be safely stored.
- Often people who are homeless will request vitamins to compensate for nutritional deficits. Understand that they are usually trying their best to follow treatment regimens. Acknowledge this fact.

Part of a healthy partnership with homeless populations is further assessment of health and social service resources. See the list below for additional community assessment information. (This is a good time to refer to your general community assessment and evaluate it in terms of information specific to individuals and families who are homeless.)

- Do shelters offer clinic services? Is the service daily or weekly? What services are on-site and what services are referred?
- Are local health departments and county hospitals within walking distance? Are bus tokens available for medical appointments? How long are the waits?
- Do mobile health vans operate in the area? Are they consistent in their delivery of health care (i.e., do they come the same day of the week to the same street corner)? What services do they offer? Some services are key to treating people who are homeless (e.g., laboratory services including HIV testing and counseling, x-ray, and dental services).
- Are services linked to a religious group? There may be expectations associated with receiving services that may or may not be acceptable to the person who is homeless.

Overcoming Barriers Related to the Education of Youth Who Are Homeless

The McKinney-Vento Homeless Education Act of 2001 legislated the reduction of barriers to enrollment, attendance, and success in school. Under the reauthorization, each homeless child/youth is ensured equal access to an appropriate public education, including public preschool. The Act also stipulates that homelessness alone is not a reason to separate children from mainstream education. See the full text of the legislation at the National Center for Homeless Education website (http://www.serve.org/nche/), a clearinghouse for information and resources on the educational rights of homeless children and youth. To escape the cycle of adult poverty, it is imperative that children and youth who experience homelessness stay in school. Furthermore, school may be the only stable factor in their lives. Unfortunately, some well-meaning school personnel may be unaware or insensitive to the educational system barriers faced by parents and their children without stable housing. See Box 18.1 for an outline of these barriers.

BOX 18.1

EDUCATION SYSTEM BARRIERS FOR THE HOMELESS

Enrollment Barriers
- Transportation
- Lack of immunizations/medical records
- Lack of previous school records
- Guardianship/residency issues
- School fees

School Success Barriers
- Frequent mobility
- Inability to complete assignments
- Poor health/inadequate medical care
- Lack of food/clothing
- Teacher/staff unawareness/insensitivity
- Isolation or stigma associated with being homeless
- Difficulty accessing services (psychological, special education, English as a second language [ESL] instruction, and so forth)

PROMOTING THE SEXUAL HEALTH OF ADOLESCENTS WHO ARE HOMELESS

Adolescents, particularly young women, constitute one of the most vulnerable groups within the homeless population. In one study by Rew, Chambers, and Kulkarni (2002), these young women reported the need for more instruction in self-care and stated that access to health care was less than adequate. The women claimed that they were routinely treated with a lack of respect and often not even called by name. These claims are particularly alarming in relation to a study of the National Cancer Institute that reported increased rates of cervical cancer in certain groups such as southern African American women, Latinas on the Texas–Mexico border, European American women in Appalachia, Native American women in the northern plains, Vietnamese American women, and Alaskan Natives. These increased rates are in sharp contrast with rates of the general U.S. population, which have decreased substantially, suggesting that cervical cancer may be an indicator of a larger issue—access to health care. Transportation and lack of financial resources were additional barriers to health care identified in Rew's study. The young women preferred to seek care in designated homeless outreach clinics, where their situation was understood and nonjudgmental medical care was usually dispensed; however, this was not always possible.

The following points are important to consider when designing a sexual health education and health care program for homeless adolescents or adolescents in general:

- When possible, conduct focus groups to allow adolescents to have a voice in planning for their sexual health needs.
- Establish trust with a respectful and nonjudgmental attitude.
- Maintain confidentiality and privacy.

- Use small media, such as brochures, to deliver health information.
- Provide sexual health information that is broad in nature and not narrowly focused on HIV (Ensign & Panke, 2002; Rew et al., 2002).

PROMOTING HEALTHY PARTNERSHIPS WITH PEOPLE EXITING HOMELESSNESS

Most people will exit their homeless state. To prevent recurrence of homelessness, it is imperative that a strong support system be in place. It is not enough merely to provide transitional housing. Preventing recurrence requires a commitment to support those exiting homelessness for long periods of time (usually several years). Health-promotion strategies to support people exiting homelessness include

- Coordination of services, such as health, social, substance abuse, and mental health
- Continuity of care
- Case management services
- Transportation
- Job training
- Child care options
- Sources for funding programs

Public health nurses working in the community can lobby for changes in legislation that can prevent homelessness at the primary prevention level. Supporting legislation to raise the minimum wage is one example. The National Coalition for the Homeless formulates a legislative agenda related to homeless populations, such as housing, benefits, income, protected class status, homeless veterans, and youth (see Internet Site: http://www.nationalhomeless.org/advocacy/index.html). Although harder to accomplish in difficult economic times, campaigns to raise the minimum wage and create adequate, affordable housing are top priorities. Lastly, one must recognize that some people choose to remain on the streets and continue their homeless existence. However, most people without housing do not want to remain homeless but are caught in a desperate situation. It is the responsibility of public health nurses to promote healthy partnership with homeless populations.

IMMIGRANTS, REFUGEES, AND MIGRANTS

Marginalization experienced by persons who are homeless or live with disability is also experienced by those who come to live in America from foreign lands, including immigrants, refugees, and migrants. These individuals and families have commonalities, but their differences are significant and central to their health status and access to care. The first step for nurses who care for these groups is to understand those differences with the objective of adapting health care to meet specific needs.

Although aliens in the United States are commonly called *immigrants*, there are important legal distinctions. The Immigration Act (INA) of 1990 excludes noncitizens living in the United States under legally recognized circumstances from the term *immigrant* (U.S. Department of Citizenship and Immigration Services, www.uscis.gov). A noncitizen recognized and documented is known as a *permanent resident alien, lawful permanent resident, resident alien permit holder,* or *green card holder.* Conversely, someone who enters the United States without proper authority or inspection is called an immigrant under the INA. Most permanent residents come to the United States for economic or social benefit. However, a person unable or unwilling to return to his or her country of origin out of fear of persecution for religious, racial, ideological, or political beliefs qualifies as a refugee. The President with Congress set annual quotas for admission of refugees. Some nonimmigrants seek temporary residence or transit through the United States for a specific purpose, and they can be accompanied by family members. International students fit this category. Migrant workers or temporary agricultural workers come to the United States to perform services or labor of a temporary or seasonal nature. Some migrants obtain permanent residence status in the United States but travel seasonally to different *colonias* in search of work. See the U.S. Department of Immigration Services for more information and resources at http://www.uscis.gov/.

The circumstances surrounding the motivation for leaving one's country of origin vary. Personal experiences have an impact on health. For example, the health needs of immigrants, refugees, or migrant workers are likely to be different, and access to health services will also differ. These groups frequently hesitate to object when health care services have been denied or to contact authorities when their human rights have been violated. Language barriers often add another layer of complexity and misunderstanding between health care providers and these marginalized groups.

Consider this true scenario of an immigrant hospitalized in four-point traction for 2 weeks. Only when a student nurse engaged a translator did his distressing story unfold. When the young man asked for wages due after several weeks of work, he was thrust out of a moving van on a major interstate. He had no family in the United States. He had family in Mexico, but no one had been contacted. Ethical arguments could focus on limited health care resources and the absence of legal authority in this case. The reality is that nurses and other health care professionals will encounter similar situations in health care settings across the nation and must understand the complexities and differences of each situation to develop and implement culturally relevant humane plans of care.

Refugees and immigrants typically experience three phases as they assimilate into the country of destination, with each phase having specific health care implications. The phases are an acute period (the immediate arrival in the new country), followed by a time of transition, and a resolution or chronic phase (Kemp, 2008). Acute health problems, such as tuberculosis, parasites, or hepatitis, may stem from conditions in the country of origin or result from travel to the new country. For example, one refugee who left Vietnam in a crowded small boat stated it was 14 days before the evacuees were rescued. Food and fresh water were scarce and nutritional concerns immediate. In addition, she was distraught at the time because several of her brothers had been killed in the war. History taking is an important step in planning care. Once the acute health needs have been identified and resolved, chronic conditions may emerge, including post-traumatic stress disorder (PTSD). The resolution phase is connected to how well the immigrant or refugee assimilates into the American culture. This includes identifying with mainstream politics and communicating in English. A special report, *Building an Americanization Movement for the 21st Century*, addresses this process and can be found at http://www.uscis.gov/files/nativedocuments/M-708.pdf (U.S. Department of Homeland Security, 2008).

PROMOTING HEALTHY PARTNERSHIPS THROUGH EDUCATION

Education is an important health-promotion strategy for working with the vulnerable population. Various educational strategies are discussed in the following sections. As you read the different sections, consider how you might change, modify, or combine the different educational programs to accommodate various marginalized populations.

Educating about Chronic Conditions

Having a chronic condition presents many challenges. The following is an educational program for diabetics who are homeless. You may choose to adapt this model to meet the specific needs of another marginalized group. You can make the necessary changes for another chronic condition, such as hypertension. The program can be presented in a cultural center for recent immigrants, a colonia for migrants, or the local health clinic for an impoverished community. Be sure to do a needs assessment and ask members of the community to participate in the planning phase.

- Arrange with shelter administration to have a diabetic teaching class in the main waiting area of the shelter.
- Emphasize the importance of foot care using posters written at the 3rd-grade level.
- Demonstrate proper foot care by having homeless people in attendance soak their feet in basins. Inspect feet with attention to any red, swollen, cracked, or infected areas. Be sure to discuss the importance of properly drying the feet.
- Discuss the importance of shoes that fit properly and dry, clean socks.
- Offer attendees socks, perhaps donated from local merchants or collected by neighborhood school children. A letter of solicitation to merchants for socks can be drafted from the educational institution with which student nurses are affiliated and with the shelter's name.
- Gather shoes in advance by placing receptacles in city or suburban fitness clubs encouraging runners to donate slightly used athletic shoes. (Runners often replace shoes every 2 to 3 months. Although the shoes may no longer be suitable for running, there is usually a lot of wear left for day-to-day use.)
- Distribute incentives in a fair, organized manner. Doing so requires detailed advance planning. Distribution is best done at the end of the program.
- Provide referrals for health needs (e.g., foot infections, ingrown toenails, fungal conditions, circulatory concerns); follow-up mechanisms must be in place.
- Offer blood pressure and glucose screening in conjunction with the educational program.

Offering Positive Parenting Sessions

To assist women and men in shelters learn better strategies for coping with children, parenting classes can be offered. Suggested topics to include are

- Advantages of breast feeding
- Normal behaviors for developmental ages
- Behaviors that indicate a child is ill
- Normal height and weight for age
- Nonviolent ways to discipline (e.g., time-out, consistency, clear rules)
- Healthy, low-cost food choices (fruit, peanut butter, cheese, eggs)
- Assertiveness and empowerment training

Organizing a Health Fair

A health fair is another way to cover a number of health promotion and education areas at once. Screening procedures such as dental, blood pressure, cholesterol, blood glucose, vision, hearing, and lead poison can be included in the agenda. Steps for organizing a health fair are listed below:

- Contact the shelter administrator.
- Set the date well in advance (6 months to 1 year, if possible).
- Decide what health-promotion areas to cover, depending on the audience (e.g., families versus only adult males).
- Invite identified organizations to participate.
- Solicit prizes from local merchants.
- Offer incentives for attendance, such as educational hours (most shelters require participation in self-help programs). Other ideas to consider when planning a health fair include the following:
  - Collaborate with other professionals, such as a dental school.
  - Offer immunizations.
  - Include screening stations, such as vision, hearing, blood glucose, blood pressure, lead, tuberculosis skin testing, HIV testing, depression, and intimate partner violence.
  - Assign booth areas, considering flow pattern.
  - Include fun activities, such as a magician for children or massage therapy for adults.
  - Have a plan for referral and follow-up.

Visit the Family and Consumer Services website for a Health Fair Planning Guide that offers national resources for health fairs for more ideas at http://fcs.tamu.edu/health/health_fair_planning_guide/objectives_and_planning.php.

Summary

Poverty impacts health. It potentially contributes to the marginalization of certain groups more than any other factor. Often these marginalized groups are underserved or not served at all. They are likely to be uninsured or underinsured. Americans must realize that this is a societal problem that requires multiple strategies to decrease and eventually eliminate disparities in health care.

Several marginalized groups were discussed in this chapter. More research is needed to identify marginalized populations and their particular problems. Persons with disabilities comprise a substantial portion of the U.S. population. The number of people who are homeless or at-risk for homelessness continues to increase, although the demographics are changing. Immigrants, refugees, and migrant workers are entering the United States by legal and illegal methods. To embrace the goal of Healthy People 2020, aimed at achieving health equity, eliminating disparities, and improving the health standards for all groups, a concerted effort should target and model already successful programs. Furthermore, the most important strategies are probably politically based. Nursing is well positioned to address disparities as related to the health of marginalized groups, and should work diligently to move health care for these groups into the mainstream.

Critical Thinking Questions

When working with marginalized groups, it is important to consider how different processes influence outcomes.

1. Identify political, economic, legal, cultural, and access to health care realities for a marginalized group in your community and explain how these factors may lead to positive or negative health outcomes.

2. Adherence to medical regimen is often very difficult or impossible for the homeless. As a nurse working in the health department clinic of a homeless shelter, you have noticed a high prevalence of hypertension among the residents of the shelter. Routinely, you advise your clients to modify their daily sodium intake. Is this a realistic expectation for someone living in a homeless shelter? What questions need to be answered? How is the food prepared? Who prepares the food? Is bulk food received from a government source? Do the residents have input into the meal planning? What steps or solutions would you implement to address this issue? Be sure to consider strategies at different levels of prevention. Who should be involved in the plan? What are some other conditions that might pose problems with adherence to a medical regimen?

3. What is the role of bias, stereotyping, and discrimination in relation to unequal treatment of marginalized groups? First, define the terms. How do these concepts impact ethnic/racial or otherwise marginalized groups in our society? What historical or contextual factors might be influential? Think of examples that have occurred in your community or health care setting. What strategies can you identify to increase awareness of health care providers?

4. Optional: Visit a homeless shelter in your town and observe or sample the food served. What did you learn?

5. Optional: Visit a community home for the disabled. What are some of the barriers the disabled face in the course of daily living?

6. Consider the scenario of the young hospitalized immigrant discussed in this chapter. What were the shortcomings of the health system in that case? What other situations can you think of that affect the care of immigrants? Refugees? Migrants? What steps can nurses delivering health services to these groups take to increase the quality of care? Visit the Internet to find advocacy groups specific to immigrant issues.

● References

Centers for Disease Control and Prevention (CDC). (2006). Disability and health. Retrieved December 5, 2009 from http://www.cdc.gov/ncbddd/dh/hp2010.htm

Cunningham, M. (2009). Preventing and ending homelessness—next steps. The Urban Institute. Retrieved February 27, 2009 from http://www.urban.org/UploadedPDF/411837_ending_homelessness.pdf

Ensign, J., & Panke, A. (2002). Barriers and bridges to care: Voices of homeless female adolescent youth in Seattle, Washington, USA. *Journal of Advanced Nursing*, 37(2), 166–172.

Flaskerud, J. H., Lesser, J., Dixon, E., Anderson, N., Conde, F., Kim, S., et al. (2002). Health disparities among vulnerable populations. *Nursing Research*, 51(2), 74–85.

Flaskerud, J. H., & Winslow, B. J. (1998). Conceptualizing vulnerable populations health-related research. *Nursing Research*, 47(2), 69–78.

Healthy People 2010: Understanding and Improving Health. (2000). Retrieved December 5, 2009 from http://www.healthypeople.gov/Document/html/uih/uih_bw/uih_2.htm#goals

Institute for Children in Poverty, National Data on Family Homelessness, (2008). Retrieved December 5, 2009 from http://www.icpny.org/index.asp?CID=7

Kemp, C. (2008). Promoting healthy partnerships with refugees and immigrants. In J. McFarlane & E. Anderson (Eds.). *Community as partner* (pp. 357–367). Philadelphia, PA: Lippincott.

National Center for Health Statistics (NCHS). Summary Health Statistics for the U.S. Population: National Health Interview Survey, 2006, Tables 3, 4. Retrieved February 28, 2009 from http://www.cdc.gov/nchs/fastats/disable.htm.

National Coalition for the Homeless. (2009a). Who is homeless? Retrieved December 5, 2009 from http://www.nationalhomeless.org/factsheets/who.html

National Coalition for the Homeless. (2009b). Why are people homeless? Retrieved December 5, 2009 from http://www.nationalhomeless.org/factsheets/who.html

National Coalition for the Homeless. (2009c). How many people experience homelessness. Retrieved December 5, 2009 from http://www.nationalhomeless.org/factsheets/How_Many.html

National Coalition for the Homeless. (2009d). Homelessness veterans. Retrieved December 5, 2009 from http://www.nationalhomeless.org/factsheets/veterans.html

National Coalition for the Homeless. Retrieved December 5, 2009 from http://www.nationalhomeless.org/advocacy/index.html

National Institutes of Health, U.S. Department of Health and Human Services. (2006). Strategic Plan: National Institute for Nursing Research (NINR), 2006-2010. Retrieved December 5, 2009 http://www.ninr.nih.gov/NR/rdonlyres/9021E5EB-B2BA-47EA-B5DB-1E4DB11B1289/4894/NINR_StrategicPlanWebsite.pdf

Institute of Medicine. (2002). *Unequal treatment: Confronting racial and ethnic disparities in health care.* Washington, DC: National Academics Press.

Nyamathi, A., Koniak-Griffin, D., & Greengold, B. A. (2007). Development of nursing theory and science in vulnerable populations research. *Annual Review of Nursing Research, 25,* 3–25.

Peragallo, N., & Gonzalez, R. M. (2007). Nursing research and the prevention of infectious diseases among vulnerable populations. *Annual Review of Nursing Research, 25,* 83–117.

Rew, L., Chambers, K. B., & Kulkarni, S. (2002). Planning a sexual health promotion intervention with homeless adolescents. *Nursing Research, 51*(3), 168–174.

Stone, J. (2002). Race and healthcare disparities: Overcoming vulnerability. *Theoretical Medicine, 23,* 499–518.

The U.S. Citizenship and Immigration Services. Retrieved December 11, 2009 from http://www.uscis.gov

The U.S. Equal Employment Opportunity Commission. Notice Concerning The Americans With Disabilities Act (ADA) Amendments Act Of 2008. Retrieved, December 5, 2009 from http://www.eeoc.gov/ada/amendments_notice.html

The U.S. Conference of Mayors. (2007). *A status report on hunger and homelessness in America's cities: A 23-city survey.* Retrieved February 23, 2009, from http://usmayors.org/HHSurvey2007/hhsurvey07.pdf

U.S. Department of Homeland Security. (2008). Task Force on New Americans, Building an Americanization Movement for the Twenty-first Century: A Report to the President of the United States from the Task Force on New Americans, Washington, DC 2008. Retrieved December 11, 2009 from http://www.uscis.gov/files/nativedocuments/M-708.pdf

U.S. Department of Health and Human Services. (2008). Phase I Report Recommendations for the Framework and Format of Healthy People 2020. Retrieved December 5, 2009 from http://www.healthypeople.gov/HP2020/advisory/PhaseI/summary.htm#_Toc211942896

Vasas, E. B. (2005). Examining the margins a concept analysis of marginalization. *Advances in Nursing Science, 28*(3), 194–202.

World Health Organization. (2008). The World Health Report: Primary health care now more than ever. Retrieved March 3, 2009 from http://www.who.int/whr/2008/whr08_en.pdf

■ FURTHER READINGS

Aday, L.A. & Bass, J. (Eds.), (2001). *At risk in America: The health and health care needs of vulnerable populations in the United States.* San Francisco: Jossey-Bass.

deChesnay, M. (Ed.) (2005). *Caring for the Vulnerable.* Sudbury, MA: Jones and Bartlett.

Halcon, L. L., Robertson, C. L., Monsen, K. A., & Claypatch, C. C. (2007). A theoretical framework for using health realization to reduce stress and improve coping in refugee communities. *Journal of Holistic Nursing, 25,* 186–191.

Kroloff, C. (1993). *54 ways you can help the homeless.* West Orange, CA: Behrman House. Available at http://www.earthsystems.org/ways/

Internet Resources can be found on the**Point** at http://thepoint.lww.com/Anderson6e.

Promoting Healthy Partnerships in the Workplace

Ann T. Malecha

LEARNING OBJECTIVES

After studying this chapter, you should be able to:

1. Assess health promotion needs in the workplace.
2. Discuss strategies for successful primary, secondary, and tertiary health promotion programs.
3. Plan, implement, and evaluate programs that teach healthy behaviors to diverse groups of employees and their families.

Introduction

*H*ealth promotion, disease prevention and control, wellness, risk factor reduction, and preventive health care are some of the terms applied to workplace health programs. In this chapter, the term *health promotion* is used to denote a process by which employees learn about primary, secondary, and tertiary prevention strategies to improve their health and quality of life. A partnership between employer and employee to promote the safety and health of the workers benefits both parties. The *Occupational Safety and Health Act of 1970* created the Occupational Safety and Health Administration (OSHA) to assure the safety and health of all American workers via partnerships and alliances with employers and other agencies (U.S. Department of Labor, 2006). OSHA establishes and enforces standards to help employers and employees reduce injuries, illnesses, and deaths on the job. Since 1970, workplace fatalities have decreased by 60% and injuries and illnesses by 40% even with U.S. employment increasing to over 115 million workers at 7.2 million worksites. Workplace health promotion programs have been developed and refined over the past 30 years and have achieved long-term behavior change and risk reduction among employees. Workplaces are ideal settings in which to implement health promotion programs because they contain groups of people usually in one location who share a common purpose and culture (Goetzel, Roemer, Liss-Levinson, & Samoly, 2008).

The process of promoting health in the workplace involves providing information and developing health education programs that encourage employees to take responsibility for their health to lower risk of disease and injury (American Association of Occupational Health Nurses, 2008). This knowledge is followed by learning new skills, implementing them in daily life, and finding a means of sustaining the learned behaviors over the long term.

The occupational health nurse is often responsible for health promotion programs at the worksite and is an excellent resource person for establishing a community partnership. If the organization does not have an occupational nurse, health programs may be the responsibility of the safety officer or an employee in the company's human resources or benefits department. Ask who coordinates health activities. For businesses with 2 to 100 employees, health promotion efforts can be facilitated by partnering with other local businesses, county extension or agricultural agents, state departments of health, or national awareness campaigns. The nursing processes for promoting health at the workplace focus on the entire population of the company and may even extend to the employees' dependents (spouses and children).

More than 81% of American businesses employing 50 or more workers are involved in health promotion activities (Azevedo, 2005). Companies integrate health promotion into employee recruitment (e.g., membership at a health club), job training (e.g., back care), safety (e.g., hearing conservation), health (e.g., risk profiles and screenings), and recreation efforts (e.g., fun runs and sports teams). Employers are interested in promoting the health and safety of their employees for multiple reasons, including increasing productivity, reducing absenteeism, maintaining safety standard requirements, improving employee morale, and lowering workers' compensation and insurance claims.

Health promotion activities at the workplace begin with assessing the health needs of the entire workforce, including management. The next step is creating an awareness of the health issues through companywide education, screening, and interventions that focus on behavior or lifestyle changes. This chapter discusses strategies for successful health promotion and safety programs, describes the steps used in implementing various programs, and lists several available resources.

TYPES OF HEALTH PROMOTION ACTIVITIES FOR THE WORKPLACE

Common workplace activities that promote health or prevent injury and disease are exercise, smoking cessation, back care, and stress-management programs. Frequently, companies offer employee health newsletters; health risk appraisals; health fairs; and screenings, such as blood pressure checks and blood lipid levels. Health risk appraisals and employee health-focused newsletters can be made available to employees via purchased printed materials or online subscriptions. Some web-based programs allow the employee to connect with discussion forums, encourage personalized goal setting and outcomes tracking, and provide the employer with confidential aggregate reports. Web-based programs are a particularly well-matched method to serve small businesses and telecommuters.

Health promotion in the workplace typically falls within three basic program types:

- *Awareness programs* increase the employees' level of knowledge and interest (e.g., flyers, seminars, and newsletters).
- *Behavior change activities* help participants develop healthier behaviors (e.g., smoking cessation, regular exercise, and healthy nutrition).

- *Supportive environments* create work opportunities that encourage healthy lifestyles (e.g., low-fat foods in the cafeteria, on-site aerobic classes, release time for health screenings, sunscreen dispenser by walking trail).

When deciding on the type of health promotion program to offer, it is important to determine how consistent that program is with the company's mission and goals. Also consider the costs and benefits of the activity for both the employer and the employee. Whereas employers are aware of the potential for financial benefits, such as reducing absenteeism or improved work output, most employees participate in health promotion programs for personal reasons (weight reduction, increased physical fitness). The worker desires to look and feel better or to have an improved quality of life. Meeting the needs of both the organization and the employees will support wide employee participation and a highly successful health program.

PLANNING A HEALTH PROMOTION PROGRAM

Needs Assessment

Questionnaires and health risk appraisals are commonly used to identify employees' interest in educational topics and to describe present health and safety behaviors. Ideas for health and lifestyle survey topics to include on a questionnaire appear in Box 19.1. To include all these topics on one questionnaire would be overwhelming. However, if a plan for the year were developed with a different focus each month that began with a brief questionnaire to establish interest, then one could be assured of success.

BOX 19.1

IDEAS FOR HEALTH AND LIFESTYLE SURVEY TOPICS

Exercise and fitness
Overweight and obesity
Nutrition and eating well
Vitamins and natural remedies
Smoking cessation
Weight management
Vision and hearing care
Men's health
Women's health
Pregnancy and care of the newborn
Pediatric fever and pain management
Menopause, osteoporosis, and estrogen replacement therapy
Safety (bicycle, motorcycle helmets, safety belts, and car air bags)
Safely traveling abroad
Violence (women, children, older adults, disabled persons, and workplace)
Depression and anxiety
Stress management and relaxation
Adult pain management (back, neck, and wrists)
Heartburn and indigestion
Heart health (blood lipid levels, hypertension, heart attack, and stroke)
Chronic disease management
Cancer (prevention, treatment, and survivors)
Allergies and asthma

Employee health and insurance records can also be used to identify prevalence of chronic illnesses of the employees that need to be addressed. Safety records, workers' compensation forms, or employee and manager interviews are additional resources for determining employee and company health promotion needs.

Once the needs have been identified, you may assist the occupational nurse or planning advisory committee in securing management support for a health promotion program. A proposal presentation or executive report is often one of the first steps in convincing management of the value of the project. A feasibility or business plan approach to communicating your program is used to establish a common language and understanding of the project by everyone in the organization. A sample business plan might include the following:

- *Executive summary:* A short summary of the health promotion plan, which includes the purpose (e.g., to decrease lower back strain); methods (e.g., three 30-minute classes); expected benefits (e.g., fewer work days missed, increased productivity); and costs (e.g., program costs, such as brochures, flyers, teaching time, and incentives, as well as avoidance costs, such as averted absenteeism and decreased insurance and workman's compensation claims).
- *Methods:* How, when, and where the plan will be put into action. List each task to be completed (e.g., brochure and flyer design and dissemination). Who is the responsible person(s)? Develop a timeline for task completion. Outline the content of the program, including use of guest speakers, demonstrations, return demonstrations, and methods to increase employee participation and adaptation of the taught behaviors. Include program goal and objectives in this section of the proposal. *A program goal might be*: Eighty percent of employees completing the back care program will report a decrease in the number of sick days related to low back pain. *A program objective could be*: After lectures and demonstrations on correct lifting procedures, 90% of participating employees will demonstrate correct lifting techniques.
- *Expected benefits:* List outcomes of program (e.g., fewer work days missed due to low back pain). This is a good point in the proposal to note the number of days missed in the last year and by what percentage the proposed program will decrease that absenteeism. This is also a place in the report to cite other companies that you have found in the literature that have implemented similar programs and the results these companies experienced.
- *Costs:* An accurate projection of program costs (materials, teachers' time, incentives), as well as profits expected due to decreased absenteeism and increased productivity.

Health Risk Appraisals

A health risk appraisal (HRA) is an easily administered, confidential instrument used to determine life expectancy based on current risk behaviors. The HRA can also calculate the amount of risk that could be avoided if lifestyle behaviors were changed. Some HRAs determine the person's readiness to change behavior. An HRA can be used as a teaching tool that gives positive feedback for healthy behaviors and encouragement and information for changing those unhealthy behaviors. An HRA is often completed on an interactive computer program and provides an accurate individualized report to each employee in a timely manner (within 2 weeks). Anonymous aggregate data are provided to the company. The usefulness of the information to the employer depends on a significant proportion of the employee population participating (hopefully at least 70% to 80% of employees). Confidentiality of HRA information and publicizing highlights of the aggregate summary may boost future participation levels.

Specific HRAs exist to assess nutritional status, weight, and general fitness status. If you are ready for a study break, stop and check out these HRAs on the Internet. (When you get the website, search for HRA). Consider how each could be used for a health promotion program at the worksite.

- Sample HRA—http://www.nationalwellness.org/TestWell/index.htm
- Centers for Disease Control and Prevention—http://www.cdc.gov/nccdphp/ dnpa/hwi/program_design/health_risk_appraisals.htm
- University of San Francisco Health Risk Appraisal—http://www.usfca.edu/hr/ wellness/appraisal.html
- American Heart Association—http://www.americanheart.org/presenter.jhtml? identifier=4528

USING STAGES OF CHANGE IN HEALTH PROMOTION PROGRAMS

Because most health promotion programs involve lifestyle behavioral change, Prochaska's change process (Prochaska & DiClemente, 1983), Pender's Health Belief Model (Pender, 1996), or your chosen model/theory can guide the process from planning through evaluation. A brief review of the stages of the change process follows.

- *Precontemplation:* In this stage, the employee is not even thinking about changing his or her behavior. The goal is to make the person aware of the benefits of change and to get him or her to start thinking about the possibility of change.
- *Contemplation:* In this stage, the employee is at least considering making an effort to change behavior. The employee is weighing the pros and the cons. The employee may not know how to change and may consider the change to be almost impossible. The attempt to change is not worth the effort if failure is to occur. The goal is to help the employee identify the benefits and to decide that putting forth an effort to change is worthwhile.
- *Preparation:* A person at this stage has decided to try and change a behavior(s). This employee desires help in making the change and is ready for information and skills to maintain the behavioral change.
- *Action:* At this stage, the employee is practicing the new behavior; however, it is not yet incorporated into his or her lifestyle. The new behavior requires lots of effort, which leaves the employee at risk for relapsing to the old behavior. The employee needs support, incentives, and sincere encouragement.
- *Maintenance:* The new behavior is ingrained in the lifestyle behaviors. A crisis or major stressor at work or personal life can become the impetus to revert to the previous behavior. The employee needs reinforcement, support, and opportunities to practice the new behavior. The employee benefits by sharing the newly learned behavior.

PROGRAM IMPLEMENTATION

Marketing is an essential part of successful program implementation. Some strategies for marketing include:

- *Must be professional looking.* Catchy words and titles are essential (e.g., "Weigh to Go" for a weight reduction program). Change posters frequently to keep attention focused.

- *Electronic mail messages.* Count down to event; offer a related health quiz question, and give the answer and rationale the following day.
- *Health newsletter.* Detail a success story, such as early detection of malignant melanoma, weight loss regimen using a walking program, or not knowing a person had high blood pressure until participating in a screening program and how simple lifestyle changes helped control the disease (without medication).
- *Letter from the company's president or benefits manager.* Offering company time for health screening, announcing that company will pay for all or a portion of smoking cessation program/health screening test, or allowing a trade-in of 2 hours of sick time for wellness program attendance would be appropriate messages.
- *Incentive gifts.* Offer incentive gifts to participating employees, such as T-shirts, hats, sunscreen samples, a healthy fruit snack, or water bottles.

PROGRAM EVALUATION

The evaluation process provides an opportunity to determine the outcomes derived by the health promotion program and directs improvement of employee health services. Evaluating the structure of the program, the process by which the program was delivered, as well as the outcomes of the program is a three-pronged approach common to quality assurance reviews.

Structural evaluation involves (1) reviewing the mechanism for reporting to management and the support given to the health promotion program; (2) determining if the physical facilities were adequate for the program; (3) identifying equipment and supplies used; (4) identifying staffing requirements and their qualifications; (5) analyzing employee demographics and their health status needs; and (6) determining if the program mission, goals, and objectives were formulated to meet both the health needs of the employee and the business needs of the employer.

Process evaluation addresses (1) whether the health promotion activity was appropriate for the setting; (2) whether the health promotion program was designed to meet workplace needs (you can measure against the initial needs assessment); and (3) whether there was documentation and record keeping.

Outcome evaluation focuses on (1) were expected goals and objectives achieved; (2) did the program lead to positive outcomes; (3) did health outcomes demonstrate prevention of illness/injury, increase compliance, increase employees' self-care knowledge, restore function, or relieve discomfort; (4) how did program benefits compare to program costs; and (5) satisfaction (of employees, employers, dependents) with the quality of health promotion services received.

Common methods for evaluation are postprogram rating scales, observation, and interviewing of employees about their opinions, attitudes, and satisfaction with the program. Chart-and-record reviews can be used to determine morbidity and mortality differences.

TIPS FOR MAINTAINING A HEALTH PROMOTION PROGRAM

To sustain a health promotion effort, always design the program according to the goals of the organization. Include from the beginning an identified, key workplace employee or manager. As part of the health promotion program, teach employees where, when, and how to use community resources. Include short- and middle-range evaluation of the program. If possible, give projections of long-range success, savings, health benefits (e.g., morbidity and costs of finding early-stage disease and averting possible surgery, pain, hospitalization, workman's compensation, and so forth). Always propose to incorporate health promotion into the employee benefits plan.

EXAMPLES OF HEALTH PROMOTION PROGRAMS

Skin Cancer Prevention

This Skin Cancer Prevention Program easily incorporates primary, secondary, and tertiary prevention strategies into the activities planned for the company's annual fun run, summer picnic, or sports event. Here is a schedule and accompanying prevention level:

- *Two weeks before event*—Add visual graphics to the event advertising that depict a runner with a hat on, a volleyball player putting on sunscreen, or other sun-appropriate activity. *(Primary prevention.)*
- *Ten days before the event*—Give a brown bag lecture or have a guest "expert" speaker from the American Cancer Society discuss skin cancer (incidence, prevalence, types of skin cancer, risk factors, warning signs, and prevention). Announce at the lecture that there will be skin cancer screening as part of the company event. *(Primary prevention.)*
- *Seven days before the event*—Set up a table-top poster display on types of sun protection describing the amount of protection offered by each product (broad-brimmed hat vs. cap, white T-shirt vs. tightly woven shirt, sun block vs. sunscreen) or multiple types and forms of sunscreens (alcohol-based, creams, waterproof, water-resistant, gels, sprays), and have samples for testing. *(Primary prevention.)*
- *Five days before the event*—Distribute an e-mail announcement that a dermatologist or skin cancer specialist will be conducting skin cancer screenings at the picnic. Have employees reserve a 5-minute time slot for each member of their family by phoning the "appointment hotline" number that you staff. *(Secondary prevention.)*
- *Four days before the event*—Distribute an e-mail quiz regarding a fact about skin cancer prevention. Have the employees respond by the end of the work day. Place the prize and a flyer of congratulations on their desks or in their mailboxes the following morning. Continue the marketing by congratulating for several days. (Award ideas: lip balm with sunscreen, sun visors, sunglasses, sunscreens, and hats). *(Primary prevention.)*
- *Event day*—Set up a booth and conduct skin cancer screenings and counseling. Distribute a list of dermatologists within the company's health benefits plan. Set up a station for demonstrating correct application of sunscreen. Dispense a medicine cup full of sunscreen to each passerby. Give the children red helium balloons imprinted with "Red balloons, NOT red children." *(Secondary prevention.)*
- *First day of work after the event*—Send short e-mail evaluation to all employees regarding use of sun-protective products, number of family members sustaining sunburns, and value of the activities to the employee and their family. *(Primary prevention.)*
- *Two and 4 weeks after the event*—Follow up on all written referrals given to employees and their families during the skin cancer screening. Determine outcomes and report to management concerning evaluation of the event. *(Tertiary prevention.)*

Intimate Partner Violence Awareness and Prevention

Each year in the United States about 1 million incidents of physical violence occur against women by an intimate partner, such as a current or former spouse or boyfriend. The effects of intimate partner violence spill into the workplace and can impact employment productivity. Working women who are being abused at home have reported being harassed by their abusive partners in person or by telephone while at work, being late, leaving work early, or missing work because of the abuse, and being reprimanded for problems associated with the abuse. Abused women have also reported losing a job because of the violence in their lives. More and more employers are recognizing that domestic violence is a major problem in the workplace and are willing to implement policies and procedures that address domestic violence prevention. The following are elements of a domestic violence awareness program that addresses primary, secondary, and tertiary prevention of intimate partner violence against women.

Primary Prevention

- Support a company policy of zero tolerance against hostility and violence against all persons.
- Support a company policy that rewards collaboration, collegiality, and teamwork, and penalizes controlling behaviors and aggression.
- Maintain a workplace environment in which all employees, regardless of gender, ethnicity, sexual orientation, and religion are treated with respect and dignity.
- Promote policies that raise the status of women in the company.
- Promote human resource policies that support men as involved coparents, sons, partners, and spouses.
- Display a poster on the "safety bulletin board" about domestic violence awareness and change to a different poster on domestic violence, such as child abuse or elder abuse, several times a year as an effective way to increase knowledge (Coker, 2005).

Secondary Prevention

- Support a company policy with a statement that clearly demonstrates concern and commitment to employees who may be experiencing violence at home. The policy must include nondiscrimination against victims in recruiting, hiring, and promoting, and sensitivity in performance evaluation.
- Offer annual manager and employee educational opportunities, such as brown bag seminars, newsletters, posters, and brochures on domestic violence, to help create a work culture that recognizes and strives to prevent intimate partner violence. October is National Domestic Violence Awareness month, and many national organizations offer resources to raise workplace awareness about domestic violence. Consider having a panel of community experts, such as a police officer, counselor, and nurse; discuss different types of domestic violence, such as stalking, abuse during pregnancy, and sexual assault; and offer available health, social, and legal services. Organizing employees to collect food and clothing for a local battered women's shelter is another way to support prevention efforts. These activities promote and maintain a work environment that supports abuse disclosure.
- Promote employee counseling and intervention. Everyone at the worksite needs to be aware of the signs and symptoms of intimate partner violence. A flexible and

empathic work environment allows abused employees to disclose the violence and seek help. A current list of telephone numbers and addresses of community resources and social service agencies specializing in domestic violence should be available at all times. Posting hotline phone numbers and steps of a safety plan in the women's restrooms with a basket or box of business-card-size listing of community resources and telephone numbers (preferably available in individual toilet stalls) is a safe method for dissemination of resource information. Companies that offer an Employee Assistance Program (EAP) need to ensure that counselors are trained to provide appropriate assistance with domestic violence.

- Implement domestic violence screening questions on preemployment and annual health examinations. Information on domestic violence, safety measures, and community resources must be part of every health fair, screening, and health education event. Examples of domestic violence screening questions are available from the Internet Resources listed at the end of this chapter.

Tertiary Prevention

- Provide adequate security to employees. All employees need to be reassured of a safe worksite even if an abuser attempts to stalk and harass an employee at work. Procedures must be in place to deal with trespassing, violence in the workplace, harassment, and accessing law enforcement. Safety plans for victimized employees may include advising coworkers of the situation and possibly supplying a photograph of the abuser, temporarily relocating the victim to a secure area, reassigning a parking place, and escorting to and from the worksite.
- Offer flexible work hours. Abused employees may need time off for criminal or civil court proceedings, health care and counseling, and safe housing relocation for themselves and their children.
- Provide financial support to employees. Examples of emergency financial assistance to abused employees include: (1) making changes in benefits at any time during a calendar year to ensure adequate health coverage for the employee and dependents; (2) expediting requests for changing the process of electronic paychecks into different bank accounts; and (3) providing emergency funds for employees in crisis.

Chronic Disease Self-Management in the Workplace

Self-management programs teach problem-solving skills in addition to health education. Self-management programs are successful in helping patients with chronic diseases such as diabetes mellitus and arthritis to make lifestyle behavior changes that improve pain, fatigue, physical function, and emotions. This type of intervention is classified as tertiary prevention; its goal is to maintain or minimize disease progression or to foster rehabilitation. Once a chronic condition has been identified, either for an individual or a subgroup of the worksite population, counseling and plans can be initiated to decrease the disease impact on life and to improve the persons' quality of life and physical functioning. This process is collaborative and often includes assessment, planning, implementation, referrals, coordination, monitoring, and evaluation. Effective chronic disease self-management tasks include:

- Taking care of the disease process—employees self-manage their diseases by knowing their medications, regimens, side effects, reporting changing symptoms to health care providers, healthy eating, and exercising, to name a few.
- Taking care of normal activities—employees self-manage type, amount, and structure of their normal social, work, and home life activities.

- Taking care of their emotions—employees self-manage emotional changes that occur with chronic illness, such as anger, uncertainty, depression, changed role expectations, and goals.

A self-management program for obesity may include group sessions and individual follow-up that includes: walking for fitness; healthy eating; setting realistic goals and weekly plans for action; pedometer and activity diary; height, weight, and BMI; community resources.

HEALTH PROMOTION FOR SPECIALIZED WORKPLACES AND WORKERS

Agricultural Workers

More than 2.25 million full-time workers are employed in the agriculture sector in the United States, and there are an estimated 4.5 million additional unpaid farm workers and family members aged 14 years and older. Farming is one of the most dangerous occupations in the United States, with over 700 work-related deaths and another 120,000 agricultural disabling injuries per year (National Safety Council, 2009). Farming is one of the few industries in which the families, who often share the work and live on the premises, are also at risk for injuries, illness, and death. Farmers and their families are exposed to many hazards, which are listed in Box 19.2. Additional factors impacting the risk for farm work–related injuries are discussed in the following sections.

Age

Injury rates are highest among children aged 15 and under and adults over 65. Approximately 1 million children and adolescents under age 15 years reside in a farming household, while another 800,000 children and adolescents live in households headed by hired farm workers. Each year, about 100 children are killed and 100,000 children and adolescents are injured in agriculture-related activities. Most deaths among children on farms result from being innocent bystanders or passengers on farm equipment. Many farm children are working in dangerous environments by the age of 10 (National Institute for Occupational Safety and Health [NIOSH], 2009a). Additional issues of the adolescent worker are presented later in this chapter.

Farmers do not usually retire at age 65, and many work well into their 70s and 80s. Senior farmers often take prescribed medications, work with physical disabilities, and may suffer from vision and hearing loss. All these factors may increase senior farmers' risk for work-related injuries and death.

Equipment and Machinery

Most farm accidents and fatalities involve machinery. Proper machine guarding and equipment maintenance according to manufacturers' recommendations can help prevent accidents. Only one half of the farm tractors used on U.S. farms are equipped with life-saving rollover protective structures (ROPs) with seat belts. Many farm tractors were manufactured before the voluntary installation of ROPs with seat belts, while some newer tractors have had their ROPs removed by the owner. Personal protective equipment (PPE) and certain injury prevention activities can reduce the number and severity of farm work-related injuries and illnesses (Table 19.1).

BOX 19.2

POTENTIAL HAZARDS FOR AGRICULTURAL WORKERS

Machinery and Equipment
- Large riding machinery (tractors, combines)
- Entanglement in machinery
- Old equipment lacking safety devices

Chemical Exposure
- Fertilizers, pesticides, fungicides
- Anhydrous ammonia, organophosphates
- Toxic gases
- Cleaning solvents

Livestock
- Unpredictable behavior (crushing, kicking, biting)
- Risk of transferable disease; zoonoses
- Animal health care work
- Exposure to animal excrement
- Cumulative trauma: noise and ergonomics
- Noise exposure
- Repetitive motions; especially hand and wrist
- Excessive stooping, kneeling, twisting
- Vibration exposure; especially with hand tools
- Heavy lifting

Elemental Exposure
- Ultraviolet rays
- Dust and molds
- Heat and cold
- Weather exposure: wind, lightning
- Electricity
- Silos, grain bins, manure pits
- Ponds, mud, ice
- Highway traffic while operating farm equipment

Physical Structures
- Lighting
- Ventilation; especially in silos
- Ladders

Farm Stress
- Weather-related; poor crop yield
- Financial uncertainty
- Fatigue
- Day care facilities rare, expensive

Source: Reed (2004).

Medical Care

Hospitals and emergency medical care are typically not readily accessible in rural areas near farms. The isolated nature of farms and ranches in our nation's rural areas creates difficult conditions for emergency medical service providers. Farmers and

TABLE 19.1

Personal Protective Equipment and Injury Prevention Objectives for Agricultural Workers

Objective	Health Hazard
Wear respiratory protection (dust masks, cartridge respirators, gas masks, air packs)	Dust, chemicals, gases, pesticides, fertilizers, mold, paint
Wear seat belts on farm machinery	Accidents such as roll-overs, collisions, falls
Wear helmets on all-terrain vehicles and when riding horses	Accidents such as roll-overs, thrown from horse, falls
Wear hard hats when performing construction work, trimming trees, repairing machinery, and doing other jobs with risk of head injury	Falling and/or airborne debris
Wear skin protection including sunscreen and sun safety hats (wide brim and neck protection)	Ultraviolet rays
Wear job-matched gloves, barrier creams, and rubber boots	Animal waste products, pesticides, fertilizers, everyday exposure
Wear hearing protection (acoustic earmuffs, earplugs)	Loud and continuous machinery and equipment noise
Use safety eyewear (safety glasses, goggles, face shields)	Chemicals, gases, pesticides, fertilizers, dust, airborne debris, other foreign particles
Keep hair away from machinery by keeping it tied back or under a cap	Power take-off devices and moving machine parts
Do not wear jewelry, scarves, dangling strings, and loose garments near machinery	
Wear safety shoes or boots with nonslip soles and heels	Wet, slippery working environment
Wear impervious garments (long-sleeved shirts, pants, coveralls) when working with irritating or toxic substances	Chemicals, gases, pesticides, fertilizers, paint
Practice safe ergonomics	Heavy lifting; overexertion; excessive stooping, kneeling, and squatting; repetitive hand and wrist work; vibrating tools

ranchers often work alone and may become entrapped, entangled, or disabled for hours before they receive medical attention.

Health Promotion Activities

Because of the multiple, varied, and serious hazards that exist in the farming community, the types of agricultural safety and health promotion activities are numerous. Box 19.3 provides a list of potential health promotion activities. Accessing and meeting with the farming community is not difficult. Nurses can reach farmers and ranchers by working with the following community partners:

- Local county extension office
- Farm Bureau committees and officers
- State Cooperative Extension Education and Research Service Office (CEERSO)
- Farm organizations
- Farm supply and equipment stores and dealerships
- County fair organizers
- Rural health care providers
- Public health department
- Churches
- Schools (Future Farmers of America, 4-H clubs)

B O X 19.3

AGRICULTURAL SAFETY AND HEALTH PROMOTION ACTIVITIES

- Work with local television and radio programs to feature spots on farm safety and health issues to promote safety throughout the year.
- Organize a safety field day for farmers and farm families that can be used to educate the whole family on farm safety and health issues.
- Organize and conduct a farm safety day camp for youth to educate the children in the community on a variety of hazards found on the farm.
- Make sure any local farm event or gathering has someone on the program speaking about a farm safety topic (e.g., combine safety, hazardous materials handling, respiratory protection, working in confined spaces). Develop a list of local events, desired topics, and possible speakers.
- National Farm Safety & Health Week is the third week of September, an opportunity for special events.
- Sponsor and promote a first responder program for farm families. Familiarize them with what to do in the event an injury occurs on the farm. Train them on farm hazards, how to turn equipment off, rescue procedures (grain entrapment, trenches, manure pit rescues), and how to summon help.
- Sponsor and promote a first aid and a CPR course for farm families in your community.
- Sponsor and promote a farm emergency response and rescue training class for emergency medical and rescue personnel in your community.
- Sponsor and promote a Defensive Driving Course for farm and rural residents in your community.
- Organize and promote a farm safety poster or coloring contest at your local grade school or community organization. Offer safety items, farm safety activity books, or coloring books as prizes.
- Work with local businesses to display farm safety and health posters and safety reminders throughout the year.
- Work with rural health professionals to provide free blood pressure and cholesterol testing at farm supply stores, equipment dealerships, etc.
- Develop a farm safety display and use it at farm field days, events and programs, county fairs, etc., to promote farm safety and health.

Source: National Safety Council (2009).

Small Business Employees

A small business is defined as a business that is independently owned and operated, is not dominant in its field of operation, and typically employs fewer than 100 workers. Of the approximately 6.5 million private industries operating in the United States, more than 6.3 million (98%) employ fewer than 100 employees, and more than 5.6 million (87%) employ fewer than 20 employees. Prevention of work-related illness and injury is often difficult in small businesses because they have few safety and health resources, cannot hire staff devoted to safety and health activities, and often lack the ability to identify occupational hazards as well as conduct periodic surveillance (NIOSH, 2009d). The best opportunity to prevent illness and injury in small business industries is for the owners, managers, and employees to identify and understand the hazards and risks that workers might encounter on the job.

In 1996, Congress passed the Small Business Regulatory Enforcement Fairness Act (SBREFA) to help small businesses incorporate health and safety prevention into their workplace. Under this act, the Occupational Safety and Health Administration

(U.S. Department of Labor, 2005) can help small businesses through a variety of tools, including partnership, consultation, compliance assistance, education and training, outreach, and plain language regulations:

Partnership: The Voluntary Protection Programs (VPP) identify worksites where employers and employees work well together to achieve safety and health excellence. Small firms can be partnered with and mentored by a VPP site that will share its experience and expertise on workplace health promotion programs.

Consultation: Small business owners may also request assistance from the OSHA Consultation Service, a program that provides on-site assistance in finding and fixing potential health and safety hazards before they occur. The consultation service offers workplace safety and health training and technical assistance. This service is completely separate from OSHA's inspection effort; no citations or penalties are issued. The employer's only obligation is to correct serious hazards.

Compliance assistance: Small business owners are to contact the OSHA area office closest to them and speak with a compliance specialist. That person can offer advice on training and educating employees on health and safety regulations. A list of offices by region can be found at http://www.osha.gov/html/RAmap.html.

Education and training: OSHA training education centers are located across the United States and provide basic and advanced courses in safety and health. The area offices offer information services such as audiovisual aids, technical advice, and speakers.

Outreach: Computer-based training software developed by OSHA, called *Expert Advisors*, is available on topics such as hazard communication, asbestos, cadmium, confined spaces, fire safety, and lead in construction.

Plain language regulations: A variety of electronic and print materials are available on the OSHA standards, interpretations, directives, compliance assistance materials, and topics specific to small businesses. Additionally, the U.S. Small Business Administration's (SBA) Small Business Development Centers have opened across the country. There are a total of 1,000 centers, with at least one center in every state. These centers provide services to small businesses that include health and safety.

Telecommuting Employees

Telecommuting is a work agreement that allows an employee to perform assigned duties at an alternative site, usually home, during some or all of his or her scheduled work hours. It is a managerial option and not an employee benefit or right, and must conform to all state laws and regulations regarding state employment. Approximately 15% of the total U.S. workforce, 19.8 million Americans, regularly works from home at some point during the work week.

The Occupational Safety and Health Act (OSHA) does not require inspections of home offices and does not hold employers responsible for injuries sustained while employees are working from home except if an employee is injured while working with job-related hazardous materials. However, because OSHA still requires employers to record all workplace injuries and illnesses, including those that occur in home offices, employers should require telecommuters to immediately report any incident that does occur. Workers' compensation carriers typically will cover occupational injuries that occur in home offices.

Employers are recognizing they have a tremendous investment in their telecommuters' home offices, not only from the standpoint of the equipment the employer might own in those remote locations, but also in terms of safety and security issues. More and more workplaces will develop telecommuting employee guidelines to promote health as well as conduct home visits to promote safety.

The following points should be part of a health and safety checklist for the telecommuter worksite:

- The telecommuter must have a dedicated work space, preferably a room with a door that can be shut or locked, because most alternative work sites are in the employee's home. The space should be large enough to accommodate the office equipment so that the worker can move freely without fear of tripping or falling.
- The work space must have adequate power and power outlets to accommodate the necessary equipment. Power cords, tools, and equipment should be safely arranged and secured.
- The work area must be clean, safe, and free of obstructions and hazardous materials.
- The work area must have ergonomic lighting and seating.
- The employee's home must comply with all building codes, and health and safety requirements, including the presence of functioning smoke detectors.
- The work area has safeguards in place against loss or theft of the employer's proprietary data and equipment.
- The work area has reasonable safeguards in place to protect the confidentiality of matters related to the telecommuter's work.
- If a telecommuter incurs a work-related injury while telecommuting, worker's compensation law and rules apply. Employees must notify their supervisors immediately and complete all necessary or management-requested documents regarding the injury.

Adolescent Workers

Approximately 2.6 million workers aged 16 to 17 years are employed. Adolescent workers are employed primarily in food preparation and service jobs; stock handler or laborer jobs; administrative support jobs; and farming, forestry, or fishing jobs (NIOSH, 2009c). This population experienced an estimated 52,600 work-related injuries that required treatment in hospital emergency rooms and 38 work-related deaths in 2007. Most injuries (54%) to these young workers occur in the retail industry (e.g., restaurants, fast-food outlets, grocery stores). The service industry (e.g., health care settings, nursing homes) accounts for 20%, and agricultural employment accounts for 7% of work-related injuries. Most of these injuries are lacerations, burns, contusions or abrasions, strains, and sprains. The majority of work-related fatalities (42%) occur in agriculture, with one half of the victims being under age 15. The retail trade accounts for the second highest number of workplace fatalities, with 63% of these deaths caused by assaults and violent acts, most of which were homicides. Handling cash, working alone or in small numbers, and working in the late evening and early morning hours increases the risk for workplace homicide. Workers under age 18 also account for 45% of the fatal work-related injuries resulting from transportation incidents such as motor vehicle accidents. Operating a motor vehicle at work is prohibited for workers age 16 years or younger. Despite current restrictions, transportation-related fatalities and injuries continue to occur among teen workers.

The primary federal law governing the employment of workers under age 18 is the Fair Labor Standards Act (FLSA) of 1938 and applies to businesses with gross annual revenues of $500,000 or more. Some state laws extend coverage of child labor laws to all businesses regardless of revenues. However, no federal law covers children working on their parents' or guardians' farms. There are also special regulations that allow children to work in their family's business.

In designing health promotion activities for the adolescent worker, nurses need to partner with various groups and address the following issues (NIOSH, 2009c).

The Teen Workers

- All workers must participate in workplace training programs offered by the employer or request training if none is offered.
- All workplace hazards must be identified to the employees before completing a task.
- All workers have the right to work in a safe and healthy work environment free of recognized hazards.
- All workers have the right to refuse unsafe work tasks and conditions.
- All workers have the right to file complaints with the Department of Labor when rights have been violated or safety has been jeopardized.
- All workers are entitled to workers' compensation for work-related injury or illness.
- Know the child labor laws. Visit http://www.youthrules.dol.gov

Employers

- Assess and eliminate hazards in the workplace.
- Make sure equipment used is safe and legal.
- Provide training in hazard recognition and safe work practices.
- Have all young workers demonstrate they can perform assigned tasks safely and correctly.
- Ensure all young workers are appropriately supervised.
- Ensure all supervisors and adult coworkers are aware of tasks teen workers may or may not perform.
- Know and comply with state and federal child labor laws.
- Develop an injury and illness prevention program.

School Educators and Counselors

- Talk to students about workplace hazards and students' rights as workers.
- Ensure all school-based work programs include safety and health training.
- Incorporate worker safety and health into junior and senior high curricula.
- Know the state and federal child labor laws.

Parents

- Know the name, address, and phone number of the child's employer.
- Ask the child about work tasks and equipment used.
- Ask the child about training and supervision.
- Be alert for signs of fatigue or stress as the child tries to balance work, school, home, and extracurricular activities.
- Know the state and federal child labor laws.
- Report unsafe working conditions to the Department of Labor.

PROMOTING A NONVIOLENT WORKPLACE

Workplace violence has emerged as an important safety issue in today's workplace with almost 2 million nonfatal violent victimizations per year (38,000 per week) occurring against persons aged 12 years and older who were at work or on duty (U.S. Department of Labor, 2002). About 800 work-related homicides occur per year; about 15 per week (NIOSH, 2009b). Homicide at the worksite is the leading cause of death for female workers and the second cause of death for male workers. It is estimated that workplace violence contributes to 18% of all violent crime in the United States.

The Occupational Safety and Health Act of 1970 (OSHAct) (U.S. Department of Labor, 2009) General Duty Clause, Section 5 (a)(1), requires employers to provide a safe and healthful workplace for all workers covered by the OSHAct. Workplace violence-prevention strategies are currently being developed and tested. However, effective interventions are still lacking as community and public health care providers and researchers learn more about workplace violence.

Defining Workplace Violence

The study of workplace violence is in its infancy stage. A variety of definitions for workplace violence exist, including:

- According to the U.S. Department of Justice, workplace violence is "nonfatal violence in the workplace, rape and sexual assault, robbery, aggravated assault (with a weapon), and simple assault (without a weapon or injury requiring less than 2 days hospitalization)" (Duhart, 2001, p. 12).
- Physical assaults and threats of assault directed toward employees with two types of workplace violence: (1) coworker initiated violence; and (2) public initiated violence (LeBlanc & Kelloway, 2002).
- According to the Federal Bureau of Investigation (FBI), workplace violence is "a continuum that includes homicide, physical assault, domestic violence, stalking, threats, harassment, bullying, emotional abuse, intimidation, and other forms of conduct that create anxiety, fear, and a climate of distrust in the workplace" (Rugala, 2004, p. 12). The FBI identifies four subtypes of workplace violence:

Type 1: Committed by criminals who have no connection with workplace
Type 2: Committed by customers, clients, patients, students, inmates, etc.
Type 3: Committed by coworkers, supervisors, manager, present or former employee
Type 4: Committed by someone who does not work at workplace but has a personal relationship with an employee; intimate partner (Rugala, 2004).

The literature on workplace violence presents a continuum of workplace violence including the following, some of which are defined below:

- Incivility
- Workplace bullying
- Horizontal violence
- Harassment
- Verbal abuse
- Threats
- Physical assault

Incivility: The conscious or unconscious behavior that violates workplace norms of courtesy or respect toward others. It may be the subtle, rude, or disrespectful behavior that demonstrates lack of regard for other employees such as interrupting others without care, not listening, disrupting meetings, inappropriate behavior at meetings, speaking with condescending attitude, or using up supplies or breaking equipment without notifying anyone or asking for help (Pearson, Andersson, & Porath, 2004).

Workplace bullying: "Status-blind" interpersonal hostility that is deliberate, repeated, and sufficiently severe as to harm the targeted person's health or economic status. This type of bullying is driven by perpetrators' need to control another individual, often undermining legitimate business interests in the process (Namie, 2003).

Horizontal violence: Nonphysical interpersonal conflict that is manifested in overt and covert behaviors of hostility. This behavior is often associated with oppressed groups and can occur in any arena where there are unequal power relations, and where one group's self-expression and autonomy is controlled by forces with greater prestige, power, and status. Horizontal violence is also referred to as workplace aggression and can be manifested as passive aggression (nondirect, subtle, talking behind a colleague's back, withholding information needed to do a job, ignoring a colleague), or active aggression (criticizing, screaming, physical assault) (Duffy, 1995; Farrell, 2001).

Harassment: Defined as any unwelcome verbal, written, or physical conduct that either denigrates or shows hostility or aversion toward a person on the basis of race, color, national origin, age, sex, religion, disability, marital status, or pregnancy. Harassment can create an intimidating, hostile, or offensive work environment; interferes with an employee's work performance; and affects an employee's employment opportunities or compensation. See Box 19.4 for signs and symptoms of workplace violence.

Addressing Violence in the Workplace

Many companies have policies and procedures on how to address violence perpetrated by strangers, customers, family members, and patients. However, violence between coworkers, supervisors, and employees is rarely addressed by policies and procedures. Workplace policies are needed not only to address physical assault but also to define and address nonphysical aggression, bullying, and harassment. There are 10 steps a workplace can incorporate to prevent workplace violence:

1. Foster a supportive, harmonious work environment. Creating a culture of mutual respect can help reduce harassment and hostility.
2. Train supervisors and employees how to resolve conflicts. Conflict on the job can be reduced by developing employees' skills in negotiating, communicating effectively, team building, and resolving disputes.
3. Develop effective policies to protect employees from harassment. A company policy should clearly denounce harassment and state that it will not be tolerated.
4. Establish procedures for handling grievances. Employees need to be aware of the grievance procedures for reporting complaints of workplace violence and believe the procedures will be followed.
5. Provide personal counseling through an EAP. Family, marital, financial, and personal issues can have a profound impact on employees' work performance, as well as their interactions at work.
6. Implement security programs that protect employees. Security guards, identification badges, monitoring systems, preemployment screening, and safety awareness and training help to ensure safety in the workplace.
7. Provide employee safety education programs.

BOX 19.4

SIGNS AND SYMPTOMS OF WORKPLACE VIOLENCE

Employee Signs and Symptoms of Being a Victim of Workplace Bullying, Harassment, or Horizontal Violence
- Anxiety, excessive worry
- Loss of concentration
- Disrupted sleep
- Feeling edgy, irritable, easily startled, and constantly on guard
- Stress headaches, migraine headaches
- Increased heart rate
- Body aches in the muscles or joints
- Stress-related fatigue and exhaustion
- Diagnosed depression
- Significant weight change (loss or gain)
- Chronic fatigue syndrome
- Panic attacks
- TMJ (jaw tightening/teeth grinding)
- Skin changes (shingles, rashes, acne)
- Use of substances to cope: tobacco, alcohol, drugs, food
- Suicidal thoughts

Departmental Signs and Symptoms That Workplace Violence May be Present
- A disproportionate turnover rate higher than industry standards.
- A higher rate of absenteeism, paid time off, workers' compensation, or disability insurance claims.
- Employees request transfers from certain departments more than from others.
- A pattern of harassment complaints about particular individuals that do not meet eligibility requirements for illegal violations of civil rights or internal policies.
- When repeated complaints about particular individuals are investigated internally, witnesses routinely refute what the complainant saw, heard, or experienced.

8. Provide job counseling for employees who have been laid off or fired. Being laid off can be traumatic, and counseling and support services can help workers develop new skills and ways of coping.
9. Train supervisors how to recognize signs of a troubled employee. Supervisors can be trained on how to recognize signs and symptoms of a potentially violent employee, such as threatening behavior or preoccupation with violence.
10. Set up a crisis plan that addresses violent incidents.

Summary

This chapter discusses many strategies for promoting healthy partnerships with people at the worksite. As you plan worksite health promotion programs, also consider programs discussed in other chapters, such as healthy partnerships with faith communities and schools (remember, many employees have children). Most adults spend about one third of each day at the worksite. This time presents an excellent opportunity for promoting healthy lifestyles. Appendix A provides an occupational and environmental assessment guide.

Critical Thinking Questions

1. An occupational nurse at a chemical and mineral plant is interested in using the results of employee HRAs to assess the need for health promotion programs at this facility.

   a. How would you implement this plan? Identify two potential employee health risk areas and design an educational and screening program for employees to address the areas.

   b. How would you promote your ideas within management? How would you generate interest among the employees to participate in the prevention offerings?

   c. Discuss several potential barriers to the success of the health screenings. What steps could be taken to counteract the barriers? How would you case-manage the illness of an employee that was first diagnosed during the health screening? What data would you need to evaluate the success of your program?

2. Think of where you live and answer the following questions. How many farms are in your area? What kind of farms are they? What do they produce? What types of machinery do they use? What kinds of chemicals do they use? When are the peak times of farm work? How many people live on a typical farm? How many people work on a typical farm? How many hours per week do they work? Are there any children living or working on the farm? How old are the children? In what types of farm activities do the children participate? What type of schooling do the children receive? What type of health coverage or insurance do the farmers have? Are immunizations current for children and adults? Does anyone have any chronic health problems? Are any existing health conditions exacerbated by farming? What types of recreational and social activities exist? Do the farmers go on vacation? How do the farmers learn about new agricultural information and technology? What other questions would you ask the farmers?

● REFERENCES

American Association of Occupational Health Nurses. (2008). The occupational and environmental health nursing profession. Retrieved May 1, 2009, from http://www.aaohn.org/press_room/fact_sheets/upload/OHN_Profession_2008.pdf

Azevedo, M. A. (2005). MEDeCOACH takes off with first customers. Retrieved May 1, 2009, from http://buffalo.bizjournals.com/industries/business_services/employee_compensation_benefits/2005/07/11/houston_daily50.html

Coker, A. L. (2005). Opportunities for prevention: Addressing IPV in the health care setting. *Family Violence Prevention and Health Practice, 1*, 1–9.

Duffy, E. (1995). Horizontal violence: A conundrum for nursing. *The Collegian, Journal of the Royal College of Nursing, 2*(2), 5–17.

Duhart, D. T. (2001). Violence in the workplace 1993–99. U.S. Department of Justice, NCJ 190076. Retrieved May 1, 2009, from http://www.ojp.usdoj.gov/bjs/pub/pdf/vw99.pdf

Farrell, G. A. (2001). From tall poppies to squashed weeds: Why don't nurses pull together more? *Journal of Advanced Nursing, 35*(1), 26–33.

Goetzel, R., Roemer, E., Liss-Levinson, R., & Samoly, D. (2008). Workplace health promotion: Policy recommendations that encourage employers to support health improvement programs for their workers. Retrieved May 1, 2009, from http://www.prevent.org/images/stories/PolicyPapers/worksite%20health.pdf

LeBlanc, M. M., & Kelloway, E. K. (2002). Predictors and outcomes of workplace violence and aggression. *Journal of Applied Psychology, 87*(3), 444–453.

Namie, G. (2003). Workplace bullying: Escalated incivility. *Ivey Business Journal*, November/December, 1–6. Retrieved July 25, 2005, from http://www. iveybusinessjournal.com/view_article.asp?intArticle_ID=449

National Institute for Occupational Safety and Health. (2009a). Childhood agricultural injury prevention initiative. Retrieved May 1, 2009, from http://www.cdc.gov/niosh/childag/

National Institute for Occupational Safety and Health. (2009b). Occupational violence. Retrieved May 1, 2009, from http://www.cdc.gov/niosh/topics/violence/

National Institute for Occupational Safety and Health. (2009c). Young worker safety and health. Retrieved May 1, 2009, from http://www.cdc.gov/niosh/topics/youth/#keyresources

National Institute for Occupational Safety and Health. (2009d). Safety and health resource guide for small businesses. Retrieved May 1, 2009, from http://www.cdc.gov/niosh/docs/2003-100/default.html

National Safety Council. (2009). Agriculture safety. Retrieved May 1, 2009, from http://www.nsc.org/resources/issues/agrisafe.aspx

Pearson, C. M., Andersson, L. A., & Porath, C. L. (2004). Workplace incivility. In P. Spector & S. Fox (Eds.). *Counterproductive workplace behavior: Investigations of actors and targets* (pp. 256–309). Washington, DC: American Psychological Association.

Pender, N. (1996). *Health promotion in nursing practice* (3rd ed.). Los Altos, CA: Appleton & Lange.

Prochaska, J. O., & DiClemente, C. C. (1983). Protection motivation theory and preventive health: Beyond the health belief model. *Health Education Research: Theory and Practice, 1*(3), 153–161.

Reed, D. B. (2004). The risky business of production agriculture: Health and safety for farm workers. *AAOHN Journal, 52*(9), 401–409.

Rugala, E. A. (2004). Workplace violence: Issues in response. Retrieved May 1, 2009, from http://www.fbi.gov/publications/violence.pdf

U.S. Department of Labor, Occupational Safety and Health Administration. (2002). Workplace violence: OSHA fact sheet. Retrieved May 1, 2009, from http://www.osha.gov/OshDoc/data_General_Facts/factsheet-workplace-violence.pdf

U.S. Department of Labor, Occupational Safety and Health Administration. (2005). Q's and A's for small business employers. Retrieved May 1, 2009, from http://www.osha.gov/Publications/OSHA3163/osha3163.html

U.S. Department of Labor, Occupational Safety and Health Administration. (2006). All about OSHA. Retrieved May 1, 2009, from http://www.osha.gov/Publications/all_about_OSHA.pdf

U.S. Department of Labor, Occupational Safety and Health Administration. (2009). General duty clause. Retrieved May 1, 2009, from http://www.osha.gov/pls/oshaweb/owadisp.show_document?p_table=OSHACT&p_id=3359

Internet Resources can be found on the**Point** at http://thepoint.lww.com/Anderson6e.

Promoting Healthy Partnerships With Community Elders

SHIRLEY F. HUTCHINSON

LEARNING OBJECTIVES

After studying this chapter, you should be able to:

1. Discuss selected health and social factors that impact health status and functional ability of the elderly.
2. Differentiate between individual- and community-based health promotion strategies.
3. Design and implement a health promotion initiative for community elders.

Introduction

*I*mprovements in medicine, science, public health, and technology have enabled older populations to live longer and healthier lives than prior generations. As society anticipates the aging of the "baby boom" population, tremendous challenges of health promotion for elders confront society. Most health care providers agree that a major concern is assisting the elderly to live healthy, independent, and productive lives in their communities. The needs of community elders are as diverse and multifaceted as the elders themselves. Building communities in which elders can live satisfying lives requires a thorough understanding of the issues facing elders as they try to maintain their independence. Elderly populations no longer want to accept disability and chronic illness as inevitable. Health promotion and disease prevention activities are an increasing priority for older adults, their families, and the health care system. This chapter focuses on developing individual-focused as well as community-based health promotion strategies and partnerships with noninstitutionalized elders. The terms *elderly, older adults, aging,* and *senior citizens* are used interchangeably to denote people aged 65 years and older.

DEMOGRAPHICS OF AGING IN THE UNITED STATES

The older population, aged 65 years and above, numbered 37.3 million in 2006, representing 12.4% of the total U.S. population (Administration on Aging [AoA], 2007a). The percentage of older Americans has more than tripled from that in 1900

(4.1%), and the number has increased more than 11 times (from 3.1 million to 37.3 million). A child born in 2004 could expect to live 77.9 years compared to about 29 years in 1900 (Administration on Aging [AoA], 2007a). This phenomenal growth has occurred as a result of reduced mortality rates of children and young adults. However, reduced death rates have occurred in the 65 to 84 age group. By 2030, the older population will more than double to 71.5 million and the over-85 population is projected to increase from 5.3 million in 2006 to 8.9 million (Administration on Aging [AoA], 2007a). Moreover, it is predicted that there will be as many people over age 65 years as there are people under 20. Of special note, the fastest-growing population of older Americans is the 85 years and older group. The older population will grow significantly between 2010 and 2030 as "baby boomers" (those born during America's post-World War II population explosion, beginning in 1946) begin to turn 65 years old (Administration on Aging [AoA], 2007a). Aging represents a challenge around the world. Rapidly expanding numbers of very old people around the world represent a social phenomenon that is without precedent. It is projected that by 2025 Asia will be home to 58% of the world's 60+ population (AARP International, 2009b).

HEALTH CHALLENGES, RISK FACTORS, AND CONCERNS OF ELDERS

Health Status

Morbidity and mortality patterns of the elderly generally follow patterns of the population as a whole, with cardiovascular disease and cancer as the leading causes of death. The majority of older persons have at least one chronic condition and many have multiple conditions. In 2004 and 2005, the most frequently occurring conditions of the elderly included hypertension (48%); diagnosed arthritis (47%); all types of heart disease (29%); any cancer (20%); diabetes (16%); and sinusitis (14%) (Administration on Aging [AoA], 2007b). In 2006, 39% of noninstitutionalized elderly assessed their health as excellent or very good, compared to 65.1% for persons aged 18 to 64 (AoA, 2007b). Elderly persons also have to cope with disabilities and activity limitations. In 2002, 52% of the older population reported having at least one disability, and over one third reported at least one severe disability. The percentage of disabilities increases with age (AoA, 2007b). As the percentage of elderly people 85 years and older grows, so will the severity and number of chronic illnesses and disabling conditions. Because chronic illness is often related to frailty in the elderly, creative, multidisciplinary approaches to chronic illness management will be needed to optimize independence and functional ability.

Access to Health Care

Accessibility and affordability of health care are challenges for the elderly, particularly for rural and poor elders. Many have not adequately planned for the medical expenses that often accompany the chronic illnesses common among older adults. Access to preventive services is often limited for the elderly. Medicare, the primary health insurance for older adults, offers very little coverage for health promotion and preventive services. Medicare coverage is often poorly understood, sometimes leaving elders paying for services that are covered by Medicare. Additionally, Medicare has many necessary health-related costs, such as prescription drugs and dental care that are not covered by Parts A or B. The elderly are among the greatest consumers of prescription drugs, many times paying for them out of pocket. With the passage of the Medicare Prescription Improvement and Modernization Act of 2003 (P.L. 108-173), eligible persons 65 and older now have access to a variety of prescription drug plans. While there are numerous Medicare Supplemental insurance plans available for purchase, many Medicare beneficiaries are unable to afford the cost of the premiums. Although state Medicaid programs provide coverage for some low-income older people, stringent eligibility requirements leave many without access to Medicaid health insurance. Although older adults have health needs that require a range of services on a continuum, not all services on the continuum are available to older adults in a variety of settings, leading to potential fragmentation of care.

Preventive services for the elderly are often neglected, because many providers do not see any point in prevention during the last years on the age continuum. A related issue is the recruitment and training of health professionals to provide medical and health care for seniors. Until the mid-1970s, medical schools placed little emphasis on geriatrics (Gelfand, 2006). However, professional nursing has been at the forefront in educating advance practice nurses in gerontology and adult nursing, as well as incorporating courses on aging in nursing curricula.

Alternative forms of health care, such as acupuncture and herbal medicine, may not be covered by insurance plans. Medicare Managed Care (Medicare Advantage Plans) is now available to older people, as is Medicare supplemental insurance, which provides coverage for certain services that are not covered by Medicare. Elderly populations often need guidance in selecting Medicare supplement plans that can best meet their needs.

Transportation is another issue that impacts access to health care by the elderly, and rural elderly are hit hardest by lack of transportation. Elderly people often rely on friends; family members; lay taxi drivers (people who use private cars and often charge high fees); church volunteers; public transportation; and other forms of community-sponsored transportation to access health services. Nurses can play a key role during debates on Medicare and Social Security reform by promoting health care coverage not only to prevent illness, but also to keep older Americans from losing their savings as they try to pay for health care and, consequently, fall into poverty or sink deeper, if already poor.

Elder Abuse

As functional status and sensory acuity begin to decline, the elderly become vulnerable to an assortment of abusive and neglectful situations. Elder abuse is an umbrella term referring to any knowing, intentional, or negligent act by a caregiver or any other person that causes harm or a serious risk of harm to a vulnerable population. According to the National Aging Information Center (NAIC, 1998), there are three basic categories of abuse: domestic, institutional, and self-neglect. Domestic elder abuse refers to the maltreatment of an older person residing in his or her own home or the home of a caregiver. Institutional abuse occurs in residential facilities. Self-neglect refers to neglect inflicted when the safety or health of older people is threatened by their living alone. Elder abuse may take the form of physical abuse, sexual abuse, emotional or psychological abuse, financial exploitation, neglect by caregiver, self-neglect (as noted above), or abandonment.

In a 2004 survey of State Adult Protective Services agencies, the National Center on Elder Abuse found a 15.6% increase in substantiated elder abuse cases from 2000 to 2004. In 20 of the states 43% of the victims were age 80 or older

(National Center on Elder Abuse [NCEA], undated). However, because elder abuse and neglect are largely hidden under the shroud of family secrecy, it is grossly underreported.

Mistreated elders are often frail, dependent, over age 70, and women. Typically, family members, not strangers, inflict abuse on elders. Elders who were abusive parents themselves are at higher risk of abuse. Elder abuse and neglect encompass a variety of events that harm older people, including trauma; swindling and fraud; unattended medical problems; poor hygiene; dehydration; malnourishment; battering; verbal abuse; forced confinement; and other types of mistreatment at the hands of family members, neighbors, and caregivers. Resolving abusive situations may require involvement of protective agencies as well as law enforcement. Community nurses need to be familiar with state abuse reporting laws and how to work with state adult protective services agencies.

Community Safety and Fear of Violence

Many community-dwelling elders are virtually prisoners in their homes because they fear becoming victims of muggings, break-ins, rapes, robberies, and scams. Rates of crime perpetrated against the elderly are different from those perpetrated against younger people. People older than 65 years are more likely to be victims of crime in or near their own homes because elderly people often lack access to transportation and do not travel great distances. The elderly are more vulnerable to crime. Due to declining physical strength to protect themselves, elderly people, especially women living alone, are easy prey for criminal victimization. Therefore, few venture outside and many take extraordinary measures to barricade themselves into their homes. This fear is compounded for the elderly poor who live in high-crime neighborhoods. The impact of criminal victimization is more devastating for the elderly than for younger adults. A low or fixed income makes it difficult for many older people to recoup from a robbery. These elderly often live in aging neighborhoods that are undergoing change and economic decline (Gelfand, 2006). Fear for their safety can be a deterrent to elderly people engaging in walking as a form of exercise. This fear can also cause social isolation. Community health nurses can facilitate neighborhood safety campaigns, such as crime watch programs.

Mental Health and Mental Wellness Challenges

Mental health is an important aspect of healthy aging. Ostir, Ottenbacher, and Markides (2004) found a link between positive emotions and frailty. They concluded that a positive outlook on life can help protect against physical and functional decline. Ostir, Berges, Ottenbaccher, Clow, and Ottenbacher (2008) further demonstrated that positive emotion is associated with gains in functional status after stroke. Mental health issues faced by the elderly include social isolation and loneliness, depression, suicide, and alcohol addiction. Tremendous loss and role transition are associated with old age, including retirement, death of friends and loved ones, loss of vitality and energy due to illness or disability, and, in many cases, less contact with children and grandchildren who may live in a different city or state. Social isolation is associated with the very old (aged 85 and older), those in frail health, and the elderly living alone.

Depression is a common problem many elders encounter as they experience health and psychosocial changes. Estimates of depression in older adults living in the community range from less than 1% to 5%, but the estimates rise to 13% for those receiving home health care and 11.5% for elderly hospital patients (National Institute of Mental Health [NIMH], 2008). Older adults are disproportionately likely to die by suicide. In 2004, people age 65 and older accounted for 16% of suicide deaths although they comprised only 12% of the population. Non-Hispanic white men age 85 and older were most likely to die by suicide (NIMH, 2008). Community health nurses and other health care providers need to be aware of the signs and symptoms of elderly depression and suicidal tendencies. A number of depression scales are available for assessing levels of depression in elderly clients. Anxiety symptoms (feeling fearful, tense/keyed-up, or shaky/nervous) have been found to be common among depressed and nondepressed older persons (Mehta et al., 2003). Additionally, anxiety has been observed to be a significant risk factor for the progression of disability in older women (Brenes et al., 2005).

Accidents

Falls are the most common accidents experienced by people over age 70. It is estimated that about two thirds of falls among the elderly are preventable. Whereas a fall in a younger person may not be problematic, a fall by an older person can have devastating results. Common risk factors for falls include use of medications or alcohol, poor physical condition, changes in visual acuity, inner ear disturbance, foot problems, gait and balance disorders, and hazards in the home and community. The presence of osteoporosis increases the likelihood of a broken bone when a fall occurs, particularly in women.

Several risk assessment tools for falls have been developed and are widely available. Scores can be calculated and reviewed with elders to plan fall-prevention strategies. Older adults are also at risk for accidental injury related to driving, fires, overmedication, and hypo- or hyperthermia. Decreased sensory acuity, impaired balance, decreased muscle strength, and decreased reaction time can diminish the ability of elderly people to interpret their environment. Community health nurses are in an excellent position to facilitate communitywide, as well as individual, injury prevention programs that target the elderly.

Disasters and the Elderly

Natural or human-made disasters, such as hurricanes and bioterrorism, can have a devastating effect on elderly populations. The terrorist acts that occurred on September 11, 2001, and the multiple large-scale weather disasters, such as hurricane Katrina, that have occurred during the past decade have heightened awareness of the special needs of elderly populations. Roughly 71% of the Hurricane Katrina deaths in Louisiana were among persons older than 60. Older persons are likely to be disproportionately vulnerable during disasters because they are more likely to have chronic illnesses; functional limitations; and sensory, physical, and cognitive disabilities than are younger persons (American Association of Retired Persons [AARP], 2006). Many elderly live alone and on limited incomes, making it nearly impossible to recover from a disaster without special assistance. The elderly are often slow to request help and are unlikely to follow through on a request. Additionally, they may have high nutritional needs, forget to take medicines, and become victims of fraudulent contractors. Recognizing the special needs of elderly populations during a disaster, the U.S. Congress passed the Older American Act, authorizing the AoA to provide assistance for the elderly through state agencies.

HEALTHY PEOPLE 2020 AND OLDER ADULTS

Healthy People 2020 provides science-based, 10-year national objectives for promoting health and preventing disease. Healthy People 2020 goals and objectives are due to be released in final form in 2010. When planning health education and health promotion programs for community elders, community nurses should incorporate priority areas and specific objectives addressed in Healthy People 2020. To stay informed, individuals can subscribe to Healthy People Listserv (http://www.healthypeople.gov/HP2020/).

Health Promotion and Health Protection Strategies for Community Elders

Health promotion and health protection are two elements of primary prevention. Health promotion denotes emphasis on helping people change their lifestyles and move toward a state of optimal health, whereas health protection focuses on protecting people from disease and injury by providing immunizations and reducing exposure to carcinogens, toxins, and environmental health hazards. The concept of health for the elderly must be revisited in planning health promotion interventions. Filner and Williams (1979) define health for the elderly as the ability to live and function effectively in society and to exercise self-reliance and autonomy to the maximum extent feasible, but not necessarily as freedom from disease. Messecar (2002) found that older people themselves define health as going and doing something meaningful, which consists of four components: (1) something worthwhile and desirable to do; (2) balance between abilities and challenges; (3) appropriate external resources; and (4) personal attitudinal characteristics. More than any other age group, older Americans are actively seeking health information and are willing to make changes to maintain their health and independence. Health promotion efforts should focus on modifiable risk behaviors, matched to the leading health problems by age (U.S. Department of Commerce, 2002). Hahn (2003) interviewed older ethnic women attending a senior center and found that they defined *healthy* as being able to perform meaningful activities, which in turn keep them healthy. It is evident from these views of health that health care goals for elderly persons must focus on improving functional ability, maintaining independence, and helping them find meaningful activities in life. To maximize health promotion for community elders, a multifaceted approach is needed. Interventions should target individuals and families as well as groups and communities.

Individual- or Family-Focused Interventions

Individual- or family-focused health promotion/health protection interventions are designed to increase the individual's or family's knowledge, skills, and competence to make health decisions that maximize health-promoting and health-protecting behaviors. The goal is empowerment of the elderly and their families to make rational health decisions. Some categories of health promotion and health protection intervention that target the individual and/or family are:

- Health screenings
- Lifestyle modification
- Health education (one-to-one or group)
- Counseling
- Support groups

- Primary health care
- Immunizations
- Home safety
- In-home care (home health, personal care, or household assistance)
- Home-delivered meals
- Social support (telephone reassurance and home visiting)
- Case management
- Home maintenance help

Community-Focused Interventions

Community-focused interventions are activities and programs that are directed toward community elders as a whole or various elderly subgroups in a community. The goal of community-focused interventions is to improve community capacity and availability of the appropriate mix of health and social services required to prolong independence and functional status of community elders. Interventions at the community level primarily involve advocacy, political action, and participation in policy making that affects community elders. Examples of community-focused interventions are:

- Communitywide health educational campaigns that emphasize older people
- Holding campaigns in May, which is designated as "Older American Month"
- Community coalitions to address specific elderly issues, such as development of local information centers, telephone hotlines, or Internet sites
- Political involvement to advocate for needs of the elderly, such as preserving or expanding Medicare coverage for in-home services
- Collaboration with universities, churches, senior centers, senior housing projects, and other established community organizations to provide comprehensive services to subgroups of elders
- Crime prevention activities
- Participation in community-based health fairs.

PARTNERSHIPS WITH COMMUNITY ELDERS

Elderly populations, in general, are open to new health practices and respond to a variety of approaches that have the potential to improve their health. To plan effective health programs, community health nurses should validate proposed goals and strategies with the targeted elderly group. Involving elders in planning health promotion and disease prevention activities is essential because older people are sensitive to potential loss of independence, and involving them increases a sense of independence. Action steps for working with older adults in the community include:

- Plan programs where elders usually congregate, such as churches, senior centers, and retirement centers.
- Incorporate outreach activities into all programs.
- Be prepared to offer transportation to group activities.
- Anticipate needs of those with poor vision (e.g., use large print, limit handouts, use a quiet room or loudspeakers).
- Maintain a slow pace for activities and allow adequate time for responses.
- Allow plenty of time for elders to share life experiences.
- Keep teaching sessions relatively short.

- Incorporate multiple repetitions and reinforcement of information.
- Structure health education activities so the elderly feel comfortable asking questions or challenging information that is new or doubtful to them.
- Encourage the involvement of families, friends, and significant others.
- Advocate for improvements in community resources and policies that affect the elderly.
- The following sections discuss selected health promotion and health protection needs of community elders.

Health Services

People over age 65 need regular primary health care services to maintain health and prevent disabling chronic illness and life-threatening conditions. Health promotion services that can form the basis for a community nursing intervention include:

- Immunizations (influenza, diphtheria, tetanus, pneumococcal vaccine)
- Screening for chronic illnesses, such as cancers, cardiovascular disease, and diabetes
- Management and control of existing chronic illnesses (health education, case management, and medication management)
- Knowledge of coverage and reimbursement practices (including alternative medicine) of Medicare/Medicare Managed Care, Medicare supplemental insurance, and specific state health insurance programs
- Community outreach and advocacy efforts to ensure linkage of elderly people to needed resources, such as health advocates, health coaches, and community gatekeepers
- Referral to existing state pharmacy assistance programs and advocacy to establish such programs where they are needed
- Education and outreach related to the Medicare Prescription Drug, Improvement and Modernization Act of 2003
- Education on medication management (scheduling, adherence, calendars, and so forth)
- Continuous source of primary care
- One-stop shopping for health care
- Connection to chronic illness support groups.

Nutrition

Adequate nutrition is important for older adults to maintain health, prevent disease, and slow down progression of existing chronic illnesses. To help the elderly improve or maintain nutritional status, it may be helpful to perform a nutritional assessment and build on existing strengths. An excellent tool that is readily available is the Nutrition Screening Checklist developed by the American Academy of Family Physicians, American Dietetic Association, and the National Council on Aging (Nutrition Screening Initiative, 1992).

Consider a nutritional health partnership program called *"Eating Healthy, Deliciously!"* Plan a class or a series of nutrition classes that focuses on basic nutrition as well as risk management nutrition (less salt, less fat, less sugar, more fiber, and so on). If special diet needs are to be covered, consider a series of classes and stratify the group according to specific dietary needs. Nutrition classes are more effective if they are highly interactive—incorporate recipe tasting and recipe sharing, build on existing positive habits, and include ethnic food preferences. Use of colorful, large-print posters and videos is appropriate. Reinforcing handouts are also helpful. Remember, many elderly people like to talk and share their experiences! Provide rewards for class attendance, such as canned goods, paper towels, macaroni, and other nonperishable, healthy food items. Enlist support of grocery stores for gifts. A major challenge is to get older people to attend these classes. Consider asking someone from the community or peer group to help with marketing and outreach.

Exercise and Fitness

The benefits of exercise are well established across the life span. Exercise activity for elders must be suitable to health and functional status. Brach, Simonsick, Kritchevsky, and Newman (2004) found that older adults who participate in 20 to 30 minutes of moderate-intensity exercise on most days of the week have better physical function than older persons who are active throughout the day or who are inactive. The following story offers a program idea for increasing exercise fitness.

While conducting a blood pressure screening clinic at a senior nutrition center, a nurse observed that the residents often arrive at the site around 8 AM. Their time was spent sitting until lunch was served at noon. A few played table games such as cards or dominoes, but there was little physical activity. While checking blood pressures, the nurse asked about physical activity and determined that most of them did not feel safe walking in their neighborhood, nor did they know of other forms of exercise. After validating the need for low-impact, chair-type exercise, a program was developed and several of the participants were trained as exercise leaders. The program was titled "Sitting Down, but Kicking High: Exercise for Seniors." Under leadership of lay exercise leaders, the program was eventually incorporated into the daily activity schedule.

Fall Prevention

As described earlier in the chapter, falls among the elderly are a major concern. You may want to team up with occupational therapists and physical therapists to conduct a fall prevention class or classes at a location where elderly people normally congregate (of course, you probably will not impact the elderly needing this class the most; they are at home because of fear of falling if they go out). Some can administer a fall assessment questionnaire, some can perform balance testing, some can demonstrate ways to prevent falls, and still others can provide individualized counseling regarding fall hazards. This collaborative, multidisciplinary project can have tremendous impact on a problem that sometimes costs the elderly their independence or even causes death. You will need to market the project and obtain space for all screening, balance testing, demonstrations, and counseling. Consider having waiver and consent forms for balance testing in the event of an accidental fall.

Community Safety

To reduce fear of violence that often haunts older people, community nurses need to work with local law enforcement agencies to develop community programs. Prototype programs include Neighborhood Crime Watch Programs, Citizens on Patrol, and other civic organization safety programs. Elders need education regarding physical and psychological self-defense programs. Population-based media campaigns should concentrate on making elders aware of their vulnerability to specific types of crimes in the community, including frequency and time of day of occurrence. Additionally, direct deposit of monthly checks should be encouraged to decrease vulnerability to violence.

Driving Safety

As the percentage of older adults in America increases, so does the number of older drivers. It is recommended that older drivers relearn to drive to accommodate neuromuscular and sensory changes that occur with aging. Older drivers should be encouraged to periodically reevaluate driving ability, including vision and hearing checkups, and evaluation of other physical changes that might affect driving. Encourage elders to ask family and friends if there are concerns about their driving ability. The AARP sponsors driver safety programs for elders to help older motorists improve driving skills, prevent car crashes, avoid traffic violations, and determine when to stop driving (AARP, 2009a). Older drivers should be referred to these resources or others that exist in the local community.

SIGNIFICANT LEGISLATION FOR OLDER AMERICANS

Finally, some important pieces of legislation merit discussion. Two important pieces of legislation that impact the lives of older Americans are the Social Security Act of 1935 and the Older Americans Act (OAA) of 1965. The Social Security Act mandated many programs to serve the elderly, including income assistance and health care. The main provisions included establishing a system of old-age benefits and enabling states to make provisions for blind people, aged people, and dependent and crippled children. The act established a Social Security Board and mechanisms for raising money for retirement income and welfare benefits. One of the most significant amendments came in 1965 and established Medicare and Medicaid health insurance programs. The OAA gave national attention to the needs of the elderly and authorized the Administration on Aging within the Department of Health and Human Services. It funded research and training in gerontology and facilitated local, state, and national programs to improve the quality of life of the elderly. Over the years, it has established many services for senior citizens, including area agencies on aging, multipurpose senior centers, nutrition services, volunteer programs, health education, transportation services, in-home health care, and preventive health activities.

Other legislation that helped to improve the quality of life for the elderly includes the Age Discrimination Act of 1974, which prevented age discrimination in employment and prevented forced retirement; the Research on Aging Act of 1974, which created the National Institute of Aging in the National Institutes of Health; and the American Disabilities Act of 1990, which ensured the rights of Americans with disabilities. More recently, the Medicare Prescription Drug Improvement and Modernization Act of 2003 requires the Social Security Administration to implement a plan to make prescription drugs more affordable for Medicare beneficiaries who qualify for the program.

Summary

Promoting healthy partnerships with community elders is an exciting venture. A comprehensive paradigm of health for the elderly, including social and environmental health, is needed. The aging population is creating tremendous opportunities for community health nurses to provide innovative, evidence-based health promotion services for the elderly population. The focus of health care for this group will continue to shift from acute medical care to self-care, chronic illness management, and services that promote independence. Additionally, health promotion strategies will emphasize quality-of-life issues as more of the elderly are expected to experience a high level of functioning well into their 80s and 90s. Community health nurses have an opportunity to develop innovative approaches to improving quality of life for elders through advocacy and service delivery.

Critical Thinking Questions

1. What impact does health promotion in younger years have on health status and functioning in older years?

2. If frail elders residing in their homes are provided "lay case management" (such as a health advocate or health coach who calls or visits in-home periodically, supervised by professional nurses), will they experience longer independent living, better health functioning, fewer falls, and fewer hospitalizations than frail elderly who do not get such support?

3. What is the appropriate mix of health and social services that can be provided through senior centers? Are such centers cost-effective?

4. Assume that you have been asked to assess the needs of the elderly population in your community. Outline the specific data that you would collect. Describe how you would collect the data.

5. Visit a senior center and ask a sample of the participants the following question: "What does being healthy mean to you?" Compare the answers to the World Health Organization's definition of health.

6. Conduct an Internet search of innovative, evidence-based health promotion programs for elderly noninstitutionalized populations. Discuss how such programs could be implemented in the local community.

● References

Administration on Aging. (2007a). AoA programs. Retrieved January 29, 2009, from http://www.aoa.gov/prof/aoaprog/aoa_programs.asp

Administration on Aging. (2007b). A profile of older Americans: 2007. Retrieved January 29, 2009, from http://www.aoa.gov/prof/Statistics/profile/2007/3.aspx.

American Association of Retired Persons (AARP). (2006). We can do better: Lessons learned for protecting older persons in disasters. Retrieved February 14, 2009 from http://www.aarp.org/research/assistance/lowincome/better.html

American Association of Retired Persons (AARP). (2009a). Driver Safety. Retrieved February 10, 2009, from http://www.aarp.org/families/driver_safety/

American Association of Retired Persons (AARP) International. (2009b). Growing old and less secure: Executive summary. Retrieved February 13, 2009 from http://www.aarpinternational.org

Brach, J. S., Simonsick, E. M., Kritchevsky, S., & Newman, A. B. (2004). The association between physical function and lifestyle activity and exercise in the health, aging, and body composition study. *Journal of the American Geriatrics Society, 52*(4), 502–509.

Brenes, G. A., Guralnik, J. M., Williamson, J. D., et al. (2005). The influence of anxiety on the progression of disability. *Journal of the American Geriatrics Society, 53*(1), 34–39.

Filner, B., & Williams, T. (1979). Health promotion for the elderly: Reducing functional dependency. In *Healthy People 2000*. Washington, DC: U.S. Government Printing Office.

Gelfand, D. E. (2006). *The aging network: Programs and services* (6th ed.). New York: Springer.

Hahn, K. (2003). Older ethnic women in faith communities; Culturally appropriate program planning. *Journal of Gerontological Nursing, 29*(7), 5–12.

Mehta, K. M., Simonsick, E. M., Penninx, B. W. J., et al. (2003). Prevalence and correlates of anxiety symptoms in well-functioning older adults: Findings from the health aging and body composition study. *Journal of the American Geriatrics Society, 5*(14), 499–504.

Messecar, D. C. (2002). Older people perceived health as going and doing something meaningful. *Evidence-Based Nursing, 5*(3), 96.

National Aging Information Center (NAIC). (1998). *Elder abuse prevention.* Washington, DC: U.S. Government Printing Office.

National Center on Elder Abuse (NCEA). (undated). The scope of elder abuse. Retrieved January 29, 2009 from http://www.ncea.aoa.gov

National Institute of Mental Health (NIMH). (2008). Older adults: Depression and suicide facts. Retrieved February 13, 2009 from http://www.nimh.nih.gov

Nutrition Screening Initiative. (1992). *Nutrition screening checklist.* A cooperative effort of the American Dietetic Association, American Academy of Family Physicians, and the National Council on Aging. Available at http://www.aafp.org/x16138.xml

Ostir, G. V., Berges, I., Ottenbaccher, M. E., Clow, A., & Ottenbacher, K. J. (2008). Associations between positive emotion and recovery of functional status following stroke. *Psychosomatic Medicine, 70*(4), 404–409.

Ostir, G. V., Ottenbacher, K. J., & Markides, K. S. (2004). Onset of frailty in older adults and the protective role of positive affect. *Psychology of Aging, 19*(3), 402–408.

U.S. Department of Commerce. (2002). An aging world. United Nations Department of Public Information, DP/2264, March.

Internet Resources can be found on the**Point**⁎ at http://thepoint.lww.com/Anderson6e.

Promoting Healthy Partnerships With Rural Communities

DAVID HARTLEY

LEARNING OBJECTIVES

After studying this chapter, you should be able to:

1. Identify health behaviors and health status issues that affect rural populations.

2. Discuss selected social and geographic factors that impact health status and health behavior of rural residents.

3. Describe environmental health promotion strategies that are appropriate for rural populations.

4. Be familiar with the Rural Assistance Center online resources, and with the most common federal programs available to address rural health issues.

Introduction

*R*ural Health has different meanings in different parts of the world. In developing countries, it often refers to basic public health services such as clean water, immunizations, and prevention of HIV. In Australia, New Zealand, and to some extent Canada and the United States, it often refers to native or aboriginal populations. In much of the United States, it is commonly used to describe issues that affect timely access to appropriate, effective, affordable services for persons who live in areas of low population density, often at a distance from specialty and tertiary care that results in a greater role for primary care as compared with urban areas. One creative approach to rural health is the concept of "clinical peripherality," which encompasses not only low population density and remoteness from tertiary and specialty care, but remoteness from the administrative offices where decisions are made that might affect quality, cost, or access to care (Swan, Selvaraj, & Godden, 2008).

When the US Office of Technology Assessment published the first comprehensive look at rural health in the United States in 1990, the question "What is rural health?" though not explicitly asked, seemed to be answered by addressing the availability of primary and acute health care services in rural America. Emphasis was placed on listing federal and to some extent state programs to address chronic shortages of personnel, to support small rural hospitals, and to support under-served populations. While rural health continues to be concerned about these issues, with the publication by the Institute of Medicine of *Quality Through Collaboration: The Future of Rural Health* in 2005, there is evidence of a shift toward a population health approach that places less emphasis on categories of services and workforce, and more emphasis on healthy communities. Specifically:

> *All rural Americans should have access to the full spectrum of high quality, appropriate care, regardless of where they live...*
>
> * *Rural communities should focus greater attention on improving population health in addition to meeting personal health care needs...*
> * *A core set of health care services (primary care, dental care, basic mental health care, and emergency medical services) should be available within rural communities...*
> * *The spectrum of services available in rural communities should be based on the population health needs of the local community.*

Institute of Medicine (2005, pp. 25–26)

This of course leaves it up to the communities, the policy makers, and the providers of care to determine what constitutes a community and what constitutes a rural community. So let us begin with a brief look at what we mean by "rural."

Newcomers to the field of rural health are often frustrated by the seemingly vast array of definitions of "rural," and cannot understand why we can't just decide on a single definition and stick with it. First, let's look at some common definitions, then let's consider why there are so many.

The most commonly used definitions of rural come from two federal agencies: the United States Bureau of the Census and the White House Office of Management and Budget (OMB). In both cases, the agency has begun by defining what is urban, leaving the definition of rural either explicitly or implicitly as "everything else." The census bureau begins by identifying *urbanized areas* as consisting of densely settled "places," often built up from census blocks that meet minimum population density requirements. When these census blocks are combined with adjacent blocks so as to encompass a population of at least 50,000 people, that is called an "urbanized area." The census bureau also identifies "urban clusters" as places that meet the population density threshold and have at least 2,500 people, but are not adjacent to an urbanized area. Many small rural towns are considered urban clusters by this definition, and, as a result, few federal programs that are intended to assist rural populations rely on this definition.

The OMB definition has been widely used for health planning and policy, because it is based on whole counties, and most of our public health data are available at the county level. The OMB approach is primarily concerned with identifying metropolitan areas (sometimes referred to as metropolitan statistical areas), which consist of one or more "urban core" counties and the surrounding counties that are economically tied to the core. The combined population of the core and surrounding counties must be 50,000 or more, regardless of the size of any of the cities. When using the OMB approach, areas not part of one of these "metropolitan areas" are considered "nonmetro," or rural.

Taking a population health perspective, whether at the local, state, or national level, neither of these definitions is adequate. As seen in Figure 21.1, the census bureau definition identifies many small communities as urban. Moreover, the kinds of health status information that help state and federal agencies target resources where they are most needed is often only available for whole counties. On the other hand, there are many whole counties in the United States that are considered "metro" by the OMB

Figure 21.1 Population-size threshold. (USDA, Economic Research Service, using data from the U.S. Census Bureau).

definition, yet have vast rural areas within their borders. For example, St. Louis County in northern Minnesota, includes Duluth, a city of nearly 100,000, yet extends to the Canadian border, and includes part of the Boundary Waters Wilderness area.

The shortcomings of certain definitions are only one reason why there are so many other definitions. At a minimum, most programs and most researchers have acknowledged that the geography of the United States is not dichotomous. Dividing populations into rural and urban denies the complexity and richness of the American experience. One approach to that complexity has been to develop a continuum from large urban core to rural counties that are adjacent to urban counties, and thence to nonadjacent counties of decreasing population along the continuum. The Educational Research Service within the United States Department of Agriculture has taken this approach with its "rural–urban continuum" and "urban influence" codes.

There are several useful references that explain these distinctions in greater detail. For the health care provider or health educator who simply wants to know if she can qualify for a recruitment incentive or grant that is restricted to rural areas, an excellent resource can be found at the Rural Assistance Center, also known as RAC online. In addition to rural definitions, this site will generate a custom report for any zip code indicating whether or not it is rural according to various definitions, and for what federal programs the area is eligible (http://www.raconline.org/funding/rural.php).

GEOGRAPHIC AND SOCIAL FACTORS THAT IMPACT HEALTH IN RURAL AREAS

Those who have made a study of rural health over the past 20 years most often have been concerned with access to services. The traditional approach has been to gather data on services that can be easily quantified, such as the number of primary care physicians, the number of hospital beds, or the number of dentists. Ratios of services to population are then calculated and the rural ratio is compared to the urban ratio. In many cases, this process leads to the conclusion that rural areas are "underserved." Note, however, that this approach does not have much to say about the health status of the population. There is an assumption that adequate health services are a necessary condition for population health.

When the National Center for Health Statistics published a study comparing urban and rural populations on population health indicators such as smoking, obesity, chronic disease, substance abuse, suicide, and child health, rural populations were found to be less healthy on nearly all indicators (Eberhardt, Ingram, & Makuc, 2001). A first response to that study by rural health advocates was to cite these disparities as evidence that more services were needed in rural areas (Morgan, 2002). Upon further reflection, however, the study led to some disturbing questions. How can more hospitals and physicians address the higher rates of smoking and obesity? Why do rural people make unhealthy choices, and continue to practice unhealthy behaviors at higher rates than urban and suburban people? Are there social and cultural factors that reinforce unhealthy behavior? (Hartley, 2004).

Population health has been defined as "an approach [that] focuses on interrelated conditions and factors that influence the health of populations over the life course, identifies systematic variations in their patterns of occurrence, and applies the resulting knowledge to develop and implement policies and actions to improve the health and well being of those populations" (Kindig & Stoddart, 2003, p. 380). A classic premise of community health is that the determinants of population health and particularly of health behaviors, are embedded in relationships that tie individuals to their family and friends, their neighborhoods, and their communities (Eng, Salmon, & Mullan, 1992). These approaches to population health and community health lead to more questions. How do rural communities differ from urban and suburban communities? What is different about those "ties that bind" in rural areas? Is there such a thing as "rural culture?"

A few recent studies make it clear that much of rural America is demographically different from urban America. In age, education, income, and health insurance status, rural is generally worse off. But even in these basic demographics, there is much diversity among rural regions. As shown in Figure 21.2, the great

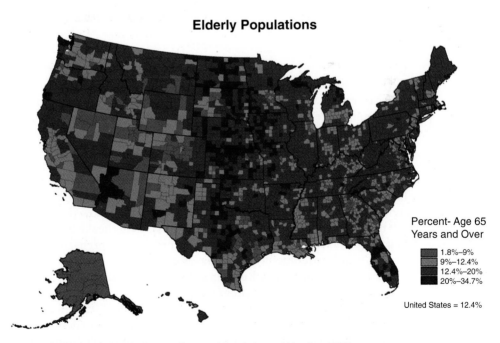

Elderly Populations

Percent- Age 65 Years and Over

- 1.8%–9%
- 9%–12.4%
- 12.4%–20%
- 20%–34.7%

United States = 12.4%

Source: United States Census Bureau, Census of Population and Housing, 2000

Note: Alaska and Hawaii are not to scale.

Figure 21.2 The aging rural population. United States Census Bureau, Census of Population and Housing, 2000. Accessed online at the Rural Assistance Center. Available at http://www.raconline.org/maps/mapfiles/elderly.jpg

County-level Variations in Life Expectancy, 1999
Both Sexes

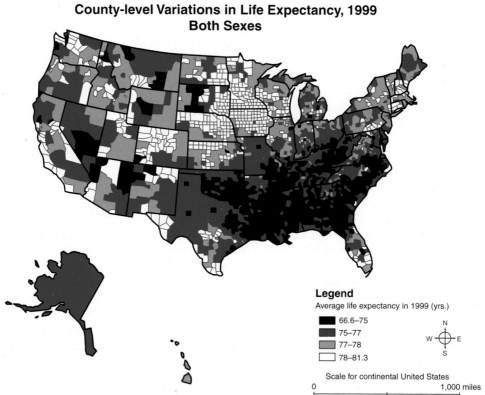

Figure 21.3   County-level variations in life expectancy, both sexes, 1999. Maine Rural Health Research Center, University of Southern Maine, Portland Maine, 2010. (Based on data from Ezzati, M., Friedman, A. B., Kulkarni, S. C., & Murray, C. J. (2008). The reversal of fortunes: Trends in county mortality and cross-county mortality disparities in the United States. *PLoS Medicine*, 5(4), e66. doi:10.1371/journal.pmed.0050066.)

plains in the heart of the country have a greater portion of the population over 65. That means more people on Medicare, and fewer people in the workforce, among other things. If we look at life expectancy, which is a very crude measure of health status to be sure, we find certain regions of the country much worse off than others, most notably, the southeastern "black belt," the Mississippi delta, and Indian country (Fig. 21.3).

Perhaps the most telling demographic marker as a determinant of health and health behavior is illustrated by Figure 21.4, which shows those counties that have been designated as experiencing "persistent poverty." These counties have been found to have 20% or more of the population living below the federal poverty level for three successive census periods (30 years). Whether delivering health services, engaging in health education and health promotion, prenatal care, dental care, or mental health care, life in these areas is qualitatively different from other parts of the country. When federal agencies such as the Health Resources and Services Administration target their programs to special populations, these areas are often included, for good reason. A simple visual inspection of Figures 21.3 and 21.4 makes it plain that poverty is strongly correlated with premature death.

Rural counties lag behind in educational attainment, too. Using data from the 2006 Current Population Survey, the Economic Research Service at USDA reports that 19% of rural residents have a college degree compared with 33% of urban residents (USDA, 2008).

Persistent poverty counties, 1970-2000

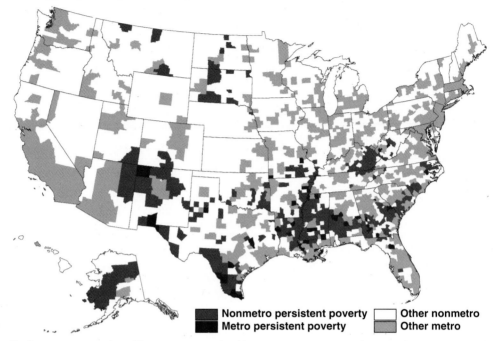

Persistent poverty counties – 20 percent or more of residents were poor as measured by each of the last 4 censuses,1970, 1980, 1990, and 2000.

Source: Economic Research Service, USDA.

Figure 21.4   Persistent poverty counties, 1970–2000. (Economic Research Service, USDA).

Not surprisingly, the disparities facing rural populations go beyond demographics to include an alarming array of health status indicators and health behaviors. A small sample of the ways in which rural populations have been found worse off than urban is depicted in Table 21.1.

Clearly, the sociodemographic characteristics of rural residents place them at risk for unhealthy behaviors and poor health status. Compounding those factors, rural residents are less likely to have health insurance than their urban counterparts. Rural counties with fewer than 2,500 persons had the highest rate of uninsured (23%) with larger rural counties adjacent to urban counties having the same rate as urban counties (19%) (Lenardson, Ziller, Coburn, & Anderson, 2009). In addition, rural communities' lack of public transportation means that those who cannot drive a car, either because they are too young, too old, disabled, or too poor to own one, may not be able to access the few services and programs that serve rural populations, and may not be able to travel to larger communities where more programs and services are available. Indeed, lack of transportation compounds many urban–rural disparities, and is often found to be a factor in designing rural programs or interventions.

It is a sad fact that, even in those rural communities where most residents have access to transportation, have a high-school education, have health insurance or access to a community health center, and, in short, have relatively fewer of these sociodemographic–geographic issues, we often observe higher rates of smoking, poor nutrition, lack of exercise, and the health problems that follow from these behaviors. That

TABLE 21.1

Urban–Rural Disparities

	Urban	Rural
Adults who smoke	22%	25%[a]
Adolescents who had 5 or more drinks in one episode	10%	15%[b]
Adults overweight or obese	23.9%	27.4%[c]
Self-rated mental health poor or fair	6%	8%[d]
Male suicide deaths per 100,000 population	17	27[e]
Total tooth loss among adults age 65 and over	28%	36%[f]

[a]Doescher, M. P., Jackson, J. E., Jerant, A., & Gary Hart, L. (2007). Prevalence and trends in smoking: A national rural study. *Journal of Rural Health*, 22(2), 112–118.

[b]Lambert, D., Gale, J., & Hartley, D. (2008). Substance abuse by youth and young adults in rural America. *Journal of Rural Health*, 24(3), 221–228.

[c]Bennett, K. J., Olatosi, B., & Probst, J. C. (2008). Health disparities: A rural-urban chartbook. South Carolina Rural Health Research Center. Available online at http://rhr.sph.sc.edu/report_by_topic. html#1–09. Accessed January 4, 2010.

[d]Ziller, E. (2010). Access to rural mental health services: Service use and out-of-pocket costs. *Journal of Rural Health*, 26(3).

[e]Advancing Suicide Prevention. (2005). Suicide the second-leading cause of death in States with primarily rural populations. Available online at http://www.advancingsp.org/Press_Release_8_11_05.pdf. Accessed December 20, 2009.

[f]Eberhardt, M. S., Ingram, D. D., & Makuc, D. M. (2001). *Health United States, 2001 Urban and rural health chartbook.* Hyattsville, MD: National Center for Health Statistics.

observation has led to the question, "Why does rural residence (culture, community, and environment) reinforce negative health behaviors?" (Hartley, 2004). There are no widely accepted answers to this question. A frank discussion of the issue can lead to stereotypes of rural culture and rural people that are simplistic, and do not lead to a solution. Often, rural communities are high in social capital, but may also be low in tolerance for diverse opinions or behaviors, leading to social pressure to conform. Changes in diet may be particularly difficult under such pressure. One rural resident, responding to this question in a personal conversation, noted that, if someone in her town started jogging every morning, it would lead others to think that she thought she was better than others in the town. In another such conversation, a rural resident commented on going to high school in a small town, where there are only 25 kids in each grade, and one must conform if one wants to have a social life. Here, too, if smoking and drinking are the norm, it is difficult to resist.

On the positive side, a rural community can come together to address a public health issue, once they accept it as something affecting their whole community, and as something that they can do something about. A great example of this phenomenon is the case of Albert Lea, Minnesota, population about 18,000. With help from AARP and the United Health Foundation, the town launched the Vitality Project, with the goal of helping citizens live longer, healthier lives. The project's strategies are simple: eat more fruits and vegetables, walk instead of drive, and stay productive and social well into old age. Some of the strategies have included sidewalk and trail construction, working with restaurants to add healthier menu options and with grocery stores to feature healthy foods. Schools eliminated sugary treats and started a "walking school bus" program that allows kids to walk to school in groups with adult supervision (Buettner, 2010). According to one report, "*the key for Albert Lea was getting the community behind a goal that was not just about weight loss, but also about fostering family relationships, a sense of purpose and healthy living habits*" (USA Today, 2009).

Health Promotion Issues that Relate to Rural Populations

Rural populations face all of the same preventable illnesses that are faced by urban populations. To a large extent, prevention of the major contributors to preventable deaths is addressed by public health systems and by primary care practices. There are practitioners in both sectors who can be effective partners in health promotion. However, in rural areas, there are typically fewer primary care practitioners than in urban areas, and they tend to be very busy. Moreover, many rural areas have no local public health department, or one that offers a limited number of services. Prevention initiatives are often undertaken by partnerships involving healthy communities coalitions, hospitals, primary health clinics, schools, social services, law enforcement, and local businesses. While state health departments and the US Centers for Disease Control offer many useful tools for prevention, it is these local partners who must ultimately decide what will work for their communities.

Two issues that challenge these prevention partnerships in rural communities are substance abuse and obesity. Both of these threats to the health of the public have been shown to affect rural populations disproportionately. Higher rates of obesity and substance abuse are particularly troubling when observed among rural youth, and in both cases, prevention initiatives that seek to modify not only unhealthy behaviors but unhealthy environments are proving to be effective. The October 2003 issue of the *American Journal of Public Health* addressed the relationship between health and the built environment (physical environment, urban design, land-use planning, urban sprawl, and housing). The articles raised many good questions about the influence of place of residence on health, but the questions were almost exclusively about urban environments. More recently, research has found that there are significant differences between the urban and rural built environment that have implications for prevention, especially for the prevention of childhood obesity (Yousefian, Ziller, Swartz, & Hartley, 2009).

Obesity

Childhood obesity rates in the United States are on the rise and the immediate and long-term medical and social consequences of childhood obesity are staggering. Over the past four decades, rates have consistently increased, and today over 33% of children and adolescents are overweight or obese in this country (Ogden et al., 2006). Childhood obesity rates are highest among low-income populations and also among racial/ethnic minorities. Research has demonstrated that this trend also applies to rural youth, where the prevalence of obesity and overweight has been shown to be higher than state and national averages and also higher than rates among youth in urban areas (Joens-Matre et al., 2008). A recent national study found that rural children are about 25% more likely to be overweight than their metropolitan counterparts (Lutfiyya, Lipsky, Wisdom-Behounek, & Inpanbutr-Martinkus, 2007). Rates of physical activity have also been found to be lower in rural areas among adults and among rural children when compared to urban and suburban populations (Patterson, Moore, Probst, & Shinogle, 2004).

Attention has been cast on the role that active living plays in obesity prevention among youth in urban and, more recently, in rural areas. The concept of active living incorporates an ecological, population-based approach to physical activity by recognizing that individual behavior, social environments, physical environments, and policies all contribute to behavior change. Active living targets entire communities to promote accessible and safe opportunities for residents to engage in physical activity during transportation, occupation, recreation, and at home (Sallis et al., 2006). Often with funding from the Robert Wood Johnson Foundation (RWJF), communities have assessed how "activity friendly" they are. This assessment process has typically involved a process of walking the sidewalks of a neighborhood with a checklist or other formal assessment tool in hand, observing the condition of the housing, sidewalks, crosswalks, intersections, recreational facilities, school areas, etc. Until very recently, the tools available for these assessments were developed for, and field tested in, urban and suburban neighborhoods. (See, for example, the SPACES instrument [Pikora et al., 2006] and the Irvine-Minnesota Inventory [Day, Boarnet, Alfonzo, & Forsyth, 2006].)

Active Living Research and Healthy Eating Research are national programs funded by RWJF providing research to address childhood obesity. In recent years, these programs have funded a small number of projects to begin exploring the needs of rural communities in this effort. A collaboration among three of their grantees has produced a set of instruments that are designed specifically for use in rural communities (Yousefian et al., 2009, 2010). Known as the Rural Active Living Assessment (RALA) tools, these instruments are especially useful for local community leaders seeking to build partnerships and to involve community members in identifying needs and designing and implementing interventions. A "codebook" has been developed that not only explains how to use the tools, but suggests ways that community members can become involved in assessing their communities' needs. Unlike the urban-based instruments mentioned above, the RALA tools treat the entire rural community as a "neighborhood," and include an inventory of resources that serve the entire town, as well as an inventory of local programs and policies that affect access to physical activity, such as late school buses, "safe routes to school," and public transportation. A Webinar (web-based seminar) presenting the RALA tools was sponsored by the Active Living Research national program office in June 2009, and was attended by approximately 400 interested people, suggesting that there is a significant need for and an interest in addressing physical activity in rural areas. The tools and codebook continue to be modified and improved as more rural communities use them. They are available from the Active Living Research web site (http://www.activelivingresearch.org/node/11947).

Substance Abuse

A second major issue that affects rural youth disproportionately is substance abuse. In most rural communities, the substance most used and abused by young people is alcohol. Recent studies have found that rural teens are more likely to use alcohol, to engage in binge drinking, and to drive while intoxicated than urban teens. Young adults living in rural areas are another population at high risk, with higher rates of binge drinking, methamphetamine, and prescription drug abuse than their urban counterparts (Lambert, Gale, & Hartley, 2008; Van Gundy, 2006). We have traditionally focused our prevention efforts for teens in the schools, with programs such as Drug Abuse Resistance Education (DARE), which seek to build self worth and autonomy in young people to empower them to make wise personal choices. In recent years, however, many states and communities have recognized that, "Holding youth solely responsible for underage drinking is like blaming fish for dying in a polluted stream" (attributed to Laurie Lieber, Marin Institute, San Rafael, CA). This realization has led to environmental or ecological approaches to prevention that seek to "purify the water in the stream." One such effort occurred in Piscataquis County, Maine, in 2006.

A statewide survey filled out by students and administered by their school systems on a biennial basis in Maine had shown that several attitudes were highly correlated with youth binge drinking. Examples of questions on the survey that reveal these attitudes:

- My parents think it is not wrong or only a little wrong for me to drink.
- My parents wouldn't catch me if I drank without permission.
- It would be easy to get alcohol if I wanted to.
- A kid in my neighborhood who drinks won't be caught by police.

MYDAUS

With help from the Maine Office of Substance Abuse, county educators, law enforcement and public health leaders determined that, if they could change these attitudes, they could begin to address youth drinking. Their three-pronged approach included addressing *norms* (what is acceptable in the community), *availability*, and *enforcement*. Enforcement was a critical part of this plan, since it would include not only reducing teen's access to booze, but also communicating the community's standards for acceptable behavior, and could be designed to focus on preventing high-risk behavior such as binge drinking at outdoor keg parties. When law enforcement "busted" a keg party, there was a zero-tolerance rule. Every teen present was escorted home by a peace officer, who then talked to the parents and impressed upon them that this behavior was not acceptable in this community. This strategy helped to engage parents as critical partners, empower them to address the problem, and begin the process of changing community norms. For the strategy to be most effective, it had to begin with a well-publicized written policy from the Sheriff's Department, endorsed by the schools. To assure the zero-tolerance rule (all treated the same), the sheriff's department developed a "call-out" system so that extra officers could be brought in to assist when breaking up a drinking party. Officers received special training in "community policing" to make their interventions effective.

Access was also addressed by issuing citations to adults who furnished alcohol to minors. In the year following the implementation of the three-part strategy, citations to adults increased slightly, from three to nine citations, but citations to minors increased from 39 to 138. More importantly, the next year that the survey was administered, attitudes had changed. Perceptions that it was easy to get alcohol had decreased from 76% to 66%, and the perception that adults in the community think teen drinking is wrong went from 61% to 68%. Most importantly, teens who admitted drinking in the last 30 days went from 44% to 36%. While these effects may not be dramatic, trends were going in the right direction, while, throughout the rest of Maine, many of these trends were going in the opposite direction. The Maine Office of Substance Abuse continues to administer the MYDAUS every 2 years, and provides guidelines to local communities to help them use the data, available online, for building local partnerships and planning prevention strategies (Maine Office of Substance Abuse, 2009).

Summary

This chapter focused on rural health, its definitions and issues surrounding attempts to measure and affect it. Geographic and social factors unique to rural populations were discussed as were major health disparities between rural and urban areas. Examples of successful programs for obesity and substance abuse, two major health issues of rural populations, were described.

Critical Thinking Questions

1. From what you know of rural communities, comment on what factors might contribute to the urban–rural differences in health behaviors. Think about the implications of such cultural factors for environmental prevention initiatives addressing substance abuse, obesity, smoking, or other major public health issues. Any statements about rural beliefs or perceptions must be backed by your own personal experience or by references—no stereotypes!

2. Consider the following statement: "Urban–rural differences in health status indicators, including neonatal outcomes, mortality rates, and health risk factors, are not true disparities, because they result from racial and socioeconomic disparities. Rural persistent poverty counties and rural African American and Hispanic populations account for most urban–rural differences." Look for evidence in favor of or against this proposition using data from the Community Health Status Indicators web site: http://www.communityhealth.hhs.gov/. Use data chosen from the following counties in making your argument: In Mississippi: Bolivar county (rural—delta), Hinds (urban), Rankin (suburban), and Jackson County (urban—gulf coast). For the Hispanic population, in West Texas, look at Presidio County (rural) and El Paso County (urban). For rural persistent poverty take a look at McDowell (rural) and Kanawha County (urban) in West Virginia. Look especially at the demographics, measures of birth and death, and the risk factors for premature death. Also, pay attention to the comparison to peer counties as well as the comparison to the US average for each of the indicators. Think about urban–rural differences within a state, as well as how rural counties compare to the US average, which is based on a population that is 80% urban. It may be helpful to prepare a table of the indicators you find most compelling.

3. How would an intervention to prevent smoking in Bolivar County Mississippi differ from an intervention to prevent smoking in Freeborn County, Minnesota (where the Albert Lea Vitality Project took place)?

● REFERENCES

Advancing Suicide Prevention. (2005). Suicide the second-leading cause of death in States with primarily rural populations. Available online at http://www.advancingsp.org/Press_Release_8_11_05.pdf. Accessed December 20, 2009.

Bennett, K. J., Olatosi, B., & Probst, J. C. (2008). Health disparities: A rural-urban chartbook. South Carolina Rural Health Research Center. Available online at http://rhr.sph.sc.edu/report_by_topic.html#1–09. Accessed January 4, 2010.

Buettner, D. (2010). The Minnesota miracle. *AARP The Magazine, 53*(1B), 42ff.

Day, K., Boarnet, M., Alfonzo, M., & Forsyth, A. (2006). The Irvine-Minnesota inventory to measure built environments: Development. *American Journal of Preventive Medicine, 30*(2), 144–152.

Doescher, M. P., Jackson, J. E., Jerant, A., & Gary Hart, L. (2007). Prevalence and trends in smoking: A national rural study. *Journal of Rural Health, 22*(2), 112–118.

Eberhardt, M. S., Ingram, D. D., & Makuc, D. M. (2001). *Health United States, 2001 Urban and rural health chartbook*. Hyattsville, MD: National Center for Health Statistics.

Eng, E., Salmon, M., & Mullan, F. (1992). Community empowerment: The critical base for primary health care. *Family and Community Health, 15*, 1–12.

Hartley, D. (2004). Rural health disparities, population health and rural culture. *American Journal of Public Health, 94*(10), 1675–1678.

Institute of Medicine. (2005). *Quality through collaboration: The future of rural health*. Washington DC: National Academies Press.

Joens-Matre, R. R., Welk, G. J., Calabro, M. A., Russell, D. W., Nicklay, E. & Hensley, L. D. (2008). Rural urban differences in physical activity, physical fitness, and overweight prevalence of children. *The Australian Journal of Rural Health, 24*(1), 49–54.

Kindig, D., & Stoddart, G. L. (2003). What is population health? *American Journal of Public Health*, *93*, 380–383.

Lambert, D., Gale, J., & Hartley, D. (2008). Substance abuse by youth and young adults in rural America. *Journal of Rural Health*, *24*(3), 221–228.

Lenardson, J. D., Ziller, E., Coburn, A., & Anderson, N. (2009). *Profile of rural health insurance coverage: A chartbook*. Maine Rural Health Research Center, Muskie School of Public Service, University of Southern Maine. Available online at http://muskie.usm.maine.edu/Publications/rural/Rural-Health-Insurance-Chartbook-2009.pdf

Lutfiyya, M. N., Lipsky, M. S., Wisdom-Behounek, J., & Inpanbutr-Martinkus, M. (2007). Is rural residency a risk factor for overweight and obesity for U.S. children? *Obesity*, *15*(9), 2348–2356.

Maine Youth Drug and Alcohol Use Survey. Maine Office of Substance Abuse. (2009). Available online at http://www.maine.gov/dhhs/osa/data/mydaus/mydaus2008.htm

Morgan, A. (2002). A national call to action: CDC's 2001 urban and rural health chartbook. *The Journal of Rural Health*, *18*, 382–383.

Ogden, C. L., Carroll, M. D., & Curtin, L. R., McDowell, M. A., Tabak, C. J., Flegal, K. M. (2006). Prevalence of overweight and obesity in the United States, 1999–2003. *JAMA*, *295*, 1549–1555.

Patterson, P. D., Moore, C. G., Probst, J. C., & Shinogle, J. A. (2004). Obesity and physical activity in rural America. *The Journal of Rural Health*, *20*(2), 151–159.

Pikora, T., Giles-Corti, B., Knuiman, M. W., Bull, F. C., Jamrozik, K., & Donovan, R. J. (2006). Neighbourhood environmental factors correlated with walking near home: Using SPACES. *Medicine and Science in Sports and Exercise*, *38*(4), 708–714.

Sallis, J. F., Cervero, R. B., Ascher, W., Henderson, K. A., Kraft, M. K., & Kerr, J. (2006). An ecological approach to creating active living communities. *Annual Review of Public Health*, *27*, 297–322.

Swan, G. M., Selvaraj, S., & Godden, D. (2008). Clinical peripherality: Development of a peripherality index for rural health services. *BMC Health Services Research*, *8*, 23. Published online at http://www.ncbi.nlm.nih.gov/pmc/articles/PMC2246121

USA Today. (2009). Minnesota town gets healthy together (October 14, 2009). Available online at http://www.usatoday.com/news/health/2009-10-14-minnesota-health_N.htm. Accessed December 28, 2009.

USDA. (2008). *Education's role in the Metro-NonMetro earnings divide*. Amber Waves, February 2008. Available online at http://www.ers.usda.gov/AmberWaves/February08/Features/EducationRole.htm

Van Gundy, K. (2006). Substance abuse in rural and small town America. *Reports on Rural America* (Vol. 1, No. 2). Carsey Institute, University of New Hampshire.

Yousefian, A., Ziller, E., Swartz, J., & Hartley, D. (2009). Active living for rural youth: Addressing physical inactivity in rural communities. *Journal of Public Health Management and Practice: Special Issue on Rural Public Health*, *15*(3), 223–231.

Yousefian, A., Hennessy, E., Umstattd, R., Economos, C., Hallam, J., Hyatt, R., et al. (2010). Development of the rural active living assessment tools: Measuring rural environments. *Preventive Medicine*, *50*(suppl 1), S86–S92.

Ziller, E. (2010). Access to rural mental health services: Service use and out-of-pocket costs. *Journal of Rural Health*, *26*(3).

Internet Resources can be found on the Point at http://thepoint.lww.com/Anderson6e.

APPENDIX A

A Guide to Nursing Assessment of the Workplace

ANN T. MALECHA AND NANCY ZAMBORAS

COMPONENTS	QUESTIONS TO ASK
THE COMPANY	
Historical development	How, why, and by whom was the company founded?
Organizational chart	What is the formal order of the system, and to whom are the health providers responsible?
Company policies	Is there a policy manual? Are the workers aware of existence of the manual?
Length of the workweek	How many days a week does the industry operate? Is the industry open year-round?
Length of the work time	Are there several shifts? If yes, describe. How many breaks? Is there paid vacation? If yes, how much? Are there scheduled paid holidays?
Sick leave	Is there a clear policy, and do the workers know it?
Family Medical Leave Act (FMLA)	Are employees paid? Are employees paid during maternity leave?
Employee Benefits	
Insurance programs	What types of insurance programs does the company offer? How much does the company pay? What are the monthly premiums? Who completes the forms?
Health	What type of coverage is offered for spouses, life partners, children, or other dependents? HMO? PPO? What is the average co-pay for an office visit or emergency visit? What are the yearly deductibles?
Dental	Is orthodontic treatment covered?
Prescription medications	What medications are covered?
Vision	What type of vision care is covered (annual exam, glasses, contacts)?
Short- and long-term disability	Does the company pay all or part? Is pregnancy covered?
Flexible spending	What type of spending is covered (e.g., childcare expenses, nonprescription medication)?
Life	What types of life insurance are offered?
Employee assistance program (EAP)	Is the EAP on-site or off-site?

Retirement program	What types of retirement programs are available and how much does the company contribute (e.g., 401K, pension plan)? How many years of employment are required before vested?
Educational program	Does the company offer continuing education on-site? Does the company financially support off-site continuing education (conferences, certification programs, college courses)?
Employee Relations	
Union representation	If a union is present, is there on-site union representation?
Shared governance	Do shared governance committees exist? How do employees voice their grievances?

THE PLANT

General physical setting	What is the overall appearance? Is the environment clean? Comment on heating, air-conditioning, overall lighting, green space, ventilation, compliance with the Americans with Disability Act (elevators, ramps, restrooms), etc.
Construction	What is the size and general condition of buildings and grounds?
Parking facilities and public transportation	How far do workers have to walk to get inside? What is the overall appearance of the parking structure: Covered? Lighting? Gated entrance? Security? Escort available to parking after-hours? Open to the public? Does the employee have to pay for parking? If yes, how much? Is vanpooling available? What type of public transportation serves the worksite?
Entrances and exits	How many people use them? How accessible are the entrances? Employee badges required? Security-monitored entrance? During what hours is security available? What are the visitor or contractor policies?
Communication facilities	Are there bulletin boards and newsletters? Common areas where all employees can gather such as inside/outside sitting areas (benches, tables)?
Housekeeping	Is the physical setting maintained adequately? Are public areas (lobbies, hallways, restrooms) clean?
Work Areas	
Space	Are workers isolated or crowded?
Ergonomics	Are work areas ergonomically safe: work stations, desk areas, chairs, lighting, computer monitors and keyboards, and work habits? Does the company conduct periodic ergonomic assessments?
Fall precautions	Is there a chance of workers falling or being injured by falling objects?
Safety signs and markings	Are dangerous areas well-marked to protect employees from slips, trips, or falls?
Safety equipment	Do the workers make use of hard hats, safety glasses, face masks, radiation badges, and so forth? Are requirements met for the OSHA standards regarding use and maintenance of personal protective equipment (PPE), as well as specific provisions on the use, design, and performance requirements for various types of PPE (eye, face, head, and respiratory protection)?

Nonwork Areas

Lockers	If the work is dirty, workers should be able to change clothes. Can workers accidentally carry toxic substances home on their clothes? Does the company supply work clothes?
Break rooms, restrooms, recreation rooms	Do workers have an area for resting and taking a break? Is it shared with the public? How accessible are the restrooms? What are the conditions of these areas? What is the policy for taking a break? Do workers feel free to use the facilities? What is the policy on break time? Can a worker who is not feeling well lie down?
Cafeteria or dining area	What types of dining areas exist for employees? Is water readily available? What kinds of food are available on-site (cafeteria, vending machines, etc.)? Are employees permitted to go off-site for meals?
Communications/technology	What are the policies on: receiving personal telephone calls? Voice mail? Use of mobile/cellular phones? Pagers? Personal e-mail? Other handheld technology?
Other nonwork areas	What is the company's smoking policy? Are there designated areas for smoking? Does the company provide on-site childcare?

THE WORKING POPULATION

General characteristics	
Demographic description of employee population	What is the total number of employees? Usually if an industry has 500 or more employees, full-time nursing services are recommended. What are the age, gender, socioeconomic, education, relationship status, and race/ethnic distributions?
Cultural considerations	What languages are spoken at the worksite? Do employees observe religious/ethnic holidays? What level of education is required? What is the percentage of skilled and nonskilled employees? What is the percentage of exempt and nonexempt employees? What percentage of employees is physically or mentally challenged?
Work status	How many employees work full-time or part-time? What is the policy on overtime? What is the policy on job sharing? What are the policies on promotion?
Absenteeism	Who keeps a record on absenteeism? What is the absenteeism policy? How many days per year are employees allowed for absences? What are the five most common reasons for absence? What is the return-to-work policy?
International travel or long-term international assignments	Do employees travel internationally for work? If yes, what type of health care is required before travel or international assignment? Whom do employees contact for health-care concerns while living out of the country? Does the worksite receive international visitors?
Physical work demands	What percentage of workers engages in physically demanding work or sedentary work?
Outdoor work	Do employees work outside? In what seasons? What health promotion interventions are addressed for outdoor work?

THE INDUSTRIAL SETTING AND OPERATIONS

Nature of the operations	What does the company produce and how? Ask for a brief description of each stage of operations so that the nurse can compare the needs and abilities of the worker with the needs of the job.
Safety committee	Is there a designated safety committee? If yes, who serves on the committee and when does the committee meet? If no committee, who oversees safety and fire issues for the worksite? Who is responsible for training of first responders? Are there specific situations or substances in the plant that pose a potential for danger and/or fire? How often are there organized fire drills? Are workers aware of what to do in other emergencies (tornado, earthquake, bomb threat, serious injury, death, etc.)?
Raw materials used	What are they and how dangerous are they? How are they stored? Check the Code of Federal Regulations and the Federal Register for guidelines on storage.
Waste products produced	What is the system for waste disposal? Are pollution-control devices in place and functioning?
Equipment used	What types of equipment are used: fans, blowers, fast-moving, wet, or dry? Is the equipment portable or fixed? Heavy or light? Ask to have each piece of large equipment marked on a scale map. What type of training do workers receive to operate equipment?
Nature of the final product	Can the workers take pride in the final product or do they make only parts?
Exposure to hazardous materials	To which hazardous materials are the workers exposed? Where are the material safety data sheets (MSDS) kept? How often do workers receive training on the MSDS? Are workers exposed to animals and/or animal products?

THE HEALTH PROGRAM

Policies and procedures	What type of policies and procedures exist? Are they up to date and written clearly?
Job descriptions for health care providers	Who provides health care to the employees? Are there job descriptions? Is health care delivered at the worksite? Off-site? Is there a medical director for the company? If yes, what are the responsibilities of the medical director (oversees standing orders, first aid/emergency policies)?
Preplacement physicals	Are they required? What types of physicals are offered? Who pays for the physical exams? Who performs the physical exams? Location?
Drug and alcohol screening	Are these screenings required? What types of screening: preplacement, DOT, for cause, random? Who pays for the screenings? Location?
First aid and personnel	What type of first-aid care is available? Who is trained to deliver first aid?
Facilities and resources	What types of space and equipment are available for delivering health care? Where is a sick or injured employee taken? Where is emergency equipment kept? Are automated external defibrillators (AEDs) available?

Supplies	What are they? Where are they kept? Who is responsible for maintenance and reordering? What is the annual budget for supplies? Make a list of the available supplies and describe the condition of each item.
Records, reports, and retention of documents	What medical records exist? Who maintains the OSHA log on work-related injuries and illnesses? Who has access to medical records? How long and where are the medical records kept?
Services provided in the past 12 months	
Clinical care provided	Acute and/or chronic care? Describe the five most common presenting complaints. Is medication dispensed at the worksite? If yes, what types? Where is the medication stored? Are immunizations provided? Who provides the clinical care services?
Work-related injuries/ illnesses	How many accidents in the past 12 months? What type of accidents? Health outcomes for injured/ill workers? Who is the workers' compensation carrier? Does the industry have a designated case manager to manage return-to-work issues?
Screening provided	What types of screenings are provided?
Referrals	What types of referrals are made? Is there a list of referral health providers, agencies, and community resources?
Health education and health promotion activities	Does the company support health promotion activities? If yes, what type? Do employees have access to physical fitness facilities either on-site or off-site?

Adapted from Serafini, P. (1976). Nursing assessment in industry: A model. *American Journal of Public Health*, 66(8), 755–760.

Postscript

It has been over 100 years since Lillian Wald coined the term *public health nurse*. It seems fitting that we "wrap up" this edition with an editorial inspired by Ms. Wald's work in New York City at the turn of the last century. As it was included in the third, fourth, fifth, and now the sixth editions of *Community as Partner*, we fervently hope that such an editorial will not be necessary at the beginning of the next millennium.

A Call for Transformation

Standing in the room where Lillian Wald once lived at Henry Street was an inspiring experience. More than 100 attendees at the American Public Health Association's annual meeting in New York came together to hear Clair Coss read her play about the woman who coined the term "public health nurse" and then visit the historic Henry Street Settlement. Each of us reflected on what public health nursing was in those early days: comprehensive health and illness care that embodied social reform and political involvement.

What happened to this once-glorious group that picketed against war, fought for the rights of women and children, aided the immigrant, initiated school health programs, and saw to it that the poor and disenfranchised received a fair wage and access to health care? In 1920, the public health nurse was described as "... one of the very greatest agents in the advancement of health, both individual and public, in this country" (1). These early professionals accomplished the goals of reducing mortality and morbidity so well that they became a threat to those in power. One of the strongest opponents of home visiting was the American Medical Association (AMA), which successfully fought against federally financed public health programs. In 1930, the AMA condemned such programs as "... unsound in policy, wasteful and extravagant, unproductive of results and tending to promote communism. ..." (2). In addition, health became a medical concern and, as a result, health problems were depoliticized. Those problems rooted in social disarray were reduced to individual, biologic, or situational factors, and the focus became the individual. Even the sacrosanct home visit became limited to the care of a medically diagnosed problem in order to carry out medically prescribed activities. Funding of programs outside the hospital was predicated on stamping out disease (always with medical prescription to back it up). Other funding was aimed at specific problems, so that we had (and still have) immunization clinics; Women, Infants, and Children programs; sexually transmitted disease clinics; and the like. But the community is not a series of fragmented risk groups. It is a collection of people who want and deserve comprehensive nursing care: primary health care given distributively whether the people are sick or well. The district nurses did that in the early part of this century. Where are they now?

Now is the time to end our focus on fragmented programs and to return to our raison d'etre, the improvement of health: not health as an end, but as a means to a full life. Health cannot occur when the means of achieving a living wage are controlled by a small minority; when agencies charged with maintaining and improving a safe environment are influenced by the polluters they are supposed to police; when the whole structure is predicated on health as a commodity to be doled out to the "deserving" (insured) by a group whose primary mission is to cure disease; when violence, from child abuse to war, is tolerated; when age defines usefulness and is given as a reason to withhold care and treatment; and when a majority of the population is relegated to second-class status because of gender, race, or ethnicity.

Community health nurses can transform our fragmented, disease-oriented "system," not by bemoaning the loss of our glorious past, but by looking into the future, by focusing on a goal and the strategies to achieve it. Health for all through primary health care means that the nurses first ask the people what they want to improve their health and then take the responsibility to work as partners with them to achieve it (empowerment). This means working with others, not just the health team, but community groups, business and education leaders, politicians, engineers, and others to overcome inequities.

Community health nurses in the model of Lillian Wald can make a difference. Let us begin immediately either to change our public health care system (now in "disarray" (3)) or forge out on our own as Ms. Wald did, get our own financing, and deliver district nursing as it should be. We know we can reduce mortality and morbidity as she did; our research has demonstrated this. What we need is a galvanizing force to do so. Our challenge is this: Join with the community to transform an unjust and failing health care system to one that reflects health for *all*, the legacy of Lillian Wald.

Elizabeth T. Anderson, Dr.P.H., R.N., F.A.A.N.
Galveston, TX

REFERENCES

1. Welch, W. H. (1920). *Papers and addresses*, (Vol. 3, p. 165). Baltimore, MD: Johns Hopkins University Press.
2. Donahue, M. P. (1985). *Nursing: The finest art* (p. 339). St. Louis, MO: C. V. Mosby.
3. Committee for the Study of the Future of Public Health, Division of Health Care Services, Institute of Medicine. (1988). *The future of public health* (p. 19). Washington, DC: National Academy Press.
Source: Anderson, E. T. (1991). Editorial: A call for transformation. *Public Health Nursing*, 8(1), 1–2.

INDEX

Note: Page numbers followed by f indicate figures; those followed by t indicate tables; and those followed by b indicate boxed material.